FINAL FRCR PART A MODULES 4–6 SINGLE BEST ANSWER MCQs

THE SRT COLLECTION OF 600 QUESTIONS WITH EXPLANATORY ANSWERS

Edited by

ROBIN PROCTOR
MA (Cantab) FRCR MRCP MRCGP
Specialist Registrar in Clinical Radiology
Southampton General Hospital
President, Society of Radiologists in Training

Foreword by

JOANNA FAIRHURST
Head of Training
Wessex Radiology Training Scheme
Consultant Paediatric Radiologist
Southampton University Hospitals Trust

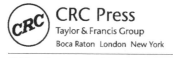

CRC Press
Taylor & Francis Group
Boca Raton London New York

CRC Press is an imprint of the
Taylor & Francis Group, an **informa** business

Radcliffe Publishing Ltd
18 Marcham Road
Abingdon
Oxon OX14 1AA
United Kingdom

www.radcliffe-oxford.com
Electronic catalogue and worldwide online ordering facility.

British Library Cataloguing in Publication Data

A catalogue record for this book is available from the British Library.

ISBN-13: 978 184619 364 4

The paper used for the text pages of this book
is FSC certified. FSC (The Forest Stewardship
Council) is an international network to promote
responsible management of the world's forests.

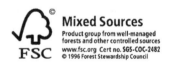

Mixed Sources
Product group from well-managed
forests and other controlled sources
www.fsc.org Cert no. SGS-COC-2482
© 1996 Forest Stewardship Council

Typeset by Pindar NZ, Auckland, New Zealand

Contents

Foreword

It is never easy to decide how best to prepare for an examination: should one concentrate on reading detailed textbooks in the hope that a sufficient proportion of the facts are retained? Are books written as examination aides enough? Should a candidate peruse the recent literature in case 'hot topics' are covered in the questions? Or in this age of increasing reliance on electronic information, should the candidate place their hopes in electronic teaching files? Whatever their personal preference, it is likely that most candidates will turn to examples of examination questions in order to help gauge their preparedness for a test and assess their progress in acquiring the necessary knowledge. The number of publications available to radiologists in training to help them prepare for the Part 2A examination for the FRCR is an indication of how popular these books are as an examination aide. Over the years these texts have been able to draw on the recollections of questions encountered by past candidates and on the expertise acquired by question-setters from a variety of backgrounds. Neither of these resources is available to the candidate about to sit the new single best answer format that the Royal College of Radiologists has adopted for the new-style 2A examination modules. This style of question has been used successfully in the medical world for a number of years, but is novel and unexplored in the context of the FRCR.

Thankfully the authors of this book have responded to the challenge of producing a volume that can provide candidates with experience of attempting to answer questions in this new format. They have collaborated to develop a large number of questions in the new style and have organised these into papers along the lines of the six 2A modules, to give readers the best chance of reproducing the feel of the new examination before sitting the real thing. This has indeed been a significant challenge: not only have the authors had to develop their own question-writing skills along new lines, but they have also had to judge how the full core curriculum will be assessed in this new format and how to therefore organise the papers to reflect likely examination topics. As a past Examiner I can testify to the difficulty in preparing questions that are sufficiently rigorous in their factual content, unambiguous in their interpretation and pertinent to the curriculum to be accepted for inclusion in the FRCR 2A exam. The authors have done an admirable job in drawing together a large number of high-quality questions that satisfy these criteria.

I have no doubt that candidates sitting the 2A exam will find this book a vital tool in their preparation. It provides a unique collection of questions, which will help familiarise candidates with the new format and demonstrate how their knowledge will need to be applied to maximise their chance of success when attempting single best answer papers. The authors are well placed to use their up-to-date knowledge of the Fellowship exam to guide future exam hopefuls through the pitfalls of the new format, and this publication should find its way onto many radiologists' bookshelves in the near future.

Joanna Fairhurst
Head of Training
Wessex Radiology Training Scheme
Consultant Paediatric Radiologist
Southampton University Hospitals Trust
June 2009

Preface

This book has been written by a large number of current trainees in Clinical Radiology and has been coordinated through The Society of Radiologists in Training (SRT). The SRT is the only national organisation of Radiology Trainees in the UK and is run by an elected committee to promote radiology training and education. The SRT organises an annual meeting for trainees and hosts an active website: www.thesrt.org.uk

This book is of particular relevance to higher trainees within radiology who are working towards the Final FRCR examination of the Royal College of Radiologists in the UK. This examination is in the process of being revised and single best answer (SBA) type questions will be introduced in Part A for the first time at the Autumn 2009 sitting. This type of question is well established in other professional examinations, but there are currently no published texts of such questions in Clinical Radiology so this book will meet a real need and aid candidates in their preparation. Candidates for other professional exams in Radiology will also find the text useful and those from other specialties will be able to explore the radiological aspects of their syllabus in greater depth.

More than 20 contributing authors, who all have very recent memory of sitting the Part A component of the Final FRCR examination, have written over 1250 single best answer questions and explanations covering the whole breadth of Clinical Radiology. As in the actual examination, readers will find that important topics have deliberately been covered by more than one author in more than one style and we hope, in addition to the factual information presented, that this will illustrate our interpretation of the various ways in which this style of question may be phrased.

The questions are grouped by topic and split into three papers of 70 questions each. This is very similar to the Royal College format of 75 questions per paper. The explanations have been separated into separate chapters so that readers may either attempt a whole mock exam paper or browse through question by question. This book is intended as a bridge between a pure revision aid and a reference text and we include a bibliography of useful references for further information. There are also references to a small number of particularly relevant journal articles within the explanations.

We thank the many colleagues who have given their time and experience in helping write the questions and thank Chuks Ihezue for his help with the genito-urinary questions. We wish every candidate success and would always be grateful for feedback, which can be submitted via the Society Website or email: president@thesrt.org.uk

Robin Proctor
June 2009

About the editor

Robin Proctor **MA (Cantab) FRCR MRCP MRCGP**
Specialist Registrar in Clinical Radiology, Southampton General Hospital

Robin read medicine at Churchill College, Cambridge where he won a college scholarship before completing his clinical studies at Balliol College, Oxford, winning the prize in Orthopaedic Surgery in the process. He subsequently completed MRCP before training as a General Practitioner and being awarded MRCGP with distinction. He then worked as a GP and Police Surgeon until returning to Hospital Medicine in 2005 as a Specialist Registrar in Radiology. He completed FRCR in 2008. He enjoys teaching medicine and has authored a number of books and articles including a randomised trial comparing teaching methods for medical students.

He has also worked as the expedition leader and medical officer on a diving expedition to the Philippines and in his spare time he enjoys the outdoors, teaches sub-aqua diving and particularly enjoys sailing on the west coast of Scotland.

He has been SRT President since 2007 and conceived this project to produce single best answer MCQs for the new Final FRCR Part A examination as part of a strategy to keep the SRT at the forefront of Radiology training.

Contributors

CHAPTER COORDINATORS

Genito-urinary, adrenal, obstetric, gynaecological and breast radiology
Helen C Addley MA (Oxon) MRCP
Specialist Registrar in Clinical Radiology, Addenbrooke's Hospital

Helen completed her medical training at Oxford University (Exeter and Green Colleges). Before starting her training in Radiology she worked at Hammersmith and Charing Cross Hospitals in General Medicine and gained her Membership of the Royal College of Physicians. She is a member of the Royal College of Radiologists (RCR), European Society of Radiology (ESR) and Radiological Society of North America (RSNA).

Paediatric radiology
Elizabeth Whittington BSc (Hons) MBBS MRCPCH
Specialist Registrar in Clinical Radiology, Southampton General Hospital

Elizabeth qualified from Imperial College School of Medicine in 2002. Following a paediatric rotation at Guy's and St Thomas' Hospitals she moved to the Wessex Deanery where she is currently in the third year of her specialist registrar training in radiology at Southampton General Hospital.

Neuroradiology, head and neck and ENT radiology
Paula McParland MB ChB MRCP FRCR
Specialist Registrar in Clinical Radiology, Southampton General Hospital

Paula graduated from Bristol University in 1999 and trained in general internal medicine in Truro and Bournemouth obtaining MRCP in 2002. Working at the Royal Prince Alfred Hospital in Sydney provided greater exposure to diagnostic imaging and she decided to pursue a career in radiology, gaining her NTN in 2005. She won the Ansell prize in 2006, the BSIR poster prize in 2007 and passed FRCR in 2008. Now in her fourth year on the Wessex training program, she aims to specialise in cardiothoracic radiology.

CONTRIBUTING AUTHORS

Genito-urinary, adrenal, obstetric, gynaecological and breast radiology

Helen C Addley MA (Oxon) MRCP
Specialist Registrar in Clinical Radiology, Addenbrooke's Hospital

Alexandra Hutchings MB ChB MRCP
Specialist Registrar in Clinical Radiology, Portsmouth Hospitals Trust

Jeremy Rabouhans BSc (Hons) MRCS FRCR
Specialist Registrar in Clinical Radiology, Guy's and St Thomas' Hospital

Peter Osborn MBBS
Specialist Registrar in Clinical Radiology, Portsmouth Hospitals Trust

Paediatric radiology

Elizabeth Whittington BSc (Hons) MBBS MRCPCH
Specialist Registrar in Clinical Radiology, Southampton General Hospital

Rajat Chowdhury MA (Oxon) MSc BM BCh MRCS
Specialist Registrar in Clinical Radiology, Southampton General Hospital

Iain DC Wilson MEng (Oxon) BM BS BMedSci MRCS
Specialist Registrar in Clinical Radiology, Southampton General Hospital

Premal A Patel BSc (Hons) MBBS, MRCS
Specialist Trainee in Clinical Radiology, Southampton General Hospital

Neuroradiology, head and neck and ENT radiology

Paula McParland MB ChB MRCP FRCR
Specialist Registrar in Clinical Radiology, Southampton General Hospital

Anita Nagadi MBBS MD MRCPCH
Specialist Registrar in Clinical Radiology, Southampton General Hospital

Mia Morgan MBBS BSc (Hons) MRCS DOHNS
Specialist Trainee in Clinical Radiology, Southampton General Hospital

Ian Pressney BSc (Hons) MBBS
Specialist Trainee in Clinical Radiology, Southampton General Hospital

Nuclear medicine

Sarah Cook MBBS MRCS FRCR
Specialist Registrar in Radiology, Southampton General Hospital

Abbreviations

ACE	angiotensin converting enzyme
AICA	anterior inferior cerebellar artery
AIDS	acquired immune deficiency syndrome
ACL	anterior cruciate ligament (of knee)
ADC	apparent diffusion coefficient map
ALP	alkaline phosphatase
AP	anteroposterior
ASD	atrial septal defect
AVM	arteriovenous malformation
AVSD	atrio-ventricular septal defect
AXR	plain abdominal radiograph
βHCG	beta human chorionic gonadotropin
bpm	beats per minute
BRCA	breast cancer, early onset (tumour suppressor gene)
CC	craniocaudal
CMV	*Cytomegalovirus*
CNS	central nervous system
CPAP	continuous positive airways pressure
CSF	cerebro-spinal fluid
CPR	cardiopulmonary resuscitation
CT	computed tomography
CVA	cerebrovascular accident
CVP	central venous pressure
CXR	chest radiograph
DaTSCAN	dopamine transporter scan
DCIS	ductal carcinoma *in situ*
DDH	developmental dysplasia of the hip
DMSA	tc-99m-dimercaptosuccinic acid
DTPA	tc-99m-diethylenetriamine pentaacetic acid
DVT	deep vein thrombosis
DWI	diffusion weighted imaging
ECA	external carotid artery
ECG	electrocardiogram

ENT	ear, nose and throat
ERCP	endoscopic retrograde cholangio pancreatography
ESR	erythrocyte sedimentation rate
FAST	focused abdominal sonography in trauma
FDG	fluorodeoxyglucose
FESS	functional endoscopic sinus surgery
FEV1	forced expiratory volume in 1 second
FLAIR	fluid attenuated inversion recovery
FNA	fine needle aspirate
FSH	follicle stimulating hormone
FVC	forced vital capacity
GBM	glioblastoma multiforme
GCS	Glasgow Coma Score
GFR	glomerular filtration rate
GOJ	gastro-oesophageal junction
GU	genito-urinary
HIDA	hepatobiliary iminodiacetic acid
HIV	human immunodeficiency virus
HMPAO	hexamethyl-propylene amine oxime
HRCT	high resolution computed tomography
HRT	hormone replacement therapy
HU	Hounsfield units
ICA	internal carotid artery
ICU	intensive care unit
ITU	intensive therapy unit
IUGR	intra-uterine growth retardation
IV	intravenous
IVC	inferior vena cava
IVP	intravenous pyelogram
IVU	intravenous urogram
KUB	X-ray of kidneys, ureters and bladder
LAD	left anterior descending (artery)
LCIS	lobular carcinoma *in situ*
LCL	lateral collateral ligament (of knee)
LDH	lactate dehydrogenase
LVH	left ventricular hypertrophy
LH	luteinising hormone
LOC	loss of consciousness
MAG3	tc-99m-mercaptoacetyltriglycine
MCA	middle cerebral artery
MCL	medial collateral ligament (of knee)
MCUG	micturating cystourethrogram
MCV	mean cell volume
MDP	tc-99m methylene-diphosphonate
MEN	multiple endocrine neoplasia

MHA-TP	microhaemagglutination treponema pollidum test
MIBG	meta-iodobenzylguanidine
MLO	medio-lateral oblique
MRCP	magnetic resonance cholangiopancreaticography
MRI	magnetic resonance imaging
MS	multiple sclerosis
MUGA	multi-gated acquisition scan
NAI	non-accidental injury
NF1	neurofibromatosis type 1
NF2	neurofibromatosis type 2
NG	nasogastric
OCP	oral contraceptive pill
OPG	orthopantomogram radiograph
PA	posteroanterior
PCOS	polycystic ovarian syndrome
PD	proton density
PDA	patent ductus arteriosus
PE	pulmonary embolus
PET	positron emission tomography
PICA	posterior inferior cerebellar artery
PID	pelvic inflammatory disease
PNET	primitive neuroectodermal tumour
PPH	post-partum haemorrhage
PSA	prostate specific antigen
PTH	parathyroid hormone
RI	resistance index
ROI	region of interest
RSV	respiratory syncytial virus
RTA	road traffic accident
SCA	superior cerebellar artery
SPECT	single photon emission computed tomography
STIR	short tau inversion recovery
SUV	standardised uptake value
SVC	superior vena cava
T1	T1-weighted MRI
T2	T2-weighted MRI
T2*	T2*-weighted MRI
TCC	transitional cell carcinoma
TNM	tumour, nodes and metastases cancer staging system
TSH	thyroid stimulating hormone
US	ultrasound
USS	ultrasound scan
VACTERL	syndrome of vertebral, anal, cardiac, tracheo-oesophageal fistula/ oesophageal atresia, renal and limb abnormalities
VDRL	Venereal Disease Research Laboratory test

VF	ventricular fibrillation
V/Q scan	ventilation/perfusion scan
VSD	ventricular septal defect
VUJ	vesicoureteric junction
WCC	white cell count

Introduction

THE NEW FRCR 2A SYLLABUS

The Royal College of Radiologists (www.rcr.ac.uk) sets the FRCR examination and will provide guidance notes and a syllabus to prospective candidates on request. These comments are our current interpretation of what the college intends but candidates should check with the college that they remain applicable.

The Final FRCR Part A syllabus has been revised and some topics have been removed, notably physics and anatomy. These remain important to Clinical Radiology and will be tested elsewhere, but it does not make sense to specifically revise them for the Final FRCR Part A examination in which they are not included. It is likely that some applied knowledge will remain applicable when directly clinically relevant, but pure anatomy and pure physics are no longer scheduled to be included.

The vast majority of the questions will be clinical questions and this is reflected in the content of this book. Do not be misled by the name of the examination modules, particularly the shortened term usually used by candidates; for example, Module 4 is 'GU' or Module 6 'Neuro'. While there will of course be genito-urinary questions in the 'GU' exam there will also be questions on renal, adrenal and breast radiology. Similarly, within the 'Neuro' module there will be questions on the jaw, teeth, eye and ophthalmology conditions, ENT and spinal pathology. While Neuroradiology questions may be the largest single group it may be that they do not even make up a majority of the exam, hence reading the syllabus and targeting exam preparation to all the topics that may be included is important.

There is also a number of general conditions that could appear in any module such as lymphoma, leukaemia, TB, HIV, NAI, melanoma, unknown primary, etc. For instance, it may be that the vignette and stem are based in the core of that module but that the question probes how that condition may extend to involve another organ or system. Consequently, a good general knowledge of such conditions may be useful.

Finally, our interpretation of the syllabus is that questions on statistics could be included and we have incorporated a handful in this book. While they are unlikely to form a large component of the exam it is likely that they will be comparatively easy marks for those who have a basic grasp of medical statistics and we hope the topics we cover will recur in the real exam.

HOW TO APPROACH SINGLE BEST ANSWER QUESTIONS

While these questions may test similar knowledge, they are different from true/ false multiple choice questions and require different skills to answer them.

In preparing both these comments and the remainder of the book in general we have studied the published advice from the Royal College regarding the planned change in format of the FRCR examination. We found McCoubrie and McKnight's article in *Clinical Radiology* an extremely useful summary of the process and would recommend it to all prospective candidates for the new FRCR 2A examination. (McCoubrie P, McKnight L. Single best answer MCQs: a new format for the FRCR Part 2a exam. *Clinical Radiology*. 2008; **63**(5): 506–10). For those who wish a more in-depth text we suggest the National Board of Medical Examiners (NBME) Item Writing Manual which is available for free download from www.nbme.org/PDF/ItemWriting_2003/2003IWGwhole.pdf While this is written for those setting questions (and NBME have been involved in the training of the regional panels who set questions for the RCR) this manual will give candidates a good background of the important issues regarding multiple choice questions of all types in the clinical setting.

Style of question

The new style question will require the candidate to read a 'vignette' – a sentence or paragraph setting the scene, which is likely to be a clinical scenario – and then to read and consider a question before picking the best answer from five possible options. These questions are widely established in other areas of clinical medicine, although they are relatively new to Radiology. They are better suited to testing more applied knowledge and compared to true/false questions it is hoped that performance will depend more on knowledge than technique. Previously, with true/false questions exam savvy candidates who may be stronger on technique than knowledge may have done much better than expected. Similarly, it will no longer be possible to associate individual words in the question and answer to work out the correct answer and it is likely that a greater command of written English will be required with single best answer questions than with the true/false style. It is also hoped that the knowledge tested will be more applied and there will be less scope for learning (or having to learn) 'just for the exam'.

The ideal question will test how to apply knowledge in a particular scenario and will require both the knowledge itself and the correct application of this knowledge to succeed rather than just the knowledge alone. The aim is for questions in the 'Who wants to be a Millionaire?' format which can almost always be answered by a good candidate before reading the possible options. (In medical education jargon, no cue is needed from the options.)

In the ideal question all the options should be 'homogeneous' or 'on the same continuum' hence while the correct option should clearly be identifiable (and should be very much more likely than the others) the other options may remain possible but much less likely and are unlikely to all be entirely wrong.

There are a number of options for how to construct good questions and after attempting a number of practice questions candidates will better appreciate how the questions are constructed. Particularly in Clinical Radiology, there is likely to be an initial description giving some combination of the clinical history, pathological, radiological and examination findings. The question part may then ask about the diagnosis, differential treatment, radiological findings (if not already given or in a different modality) or associated features. For most questions the options are likely to be presented as a list but for some questions, for instance staging lung cancer, tabulating the options works well.

When writing these questions it is possible to put a number of twists in the question or to take the question several levels away from the answer and this application of knowledge can make a question more discriminatory.

Different formats

The intention is usually to examine important information rather than what is easy to test and we suspect that the majority of questions will do this in the SBA format. There are some topics, however, which are particularly difficult to access in the new format and it remains to be seen what the Royal College Examiners will choose to do. It may be that they do not include these topics or find a novel way of approaching the information in SBA format, but we think it more likely that some topics will be examined with questions of a different format and this is the route we have chosen to take in this book where we have opted to vary the format of the questions slightly for these few topics to include particularly important information that we feel is likely to be incorporated in the College examinations.

The ideal SBA question will not be phrased in the negative and use terms such as NOT, LEAST LIKELY or EXCEPT. For some of the topics that are difficult to examine it may be that these questions are used and we have included a few in this book for this reason.

It is also possible that some questions will be phrased, 'Regarding XYZ, which of the following is true?' This is essentially a true/false question where you know that only one of the options is true, hence if you can answer any four of the options, you can answer the question correctly as even if you only know those that are false you can deduce that the remaining option must be the correct answer.

It is much easier to convert old true/false questions into these formats than proper SBA and as the RCR has a large bank of true/false questions it may be that they choose to do this to make up the number of available questions.

Similarly, there are some topics that lend themselves so well to multiple choice questions that there is always a temptation to examine them because they are easy to test rather than because they are particularly important or useful. We have tried hard to target questions to the important or useful topics and have made efforts to avoid easily constructed but largely irrelevant items, but this too would be a relatively easy way to make up the number of available questions.

No more negative marking: answer every question

You may pass with knowledge alone and the bulk of this book is dedicated to helping you do this. Some candidates, however, – whether through poor preparation, nerves, bad luck or whatever other cause – will find themselves close to passing but stumped by a number of questions and teetering close to but below the pass mark. At this point exam technique really comes into its own and it is a question of 'salvage' – getting whatever you can from the remaining questions and on balance doing better than chance. You don't need to be correct in every guess, just to skew the odds in your favour so you are more likely to be correct than with a blind guess and with each question you will continue to pull closer to the pass mark and ahead of the pack. Now that negative marking has been scrapped there is no risk of failing through bad luck from poor guessing and everyone should aim to maximise their mark even with the questions they don't understand or of which they are uncertain. Unlike with negative marking there is no longer a need to get more right than wrong and it is now quite simple – answer every question.

HOW TO GET A QUESTION RIGHT WHEN YOU DON'T KNOW THE ANSWER

You may be able to narrow the options down through your knowledge of what is being tested alone and pick between them, but even if you know nothing about the topic then you should guess intelligently.

The following methods of exam technique are likely to get you more than the expected 20% on a one from five single best answer question. These questions are difficult to construct properly and you should exploit any weakness in the question for your gain. What an examiner may consider a fault may prove helpful to a candidate with good technique and act as a marker for the right answer, even if you know nothing about the topic being examined. The following tips are presented roughly in descending order of reliability and several may be applicable to a single question.

1 Be suspicious of answers that do not follow from the stem (grammatically or temporally) as they are unlikely to be correct and are probably poor distractors.

2 If there are multiple stems that would have to be correct if one stem was correct, that stem must be wrong; that is, if option A were correct then option B would also have to be correct means that A must be wrong as there can only be one correct answer. (It remains possible that B is the correct answer unless B being correct would also imply that A had to be correct too.) See example below.

3 Compare the options and use the vignette for clues to the answer – is there a key difference between them (e.g. histiocytosis and LAM) that you remember which you can work backwards to deduce from the vignette?

4 Look for 'non-homogeneous' (to use medical education jargon) options where one answer is substantially different from the others. This item is probably an incorrect 'filler'. (Beware that it is possible but less likely that it is the correct answer and limited knowledge may help you spot this if the other four options are poor 'fillers'.)

5 You may be able to use one question to work out the answer from another; for example, a vignette may give a clinical history and a radiological finding and then later in the paper a question may ask what finding you would expect in that clinical situation.

6 Look for a cue in the options – longer options with more detail are more likely in a correct answer.

7 Terms that are repeated in question and option make that option more likely to be the correct answer.

8 Normal values or a 'null' option are probably wrong.

9 Convergence: Look for options where some component overlaps; the option with the most overlap with all the other options is more likely correct. This is particularly obvious with a table where the most frequently occurring option in a column is probably correct and by considering all the columns together it may be possible to narrow down the options to a single answer. (Note, however, that when setting the questions in this book we have deliberately drawn up tables where this is not possible, but it is an extra step to use as a possible hint and it may be that some questions creep through without this check happening.)

Option	T Stage	N Stage	M Stage
A	1	2	X
B (More likely)	2	2	0
C	3	2	1
D	1	3	0
E	2	3	0
	T1 or T2 appear twice	N2 appears 3 times	M0 appears 3 times

10 When considering tabulated data think which is the more likely clinical scenario; for example, T2N2M0 is probably more clinically likely than T1N3M0.

11 Beware of absolute terms – medicine has never been an exact science. Such terms – always, invariably, never, etc. – may well be part of a distractor that the examiner has phrased in this way to make it wrong. It is good practice to think specifically if you know about that option in the condition being tested

and whether it is a specific clue as occasionally these terms will be correct but this is often obvious and is the exception rather than the rule.

12 If you have no idea, there may even be a clue in the order of the answers. When setting the options it is tempting to put the correct option slightly more often first or last and slightly less often at B or D. Clearly, there are easy rigorous ways to overcome this (alphabetical arrangement of the answers, which will be apparent when you look at the paper or use of truly random allocation, which won't).

13 Similarly, the extremes of numerical data are probably more likely to be incorrect.

For an illustration of these features, which have been exaggerated for effect, consider the following question:

> A retired dockworker presents with shortness of breath and is assessed with a chest radiograph. This shows multiple leaf-shaped calcific opacities projected over both lungs. The underlying lungs appear normal. What is the most likely diagnosis?
> a Probably asbestos-related pleural plaques but not asbestosis
> b Asbestosis
> c Mania
> d Disseminated malignancy
> e Metastatic lung cancer

This question has a number of faults. Not only is the correct option (A) obvious but it is longer and more complete than the other options, making it distinctive. The correct option and the incorrect asbestosis are relatively similar compared to the other options, giving a hint that one of them is probably correct. The two options disseminated malignancy and lung cancer are mutually exclusive hence neither can be correct. The final distractor (mania) is entirely non-homogeneous, as the condition bears no relation to the patient's symptom and could not be diagnosed from the investigation in the question.

EXAM TECHNIQUE
Timekeeping
Single best answer questions take some time to read and time is likely to be much tighter than with the true/false format, particularly if you are not very quick at reading written English. Work out how long you have on average per question and at least on the first pass through the paper don't spend much longer than this on any one question. This method will maximise your chances of finishing the paper (and gaining any easy marks towards the end of the question paper) before you return to spend whatever time you have left on the difficult questions. Only spend the extra time on these questions as you go through if you are certain that you will, overall, still have time to complete the paper. Many people like to

take a clock and write down the time the exam started and will finish.

We chose 70 questions as the length of the papers in this book to achieve a balance between content and the time required to complete the paper before the Royal College of Radiologists confirmed their plans for the examination. They have very recently announced their intention to include 75 questions in the actual examination and we highlight this so candidates are aware that in the actual exam five more questions will need to be completed in the available time than in the papers in this book.

Order in which to answer questions

There is no obligation to answer the questions in the order in which they are presented and candidates adopt many strategies including missing out those they are unsure of and completing those of which they are certain before returning to the others. Indeed, the vast majority of candidates will miss out at least a few questions on their first pass. When doing this make sure of two things. Firstly, make sure that you make a note somewhere of which question you need to return to. You could have a blank sheet with headings such as 'Need to check' (but reasonably sure), 'It'll come back to me' and 'No idea'. Other people prefer to write on the question paper and circle the question number, draw an arrow in from the margin, or whatever. Similarly, a few will write a similar description for questions where they are so certain that they don't want to go back and waste time checking to remind them to miss out that question if they are checking the paper at the end. Secondly, and most importantly, when you miss out a question make absolutely certain that you put the answer to the next question you answer in the correct place on the answer sheet.

Writing the answers on the question paper or a blank sheet

Some candidates initially note their answers on the question paper or a blank sheet and then transfer then to the answer sheet after they have answered all the questions. This method may appeal to some people particularly if they are apt to change their minds several times and are worried they may 'make a mess' of the exam answer paper, but it is extremely high risk for two reasons. Firstly, errors when under pressure are easy and getting out of sequence with the answers will be catastrophic. Secondly, if you run out of time then rather than having, say, 99% of the paper complete you will have nothing as your answers cannot be handed in until they are transcribed. Hence we would sound a note of caution and advise that if you do choose this method, you should be exceptionally careful to keep the right question with the right answer and to complete the transcription in good time.

If you run out of time

If you run out of time, rapidly fill in any blanks and the remainder of the questions by just guessing the answer. If you really have run out of time it is critically important you mark any answer for every question as quickly as possible so do not waste time reading the question paper – just guess randomly.

Genito-urinary, adrenal, obstetric, gynaecological and breast radiology

PAPER 1

1 A 50-year-old male patient undergoes a CT examination following the administration of intravenous and oral contrast medium in the portal venous phase for investigation of persistent abdominal pain. His left adrenal gland is noted to have a 'bulky' anterior limb width measuring 2 cm with Hounsfield units of 18. What is the most likely diagnosis?
   a Adrenal haemorrhage
   b Adrenal *tuberculosis*
   c Adrenal adenoma
   d Adrenocortical carcinoma
   e Adrenal myelolipoma

2 A 45-year-old man with a spiculated mass on his chest radiograph undergoes staging CT examination following the administration of intravenous contrast medium for a possible bronchial carcinoma. There is an enlarged right adrenal mass of 2 cm found with an average density of 40 HU. What is the appropriate next investigation for characterisation of the adrenal mass?
   a PET
   b Unenhanced and delayed phase CT examination
   c MRI
   d MIBG
   e Follow-up staging CT examination in three months

3   A female neonate with a family history of an autosomal recessive lipoidosis is found to have hepatomegaly and splenomegaly on clinical examination. Punctate cortical adrenal calcification is visible on her abdominal X-ray. What is the most likely diagnosis?

   a Neuroblastoma

   b Ganglioneuroma

   c Phaeochromocytoma

   d Wolman's disease

   e Benign cystic disease

4   A 65-year-old female patient with a history of hypertension presents with acute right flank pain and shock. A CT demonstrates a right-sided adrenal mass, which is of predominately low attenuation (several areas measure –100 HU) and associated retroperitoneal haemorrhage. What is the most likely diagnosis?

   a Myelolipoma

   b Phaeochromocytoma

   c Adenoma

   d Adrenal artery aneurysm

   e Adrenocortical carcinoma

5   A 38-year-old man undergoes investigation for persistent hypertension. He is found to have an increased aldosterone and decreased renin level. What investigation is most likely to help establish the diagnosis?

   a CT examination with adrenal protocol (unenhanced and delayed phases)

   b MRI examination with fat suppression sequences

   c MIBG

   d Ultrasound

   e Adrenal venous sampling

6   A 50-year-old female presents with sweating, palpitations and uncontrollable hypertension. As part of her work-up a MIBG (metaiodobenzylguanidine) nuclear medicine scan is performed. How will this advance her management?

   a Distinguish phaeochromocytoma from carcinoid

   b Locate an extra-adrenal phaeochromocytoma

   c Distinguish between Cushing's disease and Cushing's syndrome

   d Exclude papillary thyroid carcinoma

   e Exclude Addison's syndrome

7   A 55-year-old man with acute necrotising pancreatitis was assessed with CT after being cared for on the ITU for six days. An unenhanced examination was performed due to renal impairment, which demonstrated bilateral adrenal enlargement with an attenuation of 75 HU. What is the most likely cause for this?

    a Adrenal adenomas

    b Adrenocortical carcinoma

    c Metastatic deposits

    d Adrenal haemorrhage

    e Adrenocortical hyperplasia

8   A newspaper article reports that using HRT may double the risk of breast cancer. Assuming that the report refers to the relative risk attributable to HRT and that the underlying risk in the population studied is 1.5 per 100 women over five years then what is the absolute increase in risk? (Options are per 100 women over five years.)

    a 0.003

    b 0.03

    c 0.15

    d 0.3

    e 1.5

9   A 40-year-old woman presents with a breast lump felt over the past four weeks. On examination, there is a firm, discrete, mobile mass palpable in the right upper outer quadrant. Mammography demonstrates a 1-cm well-circumscribed round soft-tissue density in the upper outer quadrant of the right breast. What is the most appropriate management of this patient?

    a Reassure that the lesion is benign in nature and discharge to primary care

    b Perform ultrasound to confirm benign appearance, provide reassurance and discharge to primary care

    c Perform ultrasound and ultrasound-guided core needle biopsy if a solid lesion is visible

    d Perform stereotactic-guided core needle biopsy

    e Discuss at MDT meeting with a view to proceeding to wide local excision

10   A 40-year-old woman presents with a palpable breast lump for several weeks. On examination, a firm, relatively mobile mass is palpable in the left upper outer quadrant. Mammograms demonstrate a well-circumscribed round soft-tissue density in the upper outer quadrant of the left breast. What feature on ultrasound would favour a diagnosis of a breast cyst above that of fibroadenoma?

    a Multiple bilateral lesions of similar appearance

    b Internal calcification

    c A round hypoechoic lesion with a smooth well-defined margin

    d A hypoechoic lesion with internal echoes homogeneously distributed within the lesion

    e A hyperechoic posterior wall

11 A 40-year-old obese woman is found to have a painless mass in the right breast by her general practitioner during a routine medical examination. What feature would favour a diagnosis of an oil cyst over that of a lipoma?

  a A history of recent lactation

  b A rounded lucent lesion on mammography

  c A surrounding capsule seen on mammography

  d Demonstration of eggshell calcification

  e Multiple areas of fatty and fibroglandular density

12 A 70-year-old woman presents with invasive ductal carcinoma. Where in her breast is it most likely to be located?

  a Retroareolar

  b Upper inner quadrant

  c Upper outer quadrant

  d Lower inner quadrant

  e Lower outer quadrant

13 A 50-year-old woman presented with fatigue and her physician was concerned she had metastatic disease of unknown origin. Her diagnostic work-up included a mammogram which demonstrated a suspicious lesion in the left upper outer quadrant. A biopsy confirmed this to be a breast carcinoma. Where is the most likely place for this lesion initially to have metastasised?

  a Brain

  b Liver

  c Bone

  d Lung and pleurae

  e Lymph nodes other than ipsilateral axillary nodes

14 A 62-year-old woman is treated for invasive ductal carcinoma with a wide local excision and axillary clearance. Which of the following is the most appropriate follow-up mammography regime?

  a Every six months until the age of 70 and then self-referral at patient's request

  b Every six months for the first year and annually thereafter

  c Every six months for the first two years and annually thereafter

  d Every year until the age of 70 and then self-referral at patient's request

  e Every year for five years then return to the breast-screening programme

15 A 51-year-old woman presents to the breast clinic with a palpable lump felt in the lateral aspect of the right breast, which had increased in size since she went through the menopause. It measures 4.5 cm and shows posterior acoustic shadowing on USS. On mammography the margins are partly well-circumscribed and partly obscured. Peripheral egg shell calcification is visible. Her menarche was at 12; she had three pregnancies and has never taken HRT or the OCP. Which of the feature makes a diagnosis other than a breast cyst more likely?

   a Margins which are partly well-circumscribed and partly obscured

   b Size greater than 4 cm

   c An increase in size in the post-menopausal period, in the absence of HRT

   d Peripheral eggshell calcification

   e Posterior acoustic shadowing

16 A 40-year-old woman with a family history of breast cancer presents with a palpable breast lump. Histology confirms a diagnosis of invasive breast carcinoma. What is the most likely pathological type?

   a Ductal carcinoma

   b Lobular carcinoma

   c Medullary

   d Sarcomatous carcinoma

   e Mucinous (colloid) carcinoma

17 A 56-year-old woman attended for routine mammographic screening. Calcification was noted on her mammograms and after further work-up she was diagnosed as having invasive carcinoma in the area of the calcifications. What is the most likely morphology of the calcifications?

   a Spherical with a radiolucent centre

   b Popcorn

   c Rounded

   d Linear, branching

   e Rod shaped (thick, linear)

18 A 51-year-old woman with a family history of breast cancer underwent a screening mammogram, which demonstrated an abnormal area of multiple microcalcifications. No other abnormality was visible and this was not seen on an ultrasound. A stereotactic-guided excision was performed which showed invasive carcinoma. How large is it most likely the calcifications were?

a <0.5 mm

b 0.5–1.5 mm

c 1.5–3 mm

d 3–5 mm

e >5 mm

19 A 65-year-old woman, who was known to have a primary malignancy elsewhere, had a mammogram which showed multiple well-defined soft-tissue opacities. These were proven to be metastases from her primary. What primary is she most likely to have?

a Lymphoma, oesophageal carcinoma, lung carcinoma, renal cell carcinoma

b Lung carcinoma, oesophageal carcinoma, renal cell carcinoma, melanoma

c Lymphoma, cervical carcinoma, colorectal carcinoma, gastric carcinoma

d Lymphoma, melanoma, ovarian carcinoma, lung carcinoma

e Oesophageal carcinoma, cervical carcinoma, ovarian carcinoma, lung carcinoma

20 A 42-year-old woman presents with a lump in the left axilla. No mass is clinically palpable in the left breast and mammography is normal. Histology demonstrates an axillary node malignancy and she is referred for an MRI of the breasts to search for an occult primary breast malignancy. Which of the following time-enhancement curves would be most likely to represent a malignant lesion on contrast-enhanced T1W subtraction sequences?

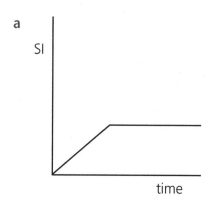

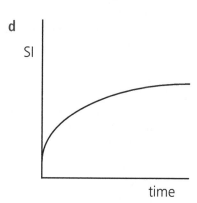

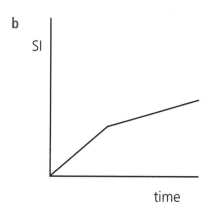

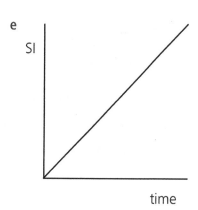

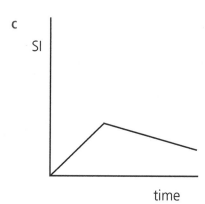

21 A 45-year-old woman presents with a rapidly increasing mass in the right breast of recent onset. Mammography shows a single well-circumscribed round, homogeneous soft-tissue opacity, measuring 8 cm in diameter with no calcification. Histology demonstrates a fibroepithelial tumour with a leaf-like growth pattern. What is the most likely diagnosis?

a Fibroadenoma

b Lipoma

c Invasive ductal carcinoma

d Papilloma

e Phyllodes tumour

22 A 65-year-old man with an abnormal karyotype presents with a left breast lump and is found to have an invasive ductal carcinoma. What karyotype is he most likely to have?

a 45 X0

b 46 XY

c 47 XXY

d 47 XXX

e 47 XY13

23 A 42-year-old woman presents with a lump in the left axilla. No mass is clinically palpable in the left breast and mammography is normal, but histology demonstrates an axillary node malignancy. What is the appropriate management?

a No further imaging, bilateral mastectomy is indicated

b Repeat mammograms

c Breast ultrasound

d Breast MRI

e Breast CT

24 A 26-year-old patient with a positive β-HCG undergoes pelvic ultrasound examination. Which finding on ultrasound is most likely to indicate a non-viable pregnancy?

a The intradecidual sign

b Non-visualisation of cardiac activity when crown–rump length (CRL) is 7 mm

c Visualisation of the yolk sac when the gestational sac is 8 mm

d Gestational sac present at 32 days

e Asymmetry of the echogenic ring surrounding the gestational sac at five weeks

25 A 60-year-old female was admitted with progressive abdominal distension and vague abdominal pain. She is found to have a 20-cm complex ovarian mass on ultrasound and a raised CA-125 level. What is the next step in management and staging?

a PET scan

b CT followed by biopsy

c Biopsy of the ovarian mass followed by MRI examination

d Primary surgery

e MRI examination followed by biopsy

26 A 45-year-old female with a complex ovarian mass and raised CA-125 level underwent staging CT examination. What are the findings consistent with her having stage III disease?

a Both ovaries involved with malignant ascites

b Extension to the fallopian tubes without malignant ascites

c Malignant ascites with implants on the uterus

d Peritoneal metastases

e Liver metastases

27 A 30-year-old female patient with pelvic pain and irregular periods underwent an ultrasound examination. In the left ovary there was a 4-cm diffuse homogeneous hypoechoic focal lesion with low-level internal echoes. What is the most likely diagnosis?

a Endometrioma

b Functional ovarian cyst

c Polycystic ovary (PCOS)

d Ovarian carcinoma

e Corpus luteum

28 A 30-year-old female with menorrhagia underwent ultrasound examination of the pelvis which demonstrated an adnexal lesion. She went on to have an MRI which, on T1-weighted images, demonstrated a low-signal mass related to the right ovary. What is the most likely diagnosis?

a Endometriosis

b Ovarian fibroma

c Dermoid

d Haemorrhagic mass

e Mucinous cystic neoplasm

29 A 35-year-old patient with a history of endometriosis presents with a number of clinical symptoms. Which of the following symptoms cannot be explained by the diagnosis of endometriosis?

a Lump at site of previous surgical scar

b Shortness of breath and pleuritic pain at onset of menses

c Haematuria

d Pelvic pain and feeling of fullness

e Aching muscles

30 A 50-year-old female with a history of bronchial malignancy underwent a PET-CT examination and was noted to have increased activity in the pelvis. Increased uptake in which organ or area would indicate sinister pathology?

a Uterine fibroids

b Ovaries

c Cervix

d Blood vessels

e Bladder diverticulum

31 A 40-year-old, pre-menopausal woman is noted to have a unilocular adnexal cyst measuring 4 cm on transvaginal ultrasound examination. What is the most appropriate management?

a MRI examination after six weeks

b Pelvic ultrasound examination after four weeks

c CA-125 blood test and referral to gynaecology

d Pelvic ultrasound examination after six weeks

e CA-125 and CT examination

32 A 50-year-old peri-menopausal female patient presents with dysfunctional bleeding. She is referred to the Gynaecology Outpatient Clinic and to Radiology for an ultrasound examination. Assuming that her symptoms are due to a gynaecological malignancy, what is the most likely site of disease?

a Endometrial

b Ovarian

c Vulval

d Cervical

e Vaginal

33 A 22-year-old female patient presented with acute pelvic pain. She had a positive β-HCG result and the gynaecologist on call has asked you to look for an ectopic pregnancy. What ultrasound appearance would reassure you there is an intrauterine pregnancy?
   a Pseudogestational sac
   b Echogenic ring-like mass outside the uterus
   c Decidual cysts
   d 'Ring of fire' on colour Doppler imaging
   e Double decidual sac sign

34 A 65-year-old patient with post-menopausal bleeding comes to ultrasound for a pelvic ultrasound examination. What risk factor on the clinical details makes the patient more at risk for developing endometrial carcinoma?
   a Multiparity
   b Early menopause
   c Late menarche
   d Hypertension
   e Diabetes insipidus

35 A 55-year-old post-menopausal patient is experiencing post-menopausal bleeding. She is not on HRT. She undergoes pelvic ultrasound examination and was noted to have an endometrial thickness of 8 mm. What is the next appropriate step in management?
   a Discharge patient with no follow-up
   b Follow-up ultrasound examination in six weeks
   c Referral to gynaecologist for Pipelle biopsy or hysteroscopy
   d MRI examination for endometrial staging and referral to gynaecology
   e CT examination for endometrial staging and referral to gynaecology

36 A 60-year-old female patient presented with post-menopausal bleeding and was found to have endometrial carcinoma. An MRI of her pelvis is performed for staging of the endometrial carcinoma. What signal would you expect normal myometrium, junctional zone and endometrium to return on T2-weighted images?

	Myometrium	Junctional zone	Endometrium
a	Low	Medium	High
b	High	Low	Medium
c	Medium	Low	High
d	Low	High	Medium
e	High	Medium	Low

37 A 75-year-old lady who had grade 2 endometrial adenocarcinoma diagnosed on endometrial sampling undergoes an MRI examination for staging. If there is cervical invasion but no further spread, what would be the correct staging?

a IC

b II

c IB

d IIIB

e IV

38 A 42-year-old female patient who is 14 weeks' pregnant has an episode of vaginal bleeding and is referred to hospital. The admitting obstetric doctor finds an enlarged uterus on examination and a raised β-HCG on blood tests. Ultrasound examination demonstrates a large echogenic mass with several small fluid-filled spaces within it within the uterus. What is the most likely diagnosis?

a Incomplete miscarriage

b Gestational trophoblastic disease

c Uterine carcinoma

d Placental abruption

e Ectopic pregnancy

39 A 65-year-old patient is noted to have a raised prostate-specific antigen (PSA) level by his general practitioner. He is referred to a urologist and undergoes biopsy which demonstrates prostate cancer. At MRI, which of the following features is suggestive of stage T3 rather than stage T2 disease?

a Extracapsular extension

b Tumour involves more than one half of one lobe but not both lobes

c Involvement of bladder neck

d Tumour involves both lobes

e Involvement of the external sphincter

40 A 73-year-old patient had a biopsy demonstrating prostate cancer and subsequently underwent MRI examination which showed an abnormality. Which of the following features suggests post-biopsy haemorrhage rather than the prostate cancer tumour?

a Low signal on T2-weighted images in the peripheral zone

b Asymmetry of the neurovascular bundle

c Low signal on T2-weighted images in the seminal vesicles

d High signal on T1-weighted images in the peripheral zone

e Obliteration of the rectoprostatic angle

41 A 38-year-old man attends his GP with testicular pain. He is referred for an ultrasound examination. This demonstrates 1–2 mm hyperechoic multiple non-shadowing foci throughout both testes. Which of the following is most likely to be associated with this finding?
a Testicular germ cell tumour
b Epididymitis
c Epididymal cyst
d Scrotal pearl
e Varicocele

42 A 42-year-old man is referred for a scrotal ultrasound examination because of a palpable lump that has been present for two weeks. This demonstrates a focal hypoechoic heterogeneous mass measuring 3 cm. What is the most likely diagnosis?
a Embryonal cell carcinoma
b Epidermoid cyst
c Teratoma
d Yolk sac tumour
e Seminoma

43 A 30-year-old man attends for a scrotal ultrasound examination having felt a lump. Ultrasound shows a well-defined 2-cm round lesion in the region of the right testis, which has rings of alternating hypo and hyperechoic echo-genicity. No blood flow can be demonstrated on colour Doppler imaging. What is the most likely diagnosis?
a Burned-out tumour of testis (Azzopardi tumour)
b Lymphoma of testis
c Epidermoid cyst
d Seminoma
e Metastasis to testis

44 A 65-year-old man with a known malignancy presents with a testicular lump that he has noticed increasing in size over the last three weeks. He is referred for an ultrasound examination. This demonstrates a heterogeneous 4-cm mass in the left testis, which was biopsied and confirmed to be a metastasis from his primary malignancy. What is the most likely site of primary malignancy?
a Brain
b Adrenal
c Thyroid
d Liver
e Lung

45 A 35-year-old man attended his general practitioner requesting a vasectomy. On examination there was a palpable scrotal mass and he was referred for an ultrasound examination. This demonstrated an 8-mm well-defined anechoic area in the head of the right epididymis. What is the most appropriate next step in this patient's management?

a Discharge the patient back to GP with no follow-up

b Discharge patient back to GP with no follow-up but recommend that vasectomy may be complicated

c Refer patient to urologist and advise follow-up ultrasound examination

d Refer patient to urologist and advise staging CT examination

e Discharge patient back to GP and advise urology referral

46 A nine-year-old boy is admitted to hospital 12 hours following the onset of acute scrotal pain and is referred for an ultrasound examination. Which of the following ultrasound appearances is incompatible with a diagnosis of testicular torsion?

a Normal grey-scale appearance of both testes

b Hydrocoele

c Scrotal skin thickening

d Diffusely hypoechoic echotexture of one testis

e Cryptoorchidism

47 A 26-year-old man presented with a testicular lump and was referred by his GP for an ultrasound examination. This demonstrated a 3-cm heterogeneous solid mass in the left testicle. What is the most appropriate next step in his management?

a Repeat ultrasound examination in three weeks following antibiotics

b Staging MRI examination

c Staging CT examination

d Bone scintigraphy

e Biopsy followed by staging examination

48 A 26-year-old male is involved in a motor vehicle accident and sustains a pelvic fracture. On ultrasound 'a bladder within a bladder' appearance is seen; that is, a bladder surrounded by a fluid collection. A diagnosis of extra-peritoneal bladder rupture is made. Where is the bladder most likely to have ruptured?

a The dome of the bladder

b The left ureteric orifice

c The right ureteric orifice

d Anterior aspect of the base of the bladder

e Diagnosis is more likely to be urethral transaction

49 A 49-year-old man is scheduled for an intravenous urogram as part of the investigation of a known transitional cell carcinoma of the bladder. His control image is normal. Five minutes following the administration of 100 mL of non-ionic low osmolar iodinated contrast medium, at which time the patient is well, there is no opacification of either renal collecting system or ureter but faint nephrograms are present. What is the most likely cause for this appearance?

a Bilateral renal artery stenosis

b Bilateral synchronous renal transitional cell carcinomas causing obstruction

c Bilateral ureteric obstruction and hydronephrosis from the bladder primary

d Contrast extravasation

e Profound hypotension related to contrast injection

50 A 27-year-old woman undergoing a contrast-enhanced CT pulmonary angiogram becomes extremely agitated immediately following the examination. She complains of intense itching, periorbital tingling and swelling, and wheeze. She has widespread urticaria, tachycardia and a blood pressure of 90/40 mmHg. Which of the following treatments is most urgently required?

a Adrenaline (epinephrine) 1:1000 0.5 mg intravenous administration

b Hydrocortisone 200 mg intravenous administration

c 500 mL 0.9% sodium chloride bolus infusion

d Adrenaline (Epinephrine) 1:1000 0.5 mg intramuscular administration

e Atropine 1 mg intravenous administration

51 Which of the following CT protocols is optimal for characterisation of a renal cortical solid mass seen on ultrasound in a 56-year-old man?

a Unenhanced scan, followed by post-intravenous contrast scans acquired at 60 and 100 seconds

b Unenhanced scan, followed by post-intravenous contrast scans acquired at 15 and 100 seconds

c Unenhanced scan, followed by post-intravenous contrast scans acquired at 90 seconds and 15 minutes

d Post-intravenous contrast scans acquired at 60 and 90 seconds

e Unenhanced scan, followed by post-intravenous contrast scans acquired at 90 seconds

52 A 27-year-old male presents with severe left loin pain, colicky in nature and microscopic haematuria. Which of the following imaging techniques is the optimal method to prove or exclude the diagnosis of ureteric colic?

  a Renal ultrasound

  b Plain abdominal radiograph

  c Unenhanced CT abdomen and pelvis, performed supine with normal mA dose protocol

  d Unenhanced CT abdomen and pelvis, performed prone with low mA dose protocol

  e Limited intravenous urogram

53 A 33-year-old female investigated for recurrent urinary infections is demonstrated to have a complete left duplex ureter on intravenous urography. Which of the following describes the classical arrangement of the duplex ureteric insertions and associated features?

  a The ureter from the superior pelvis inserts above that from the inferior pelvis, and the upper renal moiety has calyceal dilatation from distal ureteric obstruction

  b The ureter from the superior pelvis inserts below that from the inferior pelvis, and the upper renal moiety has calyceal dilatation from distal ureteric obstruction

  c The ureter from the superior pelvis inserts below that from the inferior pelvis, and is more prone to vesico-ureteric reflux

  d The ureter from the inferior pelvis is associated with a ureterocoele

  e The ureter from the inferior pelvis is associated with ectopic insertion into the urethra

54 A 43-year-old man presents with right flank pain and haematuria. A CT KUB performed to exclude renal colic is negative for an obstructing ureteric calculus but instead shows a predominantly low-density solitary right renal mass. What feature on CT would be more in keeping with this lesion being a renal carcinoma than a sporadic angiomyolipoma?

  a Presence of internal fat

  b Presence of internal haemorrhage

  c Size of 5 cm

  d Presence of internal calcification

  e Extension into peri-renal fat

55 A 21-year-old male from Nigeria presents with haematuria and urgency. A plain KUB radiograph shows bladder wall calcification. Which of the following is the most likely cause?

  a Guinea worm infection (Dracunculiasis)

  b Histoplasmosis infection

  c Taenia solium infection (Cysticercosis)

    d Schistosomiasis infection (Bilharziasis)

    e Candiru fish infestation

56 A 15-year-old boy being investigated for recurrent urinary infection under-goes Tc-99m DTPA scintigraphy which demonstrates the presence of a horseshoe kidney. What is likely to limit the isthmus?

    a Umbilical ligament

    b Urachus

    c Coeliac axis

    d Superior mesenteric artery

    e Inferior mesenteric artery

57 A 10-year-old boy is demonstrated on ultrasound to have bilateral multiple echogenic masses measuring up to 4 cm in size. A renal CT shows predomi-nantly low-density (–20 HU) masses with some heterogeneous enhancement following intravenous contrast. What underlying condition is the patient most likely to have?

    a Von Hippel-Lindau disease

    b Tuberous sclerosis

    c Neurofibromatosis type 2

    d Gorlin syndrome

    e Hurler syndrome

58 A 45-year-old male is crushed by a forklift truck palette. He complains of failure to pass urine and lower abdominal pain. A pelvic radiograph shows bilateral pubic rami fractures. Passage of a urethral catheter shows gross haematuria and the clinicians suspect a bladder injury. What investigation would you recommend to assess his injuries?

    a CT abdomen and pelvis with intravenous contrast, a clamped urinary catheter and delayed scans through the bladder

    b CT abdomen and pelvis with intravenous contrast and instilled intravesical contrast

    c Unenhanced CT pelvis

    d Pelvic ultrasound

    e Retrograde standard cystography

59 A 23-year-old female is demonstrated to have bilateral hyperdense renal masses on unenhanced CT. Following intravenous contrast administration the lesions remain homogeneous but are hypodense to normal renal cortex. There is associated retroperitoneal lymph node enlargement. What is the most likely diagnosis?

a Renal lymphoma

b Von Hippel-Lindau disease

c Adult polycystic kidney disease

d Angiomyolipomas

e Xanthogranulomatous pyelonephritis

60 A 55-year-old male is 18 months following right radical nephrectomy for an 8-cm renal cell carcinoma, which invaded the renal vein (T3b N0 M0, Stage IIIA), and is undergoing a surveillance CT scan. Where is the most likely site for distant metastatic recurrence?

a Brain

b Contralateral kidney

c Lung

d Skin

e Bowel

61 A 34-year-old male presents with left-sided renal colic and has a KUB that does not demonstrate any radio-opaque calculi. A CT is then performed and again no radio-opaque calculi are visible, but there is a small filling defect in the left ureter at the vesicoureteric junction on delayed post-contrast images. What is the most likely underlying diagnosis?

a Hyperparathyroidism

b Chronic urinary infection

c Gout

d Cystinuria

e Protease inhibitor use in HIV

62 A 35-year-old female with renal impairment is demonstrated to have bilateral renal cortical tramline calcification on CT. What is the most likely diagnosis?

a Hyperparathyroidism

b Acute cortical necrosis

c Renal tubular acidosis

d *Tuberculosis*

e Renal artery aneurysm

63 A 58-year-old male with no family history of renal cysts and no cysts in other organs is demonstrated to have multiple renal cysts on ultrasound. What is the most likely diagnosis?

a Acquired renal cystic disease

b Autosomal dominant polycystic kidney disease

c Multicystic dysplastic kidney

d Multiple simple cysts

e Von Hippel-Lindau disease

64 A 27-year-old female with a family history of nephrectomy for malignancy is demonstrated to have multiple renal cysts on a surveillance ultrasound. What is the most likely diagnosis?

a Autosomal dominant polycystic kidney disease

b Multiple simple cysts

c Acquired renal cystic disease

d Cystic renal cell carcinoma

e Von Hippel-Lindau disease

65 A 35-year-old female undergoing investigation for hypertension and renal impairment is demonstrated with ultrasound to have multiple bilateral renal cysts as well as hepatic and pancreatic cysts. What is the most likely diagnosis?

a Conn's syndrome

b Autosomal-dominant polycystic kidney disease

c Multicystic dysplastic kidney

d Multiple simple cysts

e Phaeochromocytoma

66 A 60-year-old male diabetic on haemodialysis for 10 years is demonstrated on ultrasound to have multiple small renal cysts, some of which have high echogenicity walls consistent with calcification. What is the most likely diagnosis?

a Acquired renal cystic disease

b Von Hippel-Lindau disease

c Multicystic renal cell carcinoma

d Multicystic dysplastic kidney

e Autosomal dominant polycystic kidney disease

67 A one-year-old male under investigation for an abdominal mass is demonstrated on ultrasound to have multiple left renal cysts. There is no functioning ipsilateral renal tissue on MAG3 scintigraphy. What is the most likely diagnosis?

a   Acquired renal cystic disease

b   Multicystic dysplastic kidney

c   Autosomal recessive polycystic kidney disease

d   Pelvi-ureteric junction obstruction

e   Multiple simple cysts

68 A child is demonstrated to have increased echogenicity of the renal medulla on ultrasound, and plain radiography confirms the presence of nephrocalcinosis. What is the most likely cause?

a   Renal tubular acidosis

b   Hyperparathyroidism

c   Medullary sponge kidney

d   Renal papillary necrosis

e   Primary hyperoxaluria

69 A 32-year-old male is a restrained passenger in a head-on motor vehicle collision and complains of left flank pain. He is assessed with a contrast-enhanced trauma CT. What feature on his CT would require urgent intervention (surgical/radiological), assuming no other organ injury is identified?

a   A contained leak of opacified urine into the retroperitoneum

b   Peripheral renal enhancement

c   A low-attenuation laceration extending to the medulla, but not to the collecting system

d   A low-attenuation subcapsular haematoma >1 cm in depth

e   A wedge-shaped area of low attenuation poorly enhancing renal cortex

70 A 23-year-old male motorcyclist is struck by a car at approximately 40 mph. He has bruising to the left flank and back and is tender in the left upper quadrant and lower chest wall. He is tachycardic but normotensive and has no haematuria. Which is the most appropriate imaging modality?

a   FAST ultrasound

b   Intravenous urogram

c   Unenhanced CT KUB

d   Abdominal and pelvic CT with intravenous contrast

e   No imaging is required

Genito-urinary, adrenal, obstetric, gynaecological and breast radiology

PAPER 2

1 A 39-year-old female with breast cancer detected on screening is awaiting wide local excision and sentinel node biopsy. What is the appropriate method of evaluating the site of a sentinel node?

 a 20–40 mBq of nanocolloid injected subdermally into the quadrant of the breast where the cancer is located

 b 20–40 mBq of nanocolloid subdermally into the ipsilateral axilla

 c Ultrasound-guided methylene blue injection into the most prominent node in the ipsilateral axilla

 d Injection of radio-labelled 20–40 mBq of methylene blue

 e 20–40 mBq of nanocolloid injected subdermally into the upper outer quadrant regardless of the site of the cancer

2 A 78-year-old man is being investigated by the endocrinology team for chronic primary adrenal insufficiency. As part of the endocrine investigations he undergoes CT examination of the adrenals which demonstrates small adrenal glands with calcifications bilaterally. What is the most likely diagnosis?

 a Previous *tuberculosis* infection

 b Idiopathic adrenal atrophy

 c Bilateral metastatic disease

 d Ganglioneuroma

 e Phaeochromocytoma

3 A 45-year-old female with a previous diagnosis of medullary thyroid cancer and hyperparathyroidism had an abdominal MRI which demonstrated an adrenal lesion. Which of the following are the most likely radiological findings?

   a Hyperintense areas to liver on T1-weighted images and intermediate intensity to spleen on T2-weighted images

   b Isointense/hypointense to liver on T1-weighted images and very hyperintense to spleen in T2-weighted images

   c Heterogeneously hyperintense to liver on T1- and T2-weighted images (ACC)

   d Isointense on T1-weighted images and very hypointense on T2-weighted images

   e Hypointense on T1- and T2-weighted images

4 On abdominal CT examination, which of the following appearances of the adrenal gland is unexpected and would require further evaluation?

   a Length of the adrenal limb measures 4 cm

   b Width of the adrenal limb measures 2 cm

   c Right adrenal lying behind the IVC

   d Left adrenal lying in front of the upper pole of left kidney

   e Right adrenal not seen on the same CT slice as the right kidney

5 A nine-year-old boy presents to the endocrinology team with bilateral testicular masses and precocious puberty. Which of the following are the most likely radiological findings?

   a Bilateral diffuse enlargement of the adrenals but preservation of their usual morphology

   b Normal size and appearance of the adrenals

   c Bilateral global atrophy of the adrenals but preservation of their usual configuration

   d Lack of normal adrenal tissue bilaterally

   e Unilateral enlarged adrenal with preservation of usual configuration

6 A two-year-old boy presents to the paediatric team with an abdominal mass. Ultrasound examination demonstrated a large hyperechoic heterogeneous mass on the right extending across the midline and with areas with acoustic shadowing. The right kidney could not be clearly visualised. A CT examination was then performed. Which of the following are the most likely radiological findings?

   a Centrally located heterogeneous mass arising from the right kidney with a prominent peripheral crescent-shaped subcapsular fluid collection

   b Solid intrarenal mass of right kidney with uniform enhancement of less than normal renal parenchyma with areas of low attenuation within it

c Heterogeneous solid mass with low-density areas and calcifications displacing the right kidney and encasing the IVC

d Well-defined heterogeneous partially cystic mass with a claw of right renal tissue partially extending around it

e Well-defined round mass separate to the right kidney with periadrenal fat stranding and a low attenuation centre

7 A two-year-old boy who presented with an abdominal mass and underwent ultrasound and CT examination has been diagnosed with neuroblastoma. Which of the following radiological findings would indicate that the lesion could not be fully removed surgically?

a Necrosis within the mass

b Displacement of the ipsilateral kidney

c Enlarged ipsilateral lymph nodes containing tumour

d Calcification within the mass

e Involvement of IVC

8 A 60-year-old female patient undergoes a CT examination and is incidentally found to have a heterogeneous left adrenal mass measuring 12 cm, which contains calcifications and has delayed washout characteristics. Biochemical endocrine testing is negative. What other condition is associated with the most likely diagnosis?

a Astrocytoma

b Multiple endocrine neoplasia (MEN) Type 1

c Multiple endocrine neoplasia (MEN) Type 2A

d Carney complex

e Neurofibromatosis

9 A 32-year-old woman underwent breast augmentation mammoplasty two years ago and has recently noted a change in the shape of her right breast. Her surgeon is concerned she has had an intracapsular rupture. What investigation would be most sensitive?

a MLO implant displacement mammographic view

b Breast ultrasound

c T1-weighted MRI sequence

d Standard two-view mammography.

e T2-weighted fast spin echo MRI sequences

10 A 50-year-old woman presents with a rapidly increasing mass in the right breast of recent onset. Mammography shows a single well-circumscribed round, homogeneous soft-tissue opacity, measuring 8 cm in diameter with no calcification. Biopsy shows this lesion to be a phyllodes tumour. What is the risk of malignant degeneration?

a <1%

b 1–2%

c 5–10%

d 40–60%

e >90%

11 A 65-year-old hypertensive man with diabetes and a past history of colorectal carcinoma resected seven years previously presented with bilateral breast masses situated in the subareolar region. His medication included aspirin, bisoprolol, digoxin, furosemide and metformin. He then underwent mammography which showed a triangular area of subareolar glandular tissue that points towards the nipple. What is the most likely diagnosis?

a Gynaecomastia due to furosemide therapy

b Gynaecomastia due to digoxin therapy

c Normal finding

d Bilateral metastatic disease

e Lobular carcinoma in situ bilaterally

12 A 50-year-old woman is found to have a breast mass on screening mammography. Her mammograms demonstrate a round well-circumscribed mass measuring 3 cm in diameter of mixed density with a mottled centre, reported as having a 'slice of sausage' appearance, situated in the right upper outer quadrant of the breast. The mass is surrounded by a thin smooth pseudocapsule and has a halo sign. MRI demonstrates a well-circumscribed round lesion with pseudocapsular demarcation containing a mixture of low, intermediate and high signal intensities on T1-weighted sequences and corresponding high and intermediate signal intensities on T2-weighted images. What is the most likely diagnosis?

a Fibroadenoma

b Hamartoma of the breast (fibroadenolipoma)

c Lobular carcinoma

d Lipoma

e Galactocoele

13 A 32-year-old woman who is currently breastfeeding develops a swelling in her left breast. Which of the following features would favour a diagnosis of galactocoele above that of cold abscess of the breast?

a A retroareolar location

b An anechoic/nearly anechoic area on ultrasound with posterior enhancement

c The presence of pathologic axillary lymph nodes

d A lesion of mixed density on mammography with a fat-water level on a horizontal beam view

e Secondary changes to the breast, including architectural distortion, nipple retraction and skin thickening

14 Regarding screening mammography, to which age range does the National Breast Screening Programme in the UK currently offer invitations for screening?

a 45–75 years

b 47–70 years

c 50–70 years

d 49–71 years

e 50–73 years

15 A 56-year-old woman attends the mobile mammography unit for a routine screening mammogram. Which initial view(s) are recommended in screening mammography?

a Craniocaudal

b Mediolateral oblique

c Craniocaudal and mediolateral oblique

d Craniocaudal and true lateral

e Medial and lateral

16 A 46-year-old woman underwent a left mastectomy for multicentric breast carcinoma. She noticed subsequent swelling on the left, which gradually increased in size over two weeks. A subsequent MRI of the left breast demonstrated a circumscribed area of mildly hypointense signal on T1W sequences which is hyperintense on T2W sequences and hypointense on a water-suppressed STIR sequence. Contrast enhancement was seen in the surrounding parenchyma on enhanced T1W sequences. What are these findings most likely to represent?

a Intracapsular rupture of a silicone implant

b Extracapsular rupture of a silicone implant

c Post-surgical seroma

d Residual breast carcinoma

e Autogenous tissue transplantation breast reconstruction

17 A 51-year-old woman attends for mammographic screening for the first time. An opacity is seen in the right breast and she is recalled for further views and assessment. Ultimately, she is found to have a radial scar of the breast. Which of the following statements is most accurate?

   a It characteristically arises at a site of previous surgery or trauma

   b At mammography, the lesion looks similar on both the craniocaudal and mediolateral oblique projections

   c Thickening and retraction of the overlying skin is a typical mammographic finding

   d Surgical excision is required for a definite diagnosis

   e It typically presents as a palpable breast lump

18 A 50-year-old woman presents with a three-month history of a bloody discharge from the left breast. On examination there is an erythematous, scaly rash involving the left nipple and areola, with areas of ulceration. Retraction of the left nipple is noted, which the patient reported as of recent onset. No mass is identified on palpation. What is the risk of associated malignancy?

   a Extensive invasive ductal carcinoma in 80% of cases

   b Extensive invasive lobular carcinoma in 60% of cases

   c Ductal carcinoma *in situ* in 60% of cases

   d Lobular carcinoma *in situ* in 40% of cases

   e No association with malignancy

19 A 35-year-old women presents with a swollen, erythematous and uncomfortable right breast. On mammography, there is a diffuse increase in density of the right breast, which displays a coarse reticular pattern with prominent Cooper ligaments and a skin thickness of 1.8 mm. The left breast appears normal. What is the most likely cause?

   a Inflammatory carcinoma

   b Left subclavian vein thrombosis

   c Rheumatoid arthritis

   d Congestive cardiac failure

   e Previous wide local excision for carcinoma of the right breast seven years ago

20 A 32-year-old woman underwent breast augmentation mammoplasty two years ago. She has recently noted a change in the shape of her right breast and underwent assessment with mammography. A dense area is visible contiguous with the implant on both views and an ultrasound and MRI are performed for further assessment. What finding would be in keeping with an extracapsular rupture of silicone gel-filled implants?

   a Stepladder sign on ultrasound

   b Linguine sign on MRI

   c Inverted teardrop/lasso sign on MRI

    d Snowstorm sign posteriorly on ultrasound

    e Water droplet/salad-oil sign on MRI

21 A 60-year-old woman presents with erythema of the right breast. Ultrasound demonstrates a superficial hypoechoic tubular structure containing low-level internal echoes. She is diagnosed with Mondor disease. What treatment would be most appropriate?

    a Surgical excision of this area

    b Image-guided drainage

    c Immunosuppression

    d High-dose antibiotics and lifelong prophylaxis

    e Symptomatic treatment only

22 An asymptomatic 54-year-old woman had a mammogram which demonstrates multiple long needle like dense calcifications orientated with their long axis pointing toward the nipple. The appearance in both breasts was symmetrical. What is the most likely diagnosis?

    a Phyllodes tumour

    b DCIS

    c LCIS

    d Plasma cell mastitis

    e Osteosarcoma metastases

23 A 43-year-old woman with a previously treated malignancy developed a solitary mass in the upper outer quadrant of the right breast, which is proven on biopsy to represent a haemorrhagic metastasis. What is the most likely primary?

    a Non-Hodgkin's lymphoma

    b Basal cell carcinoma

    c Choriocarcinoma

    d Ovarian cystadenocarcinoma

    e Transitional cell carcinoma of the bladder

24 A 26-year-old patient and her partner are being investigated for infertility. His semen analysis is adequate and she has been proven to be ovulating. She undergoes a hysterosalpingogram which demonstrates a uterine abnormality. What is the most likely diagnosis?

    a Bicornuate uterus

    b Unicornuate uterus

    c Septate uterus

    d Uterus didelphys

    e Arcuate uterus

25 A 33-year-old asymptomatic patient has been found to have cervical carcinoma and is undergoing a staging MRI examination. What finding on MRI is most reliable in excluding parametrial invasion?

a Absence of abnormal pelvic lymphadenopathy

b No hydronephrosis or hydroureter on either side

c Tumour volume of less than 90 cu cm

d Hypointense rim of cervical stroma

e Fine nodularity of parametrial tissue

26 A 40-year-old woman with menorrhagia is referred for possible uterine artery embolisation. Which type of fibroid would put her at highest risk of surgical intervention following the procedure?

a Submucosal fibroid

b Pedunculated submucosal fibroid

c Subserosal fibroid

d Pedunculated subserosal fibroid

e Intramural fibroid

27 A 40-year-old patient is undergoing MRI examination for possible adenomyosis. Which finding on the MRI would be inconsistent with this diagnosis?

a Junctional zone greater than 12 mm

b High signal intensity spots on T2-weighted imaging in the myometrium

c Distinct hypointense transient bulge in the myometrium on T2-weighted images

d Junctional zone: myometrial thickness ratio >40%

e Persistent focal ill-defined round area of low signal in myometrium in contact with the junctional zone on T2-weighted images

28 A 35-year-old female patient with cervical carcinoma undergoes MRI examination for local staging. What radiological finding would be consistent with the patient having stage IIB disease?

a 4 cm tumour confined to the cervix

b Parametrial invasion

c Extension into the vagina except the lower third

d Extension to the lower third vagina

e Pelvic side wall invasion

29 A 60-year-old female patient with pelvic pain and distension has had a 15-cm cystic and solid mass demonstrated on ultrasound examination, which is arising from her right ovary. The solid septations within it measure >5 mm. The CA-125 level is within the normal range. What is the most likely diagnosis?

a Epithelial ovarian carcinoma

b Endometriosis

    c Secondary deposit from another malignancy

    d Benign cyst

    e Fibroma

30 A 29-year-old female three days post partum is unwell with pelvic pain and fever. On clinical examination she has a palpable rope-like abdominal mass. What is the most likely diagnosis?

    a Right ovarian thrombosis

    b Left ovarian thrombosis

    c Bilateral ovarian vein thrombosis

    d Ruptured uterus

    e Tubo-ovarian abscess

31 A 25-year-old has an ultrasound at 39 weeks gestation of a singleton pregnancy. The amniotic fluid volume is less than 500 mL. What is the most likely underlying cause for this?

    a Severe growth restriction

    b Maternal diabetes mellitus

    c Trans-oesophageal fistula (TOF)

    d Duodenal atresia

    e Cystic adenomatoid lung

32 A 39-year-old female patient is pregnant with her fourth baby. She undergoes routine obstetric ultrasound examination which demonstrates a thickened placenta with a thickness of 6 cm. What is the most likely diagnosis?

    a Maternal diabetes mellitus

    b IUGR

    c Increasing maternal age

    d Multiparity

    e Maternal hypertension

33 A 24-year-old patient had an IUCD fitted two days ago by her general practitioner. She returned to the GP as she could not find the threads and was referred for an ultrasound. Both transabdominal and transvaginal ultrasound examination show an empty uterine cavity with no coil seen within it. There is a small amount of pelvic free fluid and possibly an echogenic linear structure, which may represent the coil outside the uterus in the right adnexa. What is the next most appropriate investigation?

    a CT

    b MRI

    c Repeat ultrasound examination in one week

    d Hysterosalpingogram

    e Abdominal radiograph

34 A 17-year-old female patient with irregular periods and occasional pelvic discomfort undergoes transabdominal pelvic ultrasound examination. This shows a right ovarian volume of 17 mL and left ovarian volume of 15 mL. Both ovaries have several small cysts seen within them measuring approximately 5 mm in a peripheral location. What is the most likely diagnosis?

   a Normal findings in this age group

   b Patient currently on the oral contraceptive pill

   c Polycystic ovary syndrome (PCOS)

   d Ovarian hyperstimulation syndrome (OHSS)

   e Endometriosis

35 A 28-year-old female patient who is under gynaecological follow-up for a cystic ovarian mass is admitted as an emergency with sudden onset of severe lower abdominal pain. A mass is palpable in the right iliac fossa. Abdominal and pelvic ultrasound examination demonstrates an enlarged hypoechoic midline mass in addition to the cystic mass and there is free fluid in the pouch of Douglas. What is the most likely diagnosis?

   a Enlargement of her existing cystic mass

   b Haemorrhage of the cyst

   c Malignant change of the cyst

   d Torsion of the ovary

   e Rupture of the cyst

36 A 38-year-old patient has chronic pelvic pain on the right side. She undergoes transabdominal and transvaginal ultrasound examination. This demonstrates a 3 cm cyst on the right ovary. What radiological findings would suggest a diagnosis of haemorrhagic cyst rather than a simple cyst?

   a Posterior acoustic enhancement

   b A 'ground-glass' pattern

   c Doppler flow in cyst wall

   d Sharply defined wall <3 mm

   e Unilocular

37 A 34-year-old patient has had previous investigations for dysmenorrhoea and menorrhagia and was found to have multiple leiomyomas. What radiological sign would be concerning for sarcomatous transformation?

   a High signal intensity on T2-weighted sequences

   b Hyperintense rim on T2-weighted sequences

   c Rapid change in size

   d Enhancement following intravenous contrast medium

   e Low signal intensity on T2-weighted sequences

38 A 19-year-old girl complains of a pelvic mass and pressure symptoms. Transabdominal ultrasound examination reveals an adnexal mass. What additional finding would suggest a diagnosis of mature teratoma from another type of germ cell tumour?

a Fat density on plain film

b Elevated βHCG

c Calcification seen on ultrasound imaging

d Elevated alpha-fetoprotein

e Complex mass on ultrasound imaging

39 A 60-year-old female with poorly controlled diabetes presents with urinary frequency, dysuria and offensive urine. She has also noticed pneumaturia. On examination she is unwell and is tender in the suprapubic region. On plain film an air-fluid level is noted within the bladder lumen. What is the most likely causative agent?

a *Actinomycosis*

b *Klebsiella*

c *Tuberculosis*

d *Escherichia coli*

e *Salmonella*

40 A 35-year-old man was involved in a road traffic accident and sustained chest and pelvic injuries. An enhanced CT scan was performed which shows pelvic fractures and an elliptical extravasation of contrast adjacent to the bladder. Which is the most likely diagnosis?

a Extraperitoneal bladder rupture

b Intraperitoneal bladder rupture

c Subserosal bladder rupture

d Retroperitoneal bladder rupture

e Intraluminal bladder rupture

41 A 42-year-old man who has recently returned from holiday to Egypt presents to the genito-urinary clinic with dysuria and a urethral discharge. He also gives a history of joint pains and intermittent eye pain and irritation. While awaiting the result of penile swab microbiology, a retrograde urethrogram is performed which shows stricture formation and luminal irregularity in the penile urethra. What is the most likely diagnosis?

a Gonococcal urethritis

b Sarcoidosis

c Reiter's syndrome

d Schistosomiasis

e *Escherichia coli* infection

42 A 25-year-old male presents with fever and increasing left-sided scrotal pain over a period of three days. He has also noticed clouding of his urine and complains of dysuria and frequency. Ultrasound of the left hemiscrotum demonstrates thickening and enlargement of the epididymis and testis on the left. The left testis is hypoechoic compared to the right. Which of the following appearances on radionuclide imaging would favour a diagnosis of epididymo-orchitis above testicular tumour?

   a Increased perfusion with decreased uptake centrally

   b Curvilinear increased activity medially and centrally in the left hemiscrotum on static images

   c A 'nubbin' sign; that is, a bump of activity extending medially from the iliac artery

   d Markedly increased perfusion through spermatic cord vessels with increased activity of scrotal contents on static images

   e Slight increase in perfusion with increased uptake in the testis alone on static images

43 A 26-year-old male has a history of recurrent episodes of urinary tract infections and as part of a diagnostic work-up for abdominal pain he underwent excretory urography. An IVP demonstrates early filling of a bulbous terminal right ureter which protrudes into the bladder lumen at the ureteral insertion with a surrounding radiolucent halo. There is prominence of a single proximal ureter and mild pelvicalyceal dilatation seen on the right. A MCUG demonstrates a round lucent filling defect near the trigone, which effaces with increased bladder distension. Ultrasound demonstrates a cystic mass at the right ureteral orifice at the trigone. The right kidney looks normal. During the scan, this is seen to periodically fill and empty with ureteral peristalsis. What is the most likely diagnosis?

   a Ectopic ureterocoele

   b Simple ureterocoele

   c TCC at the VUJ

   d Ureteral oedema due to an impacted calculus

   e Bladder diverticulum

44 A 30-year-old male mountain biker sustained a 'straddle injury' during a race. He noticed some blood in his urine for a few days subsequently but decided against consulting a doctor. A few months later he noticed increasing difficulty in passing urine. His urinary stream was weak and he had started suffering from dysuria, urgency and suprapubic discomfort. Which of the following appearances are most likely to be seen on retrograde urethrography?

   a An abrupt short segment of narrowing in the bulbous urethra

   b A short segment of narrowing in the membranous urethra

   c A long segment of narrowing involving the junction of the membranous and prostatic urethra d A long segment of narrowing of the penile urethra

    e A short segment of narrowing involving the posterior urethra

45 An eight-year-old boy presents acutely with a swollen, inflamed and very tender right testicle. An ultrasound scan shows a rounded mass of variable reflectivity at the superior aspect of the right testis with surrounding increased Doppler flow and a small hydrocele. What is the most likely diagnosis?

    a Right testicular torsion

    b Acute epididymitis

    c Torsion of the appendix testis

    d Spermatic cord torsion

    e Haemorrhagic epididymal cyst

46 A 30-year-old man presents with a two-month history of painless right scrotal swelling. An ultrasound scan shows a well-defined hyporeflective paratesticular mass which shows hypervascularity on colour Doppler. What is the most likely diagnosis?

    a Paratesticular lipoma

    b Adenomatoid tumour

    c Scrotal haemangioma

    d Epididymal papillary cystadenoma

    e Malignant fibrous histiocytoma

47 A 65-year-old man represented three years after a prostatectomy for prostate cancer with an increasing prostate-specific antigen (PSA) and an MRI of the pelvis was performed. What feature best denotes local disease recurrence?

    a Low signal intensity in the prostate bed on axial T2 sequence

    b High signal intensity in the prostate bed on axial T1 sequence

    c High signal intensity in the prostate bed on axial T2 sequence

    d Low signal intensity in the prostate bed on axial STIR sequence

    e Low signal intensity in the prostate bed on axial T1 sequence

48 A 42-year-old man with a history of infertility, recurrent urinary infections and haematuria was assessed with a trans-rectal ultrasound scan (TRUS) which shows a midline cystic mass in the prostate gland which does not communicate with the urethra. What is the most likely diagnosis?

    a Ejaculatory duct cyst

    b Prostatic abscess

    c Retention cyst

    d Mullerian duct cyst

    e Cystic degeneration of benign prostatic hypertrophy

49 A three-month-old male presents with a large palpable left flank mass. Ultrasound shows a solid lesion arising from the left kidney involving the renal sinus but not invading the collecting system or renal vein. What is the most likely diagnosis?

a Nephroblastomatosis

b Wilms' tumour

c Lobar nephronia

d Mesoblastic nephroma

e Multilocular cystic nephroma

50 A 75-year-old man presents with haematuria and is found to have transitional cell carcinoma of the bladder. Which of the following would it be possible to confirm on contrast-enhanced CT chest, abdomen and pelvis alone?

a T1 (lamina propria invasion) N0 M0

b T2 (superficial muscle invasion) N0 M0

c T3a (deep muscle invasion) N0 M0

d T3a (deep muscle invasion) N1 (single node <2 cm) M1

e T3b (perivesical fat invasion) N1 M1

51 A 65-year-old woman becomes acutely short of breath one day following coronary angiography. A CTPA is performed and is negative for pulmonary embolism. Within two days her serum creatinine has risen. What would allow the diagnosis of contrast-induced nephrotoxicity to be made?

a Rise in serum creatinine from 80 μmol/L to 124 μmol/L

b Rise in serum creatinine from 100 μmol/L to 120 μmol/L

c Rise in serum creatinine from 100 μmol/L to 144 μmol/L and documented hypotension during coronary angiography

d Rise in serum creatinine from 80 μmol/L to 160 μmol/L with a large iatrogenic retroperitoneal haematoma

e Rise in serum creatinine from 200 μmol/L to 244 μmol/L with commencement of an angiotensin-converting enzyme inhibitor

52 A 74-year-old man is undergoing staging for renal cell carcinoma. In the assessment of which of the following might MRI be superior to CT?

a Local lymph node spread

b Parenchymal lung metastases

c Inferior vena caval invasion

d Characterisation of the primary tumour

e Differentiation between T1 and T2 disease

53 A 79-year-old woman is undergoing staging for a suspected renal primary malignancy. In the assessment of which of the following might [18]FDG PET-CT have an additional role over other imaging modalities?

a Differentiating between transitional cell and renal cell carcinoma
b A 3-cm short axis regional lymph node
c Lytic bone metastases
d Inferior vena caval invasion
e Detection of synchronous primary tumours

54 A 67-year-old man has a carcinoma of his bladder diagnosed on cystoscopy. In which of the following situations is MRI the imaging modality of choice for staging?
a Multiple pulmonary nodules are visible on his chest radiograph
b Possible obstructive uropathy; for assessment of upper tract disease
c He complains of passing urine per rectum
d Further assessment of markedly abnormal liver function tests
e Further assessment during consideration of a cystectomy

55 A 23-year-old male with acute ureteric colic undergoes intravenous urography. Two days later he has an unenhanced CT-KUB for further delineation of renal calculi. CT shows vicarious excretion of contrast medium within the gallbladder. What is the most likely cause for this appearance?
a Use of high osmolar ionic contrast medium
b Iodinated impurities in the injected contrast medium
c Unilateral acute ureteric obstruction
d Pre-existing renal impairment
e Disturbed enterohepatic circulation of bile salts

56 A three-year-old female is diagnosed with juvenile onset autosomal recessive polycystic kidney disease. Which of the following pathological features of the disease is responsible for the majority of the morbidity in this group?
a Dilated and ectatic renal collecting tubules
b Pulmonary hypoplasia
c Renal interstitial fibrosis
d Hepatic fibrosis
e Systemic arterial hypertension

57 An adult diabetic woman who is a surgical inpatient is demonstrated to have gas within the urinary bladder on CT performed for investigation of suspected intra-abdominal collection. What is the most likely cause for this finding?
a Vesicointestinal fistula
b Recent bladder catheterisation
c *E. coli* urinary tract infection
d Emphysematous cystitis
e Ureteric diversion

58 An adult patient is demonstrated to have a normal-sized right kidney with an irregular apparently scarred cortex. Which one of the following sonographic features would indicate the presence of persistent foetal lobulation?

a Dromedary hump
b Broad cortical depression over a normal calyx
c Lateral indentation of the renal sinus
d Cortical depressions between calyces
e Multiple cortical depressions over dilated calyces

59 A 51 year old has an ultrasound for non-specific abdominal pain and the renal cortex is noted to be hypoechoic relative to the liver parenchyma. What is the likely diagnosis?

a Cirrhosis
b Fatty liver
c Normal finding
d Diffuse metastatic disease
e Haemochromatosis

60 Which of the following radiopharmaceuticals has high cortical binding and is therefore the agent of choice for evaluation of the renal cortex?

a I-131-orthoiodohippurate (Hippuran®)
b Cr-51-ethylenediaminetetraacetic acid (EDTA)
c Tc-99m-dimercaptosuccinic acid (DMSA)
d Tc-99m-diethylenetriamine pentaacetic acid (DTPA)
e Tc-99m-mercaptoacetyltriglycine (MAG3)

61 A 15-year-old previously asymptomatic female presents with persistent thin discharge from the umbilicus following navel piercing. Ultrasound shows a fluid filled tubular structure in the anterior abdominal wall. What is the most likely diagnosis?

a Traumatic umbilical sinus with granulation tissue
b Patent vitello-intestinal duct
c Umbilical-urachal sinus
d Vesico-urachal diverticulum
e Umbilical-peritoneal fistula

62 A 79-year-old male has locally advanced prostate cancer causing left distal ureteric obstruction and retrograde stent insertion has failed. You are to perform an emergency percutaneous nephrostomy to relieve the acute obstruction and you plan to replace this electively with an anterograde ureteric stent. What is the ideal site of puncture into the collecting system?

a Anterior upper pole calyx
b Posterior upper pole calyx

    c Anterior lower pole calyx

    d Posterior interpolar calyx

    e Renal pelvis

63 A 22-year-old female with a history of childhood urinary tract infections underwent an ultrasound for assessment of renal parenchymal disease. This demonstrated focal loss of renal parenchyma with underlying clubbed calyces in the right upper pole with normal appearances elsewhere. What is the most likely diagnosis?

    a Glomerulonephritis

    b Acute cortical necrosis

    c Papillary necrosis

    d Focal reflux nephropathy (chronic atrophic pyelonephritis)

    e Focal infarction

64 A 26-year-old male with a history of recurrent haemoptysis and impaired renal function underwent an ultrasound for assessment of renal parenchymal disease. This demonstrated smooth small kidneys with no calyceal abnormality. What is the most likely diagnosis?

    a Focal infarction

    b Glomerulonephritis

    c Amyloidosis

    d *Tuberculosis*

    e Papillary necrosis

65 A 56-year-old male on long-term antiretroviral medication presents with lower urinary tract symptoms, haematuria and sterile pyuria. Unenhanced CT shows unilateral focal high attenuation 'cloudy' dilated calyces with no associated cortical loss and delayed post-contrast imaging demonstrates poor opacification of the ipsilateral collecting system. What is the most likely diagnosis?

    a Xanthogranulomatous pyelonephritis

    b Renal stone disease

    c *Tuberculosis*

    d Acute papillary necrosis

    e *Candida albicans* infection

66 A 65-year-old male with chronic loin pain and recurrent urinary tract infections underwent an ultrasound which showed an enlarged left kidney with dilated calyces and low echogenicity parenchyma. A CT was then performed, which demonstrated multiple rounded fat attenuation masses replacing the renal parenchyma with associated perinephric fat stranding. Which of the following additional findings strongly suggests xanthogranulomatous pyelonephritis as the cause?

    a Avid cortical enhancement following contrast

    b A heterogeneously enhancing focal renal mass

    c Punctate renal calcification

    d Hydronephrosis and hydroureter

    e A renal pelvic calculus

67 A 50-year-old patient is undergoing investigations for acute renal failure. Which is the following is a contraindication to renal biopsy?

    a Warfarin therapy

    b Presence of large renal cysts

    c Hydronephrosis

    d Platelet count of 150 000/mL

    e Single kidney

68 A 25-year-old female patient is under follow-up for post-operative surveillance of a live donor kidney transplant in the right iliac fossa and an ultrasound scan is being performed. What is the most likely anastomosis of the transplant renal artery?

    a Aortic patch anastomosis to the external iliac artery

    b End-to-side anastomosis to the external iliac artery

    c End-to-end anastomosis to the external iliac artery

    d End-to-side anastomosis to the common iliac artery

    e End-to-end anastomosis to the internal iliac artery

69 A 35-year-old female diabetic on dialysis undergoes a cadaveric renal transplant. Post-operatively there is primary non-function of the graft with no reduction in serum creatinine. Which of the following investigations reliably differentiates acute tubular rejection from acute rejection?

    a Tc-99m-diethylenetriamine pentaacetic acid (DTPA) renal scintigraphy

    b Duplex Doppler renal ultrasound

    c MRI

    d Renal angiography

    e Percutaneous renal biopsy

70 A 42 year old with a live donor renal transplant undergoes Duplex Doppler US assessment for investigation of rising creatinine. The calculated resistance index (Pourcelot Index), RI is 0.9. How is this index calculated?

a Peak systolic velocity/End diastolic velocity

b (Peak systolic velocity – End diastolic velocity)/End diastolic velocity

c (Peak systolic velocity – End diastolic velocity)/Peak systolic velocity

d Peak systolic velocity/(Peak systolic velocity – End diastolic velocity)

e (Peak systolic velocity – End diastolic velocity)/Temporal mean velocity

Genito-urinary, adrenal, obstetric, gynaecological and breast radiology

PAPER 3

1   A neonate of a diabetic mother is born following a difficult labour via forceps delivery. An ultrasound examination performed in the first week demonstrated a right-sided complex solid echogenic mass in the region of the right adrenal. The remainder of the abdominal ultrasound examination was unremarkable. What is the most likely diagnosis?

   a Non-hyperfunctioning adrenocortical adenoma

   b Hyperfunctioning adrenocortical adenoma

   c Traumatic adrenal haemorrhage

   d Non-traumatic adrenal haemorrhage

   e Adrenocortical hyperplasia

2   A 45-year-old patient underwent CT and is incidentally found to have an adrenal mass. What additional finding would suggest a diagnosis of phaeo-chromocytoma rather than adrenal adenoma?

   a Calcification

   b Size <2 cm

   c Attenuation >30 HU

   d Arterial phase enhancement

   e Homogeneous enhancement

3   A 41-year-old patient undergoes CT examination and is found to have an incidental adrenal mass. What additional finding would suggest a diagnosis of myelolipoma rather than an adrenal adenoma?

   a Presence of large amount of mature fat

   b HU<10 on unenhanced CT

   c Calcification

   d Unilateral

   e Size >5 cm

4 A 40-year-old woman with paroxysmal hypertension was diagnosed with a phaeochromocytoma of her left adrenal. As part of the work-up a mass on her right adrenal was also discovered that was of a similar appearance on CT. An MRI was then performed. What feature would favour the right-sided lesion being an incidental adrenal adenoma?

  a Heterogeneous enhancement

  b Slow washout following enhancement

  c Extremely high signal on T2-weighted images

  d India ink effect on chemical shift MRI

  e Low signal on T1-weighted images on MRI

5 A 62-year-old patient presented with a cough and a CXR showed a possible mass in the left lung. He then underwent further evaluation with contrast-enhanced CT. This confirmed the presence of a pulmonary mass but also showed an adrenal mass. What additional finding would suggest a diagnosis of adrenal adenoma rather than an adrenal metastasis?

  a Calcification

  b Attenuation of 50 HU on portal venous phase images

  c Attenuation of 26 HU on delayed images 15 minutes after contrast injection

  d Contralateral gland atrophic

  e 1-cm low-density lesion on contralateral adrenal

6 A 43-year-old man has had a diagnosis of phaeochromocytoma given by the endocrine team. Which of the following tests would be dangerous due to risk of precipitating life-threatening hypertension? (He is not on alpha- or beta-blocking drugs.)

  a Contrast-enhanced CT with non-ionic intravenous contrast medium

  b MIBG scan

  c Abdominal MRI scan with gadolinium

  d CT-guided core biopsy

  e FDG-PET scan

7 A 67-year-old woman with metastatic breast carcinoma is noted to have adrenal metastases that are of increased uptake on a PET examination. In which part of the adrenal do these characteristically occur?

  a Outer adrenal cortex

  b Medulla

  c Inner adrenal cortex

  d Corticomedullary junction

  e Adrenal capsule

8   A 50-year-old female patient undergoes CT examination and is found to have
    an incidental adrenal lesion. This area is cystic in appearance and measures
    4 cm. The wall is thin at 2 mm and the contents are homogeneous with almost
    water attenuation. There is no enhancement following the administration of
    intravenous contrast medium. What is the most likely diagnosis?
    a   Cystic phaeochromocytoma
    b   Cystic adrenocortical carcinoma
    c   Adrenal adenoma
    d   True adrenal cyst
    e   Lymphangioma

9   A 65-year-old woman presents with a palpable breast lump, which on mam-
    mography corresponds to a spiculated/stellate soft-tissue density seen on
    both MLO and CC views with associated pleomorphic microcalcification.
    Wide bore core needle biopsy confirms a malignant lesion. She has no family
    history of breast cancer. Which of the following histological types is most
    likely in this case?
    a   Intracystic carcinoma
    b   Mucinous tumour
    c   Invasive ductal carcinoma
    d   Medullary carcinoma
    e   Papillary carcinoma

10 A 54-year-old post-menopausal woman attends for routine mammographic
    screening and is found to have a well-defined 10-mm mass in the left upper
    outer quadrant. What additional feature would raise the likelihood of this
    malignancy in this lesion?
    a   The presence of a central lucency in the mass
    b   A fatty peripheral notch in the border of the mass
    c   Predominantly peripheral microcalcification within the mass
    d   A normal mammogram three years previously
    e   Lack of clear delineation of the posterior border of the mass on standard
        views, which appears well-defined on cone-down compression magnified
        views

11 A 52-year-old woman presents with a mass in the left axilla which is found
    to have malignant cytology on FNA. No mass is palpable in the left breast
    and mammography is normal. An MRI is arranged. Which of the following
    findings on MRI are strongly suggestive of malignancy?
    a   Increased signal on T2-weighted images
    b   Peripheral wash-in on contrast-enhanced T1-weighted images
    c   Signal intensity increase up to 50% of baseline steadily over the first
        three minutes following contrast-enhanced T1-weighted images
    d   Gradual washout phase on contrast-enhanced T1-weighted images

e Spiculated lesion with a plateau in the post-initial phase on contrast-enhanced T1-weighted images

12 A 42-year-old woman with previously treated lobular carcinoma, undetectable on mammography, is scheduled for MRI follow-up. Which of the following represents optimal timing of the MRI scan?
a First seven days of the menstrual cycle
b Last seven days of the menstrual cycle
c Six months after radiation therapy
d Six months after open biopsy
e Nine months after neoadjuvant chemotherapy

13 A 39-year-old woman presents with a palpable breast lump, which has a benign appearance on both mammography and ultrasound imaging. A biopsy confirms the diagnosis of a fibroadenoma. What is the most common site of benign breast masses?
a Upper inner quadrant
b Upper outer quadrant
c Retroareolar
d Lower inner quadrant
e Lower outer quadrant

14 A 46-year-old woman undergoes lumpectomy for a breast mass. Malignant involvement is found to extend to the resection margins on histological examination of the specimen. An MRI is performed 10 days later which shows an ill-defined distorted mass of low-signal intensity on both T1- and T2-weighted images with a peripheral ring of high signal on T1 and low signal on T2. Post-contrast T1 images demonstrate a moderate diffuse reactive enhancement surrounding the lesion with continuous post-initial increase in enhancement. No central uptake is demonstrated within the lesion itself. What is the most likely explanation for these findings?
a Seroma
b Residual tumour mass
c Post-surgical haematoma
d Fat necrosis
e Breast abscess

15 A 31-year-old woman, who is currently breastfeeding her three-month-old daughter, presents with a painful right breast. She has a temperature of 38°C. WCC is raised. Ultrasound demonstrates a nearly anechoic area in the central subareolar region with posterior acoustic enhancement. She rapidly improves with a course of antibiotics. Which of the following best describes the expected MRI findings?

    a Low signal on T1, high on T2-weighted images with moderate peripheral enhancement on contrast enhanced T1 images

    b High signal on T1- and T2-weighted images with avid enhancement of entire lesion and surrounding adjacent tissue on contrast-enhanced T1 images

    c Low signal on T1- and T2-weighted images with no enhancement seen on contrast-enhanced T1 images

    d High signal on T1- and T2-weighted images with avid peripheral enhancement without central uptake on contrast-enhanced T1 images

    e High signal on T1- and low on T2-weighted images with moderate centripetal enhancement on contrast-enhanced T1 images

16 A 62-year-old woman has declined her previous routine screening mammograms and presents with a palpable mass, which is diagnosed as invasive ductal carcinoma on biopsy. What is the approximate cancer detection rate of the NHS Breast Screening Programme?

    a 0.3 per 100 women screened

    b 2 per 100 women screened

    c 6 per 1000 women screened

    d 13 per 1000 women screened

    e 30 per 10 000 women screened

17 A 35-year-old woman presents with a history of cyclical breast fullness, tenderness and pain. On examination there is generalised thickening of the breast tissue with palpable nodules. An enlarged nodular pattern is seen on mammography. A ductal pattern is seen on ultrasound, with duct ectasia, cysts and ill-defined lesions. Which of the following statements relating to this condition is most accurate?

    a It tends to be asymptomatic in microcystic disease

    b Symptoms occur during menstruation

    c Symptoms are aggravated during pregnancy

    d It is detected in 35% of the screening population >55 years

    e Calcification may be present

18 A 39-year-old woman who had a reduction mammoplasty one year previously presents with a lump in her right breast. This corresponds to an irregular spiculated lesion on mammography and was found to be of low reflectivity with poorly defined borders on ultrasound. An attempted biopsy yielded a small amount of yellow fluid and an area of fat necrosis is suspected. What is the risk of malignant transformation in this area?

a 0% It is not pre-malignant

b 5–15%

c 20–40%

d 45–55%

e 85–95%

19 A 30-year-old woman presents with a spontaneous serosanguinous nipple discharge. She has also noticed an intermittent mass which disappears with discharge from the nipple. The nipple discharge is produced on compression of a specific trigger point in the areolar region. A mammogram demonstrates subareolar amorphous coarse calcifications. On ultrasound a hypoechoic mass is identified within an isolated dilated duct. A MRI shows round lesion with signal isointense to parenchyma on T1-weighted images. Following contrast there is homogeneous enhancement above that of parenchyma on T1-weighted images with a continuous post-initial increase. What is the most likely diagnosis?

a Paget's disease of the nipple

b Central solitary papilloma

c Fibroadenoma

d Galactocoele

e Papillary carcinoma

20 An 11-year-old girl who has not started menstruating yet is admitted to hospital with urinary retention. A urinary catheter is inserted in the Emergency Department which drains 1 litre of urine. The paediatric doctor can feel a palpable pelvic mass and ultrasound examination demonstrates a midline pelvic mass which is hypoechoic with low-level echoes within it. The ovaries have normal ultrasound appearances. What is the most likely diagnosis?

a Tubo-ovarian abscess

b Haematocolpos

c Perforated appendix with pelvic collection

d Endometriosis

e Uterine anomaly

21 A 31 year old is pregnant with her first child. At 16 weeks' gestation the corrected alpha-fetoprotein level is noted to be raised. What is a possible cause for this?

    a Wrong dates – a normal pregnancy that is less advanced that originally dated

    b Greater than average birth weight

    c Ectopic pregnancy

    d Trisomy 21

    e Neural tube defect

22 A 27-year-old patient with pelvic pain underwent an MRI examination for further assessment of a discrete lesion on her right ovary. What additional finding would suggest a diagnosis of endometriosis rather than haemorrhagic cyst?

    a Increased signal intensity on T1-weighted images

    b Increased signal intensity on fat-suppressed T2-weighted images

    c Multiple further lesions in the pelvis

    d Fluid-debris layer on T2-weighted images

    e A thin wall

23 A 58-year-old female patient with post-menopausal bleeding is referred for an ultrasound examination of the pelvis. This demonstrates a focal thickening of the endometrium. What additional finding would suggest a diagnosis of endometrial polyp rather than primary carcinoma of the endometrium?

    a Increased echogenicity in the myometrium

    b Doppler waveform with resistive index <0.7

    c Location at the uterine fundus

    d Irregular poorly defined endometrial-myometrial interface

    e Vessel visualised within stalk on colour Doppler

24 A 52-year-old patient who is perimenopausal was referred for investigation of menorrhagia and increased frequency of menstruation. A blood sample showed elevated levels of oestrogen and a pelvic ultrasound examination was arranged. On this examination the endometrium measured 3 mm and there was a multilocular cystic adnexal mass measuring 30 cm with thick irregular septations but no intracystic papillary projections. What is the most likely diagnosis?

    a Adult granulosa cell tumour

    b Germ cell tumour

    c Krukenberg tumour

    d Clear cell carcinoma

    e Brenner tumour

25 A 35-year-old female patient with post-coital bleeding has a pelvic MRI scan as part of her work-up which demonstrates a focal mass in the cervix. What additional finding would suggest a diagnosis of prolapsed submucosal fibroid rather than cervical carcinoma?

a Hypointensity on T1-weighted images

b Hypointensity on T2-weighted images

c Blurring and widening of the junctional zone

d Early contrast enhancement on fat-saturated T1-weighted images

e Disruption of hypointense vaginal wall

26 A 38-year-old female in her third trimester has an episode of painless vaginal bleeding. She is referred to the obstetric team and ultrasound examination is performed. This demonstrates the placenta is completely covering the internal os. What is the most likely diagnosis?

a Low-lying placenta

b Partial placenta praevia

c Placenta accreta

d Central placenta praevia

e Placenta increta

27 A 21-year-old Afro-American patient is being investigated for menorrhagia and dysmenorrhoea. Ultrasound examination demonstrated several intra-mural fibroids and also a well-defined adnexal mass. MRI examination showed this to be attached to the uterus and likely to be a subserosal fibroid. What is the most typical signal characteristic on MRI of a subserosal fibroid?

a High signal on T1-weighted images

b Low signal on T1-weighted images

c Intermediate signal on T2-weighted images

d High signal on T2-weighted images

e Low signal on T2-weighted images

28 A pregnant patient with a family history of Beckwith-Wiedemann syndrome has an obstetric ultrasound examination which demonstrates that the foetus is growing along the 99.6th percentile and that there is polyhydramnios. What other condition is associated with the most likely diagnosis?

a Wilms' tumour

b Neuroblastoma

c Neurofibromatosis

d Von Hippel-Lindau

e Down's syndrome

29 A 37-year-old pregnant woman has been found to have a raised alpha-feto-protein level and an ultrasound anomaly scan is performed. The appearance of the foetus is abnormal with a flat inwardly scalloped contour of both frontal bones and a posterior curve of the cerebellum. What is the most likely diagnosis?

a Holoprosencephaly

b Lissencephaly

c Choroid plexus cyst

d Vein of Galen aneurysm

e Spina bifida

30 A 22-year-old female patient is referred to gynaecology with a palpable mass behind the labia minora. She undergoes MRI examination which demonstrates a small mass which is of high homogeneous signal on T2-weighted images. What is the most likely diagnosis?

a Bartholin's gland abscess

b Bartholin's gland squamous cell carcinoma

c Bartholin's gland cyst

d Bartholin's gland neuroendocrine carcinoma

e Bartholin's gland adenocarcinoma

31 A 79-year-old female patient who has previously had a malignant melanoma excised on her thigh presents to the gynaecology team with a vulvular mass. She undergoes MRI examination which demonstrates a 6 cm mass. What additional finding would suggest a diagnosis of malignant melanoma rather than carcinoma?

a High signal on T1-weighted images

b High signal on T2-weighted images

c Enhancement following intravenous gadolinium

d Heterogeneity

e Infiltration of surrounding structures

32 A female patient has been referred to gynaecology with pelvic pain and the gynaecology team are concerned about salpingitis. What finding would be most suggestive of *tuberculosis* rather than another cause?

a Tubal content low signal intensity on T2-weighted images

b Bilateral disease

c Thickened wall of fallopian tube

d Dilated fallopian tube

e Haemorrhage within tubes

33 A 25-year-old male presents with fever and increasing left-sided scrotal pain over a period of three days. He has also noticed clouding of his urine and complains of dysuria and frequency. Ultrasound of the left hemiscrotum demonstrates thickening and enlargement of the epididymis and testis on the left. The left testis is hypoechoic compared to the right. Radionuclide imaging demonstrates markedly increased perfusion through spermatic cord vessels with curvilinear increased activity medially and centrally in the left hemiscrotum on static images. Which of the following statements is most accurate regarding this condition?

a The commonest causative organism in this age group is *E. coli*

b It is the commonest cause of acute scrotal pain in males under the age of 20

c It is frequently associated with prostatic tenderness

d *Tuberculosis* is the second commonest cause

e Leads to testicular infarction in approximately 3% of cases

34 A 40-year-old South African male presents with painless haematuria. On IVP, control films demonstrate thin curvilinear, floccular calcification outlining a bladder of normal size and shape, as well as calcification of the distal ureters. There is an area of discontinuous calcification noted, which corresponds to an irregular filling defect seen on cystography. On cystoscopy, this corresponded to an area of abnormal-appearing mucosa on the posterior bladder wall. On physical examination, he has signs of portal hypertension. He describes episodes of haematemesis in the past. What is the most likely diagnosis?

a Transitional cell carcinoma (TCC) of the bladder

b Uncomplicated schistosomiasis

c Squamous cell carcinoma (SCC) of the bladder

d Neurofibromatosis of the bladder wall

e Bladder tuberculosis

35 One of the most common causes of non-prostatic urinary outflow obstruction in a male is a posterior urethral valve. When is it usually diagnosed?

a Prenatally

b First year of life

c Early childhood

d Late childhood

e Young adult life

36 A 22-year-old man reluctantly presents to the Emergency Department with a persistent painful erection. What is the appropriate management?

a Reassurance that it will resolve without active management

b Arterial Doppler to look for abnormal inflow

c Cavernosal aspiration/irrigation

d Angiogram

e Passage of a urethral catheter to allow urination

37 A 50-year-old man presented with difficulty passing urine and had a retrograde urethrogram as part of his work-up. This demonstrates a urethral stricture. What is the most likely cause?

a Secondary to previous trauma

b Secondary to previous gonococcal infection

c Congenital

d Malignant stricture

e Secondary to previous tuberculous infection

38 A 90-year-old man is brought to hospital from his nursing home generally unwell and with a painful scrotum. Ultrasound imaging of the testes is difficult because of tenderness and hazy echogenic shadowing. The operator also notices skin crepitus. What is the most likely diagnosis?

a Testicular tumour

b Yeast infection

c DVT

d Fournier gangrene

e Scrotal hernia

39 A 34-year-old man noticed his scrotum appeared swollen and was referred for an ultrasound scan which demonstrated an anechoic region around the right testis with posterior acoustic enhancement. Both testes were of normal appearance. What is the most appropriate management?

a Urgent urological referral

b Routine urological referral

c MRI pelvis

d CT pelvis

e Aspiration of fluid

40 An 85-year-old man presents with a swelling in his scrotum and is referred for an ultrasound. This shows a right-sided simple hydrocele. The left testis appears normal and the right testis, while of normal morphology, appears abnormally bright when imaged through the hydrocele. What technical feature of ultrasonography is responsible for this appearance?

a Time gain compensation

b Compound imaging

c Harmonic imaging

d Refractive shadowing

e Non-linear waveform propagation

41 A 65-year-old man, who used to work in a rubber manufacturing plant and has a strong smoking history, presents with frank painless haematuria. An IVP demonstrates an irregular filling defect with a broad base, situated at the base of the bladder. Cystoscopy demonstrates a papillary, frond-like tumour and endoscopic biopsies are taken for histological analysis. What sequence would be best for detection of extension of the tumour through the bladder wall?

a T1-weighted images

b T2-weighted images

c T2-weighted images with fat saturation

d STIR images

e Diffusion weighted images

42 An 83-year-old man complains of hesitancy, poor urinary flow, terminal dribbling and double micturition. On direct questioning he describes nocturia at least five times per night. His prostate feels enlarged on examination, his PSA is measured to be 9 ng/mL and he is referred for a transrectal prostate ultrasound with biopsy. What feature would be most in keeping with benign prostatic hypertrophy (BPH)?

a Measured volume of 43 cu cm

b Irregular prostatic outline

c Peripheral enlargement predominately of low reflectivity

d Peripheral enlargement with calcium and mixed echogenicity

e Central enlargement with calcium and mixed echogenicity

43 A 43-year-old woman with a renal transplant presented with recurrent urinary tract infections. An ultrasound revealed no abnormality of the transplanted kidney but a thickened section of the bladder wall was noted. She then had a pelvic MRI which confirmed the thickening which was of intermediate signal on T1-weighted and T2-weighted images. She finally had a cystoscopy and a yellowish plaque-like area was found and biopsied. What is the most likely diagnosis?

a Histiocytosis X

b Malakoplakia

c Haemangioma

d Chagas disease (South American trypanosomiasis)

e *Actinomycosis*

44 A 21-year-old man presented with a dull ache in the left side of his scrotum and was found to have a varicocele. He is considering embolisation as a treatment. What should be discussed during the process of obtaining consent?

a Risk of testicle infarction in 3%

b Infertility risk

c No symptom improvement in approximately 10%

d Sedation as it is usually required

e Need for three weeks of prophylactic antibiotics post procedure

45 A 29-year-old female with a previous history of renal stone disease presents with acute left loin pain while 19 weeks' pregnant. Ultrasound shows (maternal) left hydronephrosis. What is the best next line investigation?

a T2-weighted static fluid MR urography

b T1-weighted contrast-enhanced excretory MR urography

c Contrast-enhanced CT urography

d Unenhanced low-dose CT abdomen and pelvis

e Intravenous urography

46 A 35-year-old woman with loin pain, dysuria and fever is diagnosed with acute uncomplicated ascending bacterial pyelonephritis. What appearance is likely to have been seen on CT?

a Cortical thinning

b Perinephric fat stranding

c Alternating bands of hypo- and hyperattenuation of the renal parenchyma

d Round peripheral hypoattenuating renal lesions

e Geographic low-attenuation lesion with peripheral enhancement

47 A 15-year-old male presented with flank discomfort and was found to have renal cysts. What additional finding would be diagnostic of Von Hippel-Lindau (VHL) syndrome in this patient?

a A single pancreatic cyst

b Multiple pancreatic cysts

c Renal cell carcinoma

d A single central nervous system haemangioblastoma

e A phaeochromocytoma

48 A patient is being followed up after receiving a renal transplant. They are noted to have a dilated collecting system and rising creatinine. What is the most likely cause?

a Denervation of the renal collecting system

b Extrinsic compression from a perinephric fluid collection

c Ureteral calculi

d Ureteral ischaemia

e Ureteral kinking

49 A 65-year-old man complained of several months of progressively worsening left flank pain and swelling. CT demonstrated a heterogeneously enhancing soft-tissue density mass arising from the perirenal space, displacing the kidney and containing internal foci of calcification. The MR appearances were of a predominantly low intensity mass on T1-weighted images, with internal areas of high signal thought to represent haemorrhage. On T2-weighted images there was predominantly very high signal intensity with a 'bowl of fruit appearance' of intermixed low and intermediate signal. There was early heterogeneous enhancement with slow washout following contrast. High T2/low T1-weighted lesions within the vertebral bodies are also present. What is the most likely diagnosis?

a Lymphoma

b Well-differentiated liposarcoma

c Malignant fibrous histiocytoma

d Desmoid tumour

e Malignant rhabdomyosarcoma

50 An 18-month-old boy is confirmed to have a large multicystic renal mass on ultrasound arising from the kidney. On CT the mass appears to project into the renal collecting system, has enhancing septa and no nodular components are identified. Claw-shaped adjacent normal parenchyma is seen to enhance and there is no delayed opacification of the cystic spaces. What is the most likely diagnosis?

a Wilms' tumour

b Cystic partially differentiated nephroblastoma

c Cystic renal cell carcinoma

d Cystic mesoblastic nephroma

e Multicystic dysplastic kidney

51 A 35-year-old patient is undergoing investigation of renovascular hypertension with MR angiography. The distal part of the renal artery is abnormal and the appearance is like a 'string of beads'. The patient is diagnosed with fibromuscular dysplasia (FMD). What is the most appropriate treatment?

a Conservative management: spontaneous regression is the norm

b Surgical excision of involved segment

c Angioplasty without stenting

d Angioplasty and stenting

e Intravascular high-intensity focused ultrasound

52 A 52-year-old woman underwent radiofrequency (RF) ablation of a small renal tumour three months previously and has a follow-up CT scan. What are the expected findings?

a Low attenuation central mass with peripheral nodular enhancement

b An enhancing mass of similar appearance to before ablation

c Bull's-eye appearance of central treated tumour surrounded by a thin soft-tissue rim, with thin halo of fat separating the two

d Non-enhancing central mass with a thin uniform rim of enhancement

e No detectable ablated mass

53 A 33-year-old male pedestrian is hit by a car. His pelvic trauma radiograph demonstrates an anterior compression fracture pattern. He complains of dysuria, gross haematuria and has a swollen bruised perineum and scrotum. Retrograde urethrography does not show urethral injury and he undergoes retrograde CT cystography. What type of bladder injury is he most likely to have sustained?

   a Type 1: Simple bladder contusion
   b Type 2: Intraperitoneal bladder rupture
   c Type 3: Partial thickness bladder wall laceration with intact serosa
   d Type 4: Extraperitoneal bladder rupture
   e Type 5: Combined intraperitoneal and extraperitoneal bladder rupture

54 A 45-year old woman with tinnitus is referred for a contrast enhanced MRI for investigation of suspected acoustic neuroma. She is concerned regarding a 'killer skin disease' which she has read in the popular press is caused by MR contrast agents. Which of the following statements regarding nephrogenic systemic fibrosis (NSF) and the administration of gadolinium-based MR contrast media is correct? (as of February 2009)

   a Gadolinium-based media have been proven to be responsible for causing NSF
   b The incidence of NSF in at risk subjects given Gadodiamide (Omniscan®) is 25%
   c Gadodiamide is contraindicated in patients with chronic kidney disease (stages 4 & 5) with a glomerular filtration rate (GFR) of <30 mL/min
   d Gadolinium-based media can be safely used as a replacement for iodinated contrast media to reduce contrast nephropathy
   e Immediate dialysis following administration of gadolinium-based media prevents the development of NSF

55 A 35-year-old African male with AIDS and renal impairment has an ultrasound which shows bilateral enlarged echogenic kidneys with pelvicalyceal thickening. What is the most likely cause of his renal impairment?

   a Hypertension unrelated to HIV status
   b HIV-related nephropathy
   c Highly active antiretroviral therapy (HAART) related renal side-effects
   d Opportunistic infection with *Pneumocystis jirovecii* (*carinii*)
   e HIV-related malignancy (lymphoma/Kaposi sarcoma)

56 One week following a left laparoscopic partial nephrectomy a 55-year-old male has a CT for persistent pain at the surgical site. Which of the following findings would be most suspicious for a significant post-operative complication?

   a Adherence of the kidney to the posterior abdominal wall, and surrounding reactive change

   b Presence of a fat attenuation mass within the surgical bed

   c Presence of a low-attenuation mass containing gas bubbles limited to the surgical bed

   d Presence of a mass with attenuation of 50–60 HU limited to the surgical bed

   e A wedge-shaped non-enhancing parenchymal area

57 A 50-year-old man was found on CT scan to have an incidental renal mass. Biopsy subsequently showed this to be papillary renal cell carcinoma (RCC). What features are typical of this condition?

   a It is one of the rarest forms of renal cell carcinoma

   b It is typically less homogeneous and more avidly enhancing on CT than clear cell (conventional) RCC

   c It is less frequently bilateral and multifocal than clear cell RCC

   d It has a much better prognosis than clear cell RCC

   e It arises from the epithelium of the medullary collecting duct

58 A 54-year-old female with a history of chronic urinary tract infection undergoes excretory urography that demonstrates multiple nodular filling defects of the bladder mucosa. Which of the following conditions does not belong in the differential diagnosis for this appearance?

   a Malakoplakia

   b Cystitis cystica

   c Bullous oedema

   d Ureterocoele

   e Transitional cell carcinoma

59 A 40-year-old male motorcyclist sustained a straddle injury and blood was noted at his urethral meatus. A urethrogram was performed, which confirmed a urethral injury. What part of the urethra is he most likely to have injured?

   a Pre-prostatic urethra

   b Prostatic urethra

   c Membranous urethra

   d Penile urethra

   e Fossa navicularis

60 An eight-month old boy is referred for voiding cystourethrography (VCUG) to assess for reflux. He is known to have a duplex left-sided kidney with a ureterocoele. When would the ureterocoele be most likely to be visible?

a Early filling images

b Late filling images

c Early voiding images

d Late voiding images

e Post-void images

61 A one-year-old girl is referred for VCUG in the assessment of recurrent urinary tract infection which demonstrates reflux during voiding on the right into a normal calibre ureter and pelvicalyceal system. No left-sided reflux is visible. What management is appropriate?

a Normal finding – no treatment needed

b Prophylactic antibiotics

c Indwelling catheter

d Surgical reimplantation of ureter

e Retrograde pyeloplasty

62 A 30-year-old female is being worked up for living donor laparoscopic nephrectomy. She asks why she needs further imaging after her contrast-enhanced CT scan. What further information is required that cannot be obtained from the CT?

a Number of renal arteries

b Length of the renal vein

c Split renal function

d Ureteral anatomy

e Presence of fibromuscular dysplasia

63 A 50-year-old man presents with chronic progressive back pain, lower extremity swelling and mild renal impairment. A renal US demonstrates mild bilateral hydronephrosis. Excretory urography is performed which shows abnormal peristalsis in the upper ureter with medial deviation of the middle third of both ureters associated with gradual tapering. What is the most likely diagnosis?

a Retroperitoneal fibrosis

b Aorto-caval fistula

c Retroperitoneal sarcoma

d Aortic aneurysm

e Schistosomiasis

64 You are asked to develop a protocol to minimise the incidence of contrast-induced nephropathy (CIN). What intervention has been proven to be of most benefit in its prevention?

a No treatments are proven to be effective

b N-acetylcysteine

c Monitoring of serum creatinine for 72 hours post procedure

d Periprocedural intravenous hydration

e High osmolar iodinated contrast media

65 An 82-year-old male with bilateral ureteric stents *in situ* for localised prostate cancer for which he was treated with radiotherapy presents with intermittent gross haematuria. What condition would be the most immediately life threatening?

a Stent migration irritating bladder mucosa

b Local disease progression

c Chronic urinary tract infection secondary to stent presence

d Radiation cystitis

e Ureteral erosion

66 A 43-year-old woman presents with a subarachnoid haemorrhage and a berry aneurysm is found, which is treated with endovascular coiling. She is incidentally discovered to have renal impairment and a renal ultrasound showed bilateral renal enlargement with multiple cortical cysts. Her father is known to have polycystic kidney disease. What is the likely method of inheritance of her condition?

a X-linked dominant

b X-linked recessive

c Autosomal dominant

d Autosomal recessive

e Mitochondrial

67 A 19-year-old man presents with a suprapubic mass and haematuria. After investigation he is found to have a tumour originating within a patent urachus. What is the most likely diagnosis?

a Adenocarcinoma

b Sarcoma

c Transitional cell carcinoma

d Squamous cell carcinoma

e Lymphoma

68 A 17-year-old male was hit by a car and a contrast-enhanced trauma CT reveals a number of right-sided injuries. Images of his kidney show a lenticular-shaped area peripherally with a density of 50 HU. The remainder of the kidney enhances normally. What is the appropriate management of his renal injury?

a Conservative management

b Endovascular embolisation/coiling

c Surgical revascularisation

d Endovascular stenting of renal artery

e Nephrectomy

69 A 33-year-old female with systemic lupus erythematosus (SLE) presents with a painful mass in her left flank and haematuria. CT demonstrates non-opacification of the left renal vein. What is the likely appearance on ultrasound?

a Small kidney with enhanced cortico-medullary differentiation

b Small kidney with loss of cortico-medullary differentiation

c Normal-sized kidney with loss of cortico-medullary differentiation

d Enlarged kidney with enhanced cortico-medullary differentiation

e Enlarged kidney with loss of cortico-medullary differentiation

70 A newborn male infant had bilateral hydronephrosis detected in utero. VCUG demonstrated a bullet-nosed dilatation of the posterior urethra with a trabeculated bladder and vesicoureteral reflux on the left. What is the most likely diagnosis?

a Prune belly syndrome

b Primary megaureter

c Posterior urethral valves

d Ureterocoele

e Congenital urethral diverticulum

Paediatric radiology

PAPER 1

1   A three-week-old full-term infant presents with abdominal distension and bilious vomiting. An abdominal radiograph shows generalised distension of bowel loops and no evidence of free intraperitoneal air. Barium enema shows a normal-calibre segment of distal sigmoid colon and a dilated proximal colon with an inverted cone shape at the transition between the two. What is the most likely diagnosis?

  a   Intussusception
  b   Volvulus
  c   Hirschsprung disease
  d   Necrotising enterocolitis

2   A six-year-old girl presents with a three-day history of irritability, headache and high fever. On examination she is lethargic and pyrexial with no evidence of a purpuric rash. The paediatricians suspect that the patient has herpes encephalitis. An MRI brain is performed. What imaging findings are most likely to be seen?

  a   Nothing, it is too early
  b   Temporal lobe high signal on T2-weighted images; low signal on T1-weighted images
  c   Periventricular high intensity on T1-weighted images
  d   Temporal lobe low signal on T2-weighted images; low signal on T1-weighted images
  e   Hyperintense signal in the brain stem

3 Anteroposterior and frog-leg lateral hip radiographs of a 10-year-old girl demonstrate bilateral posterior and inferior displacement of the femoral heads with respect to the femoral shafts. Which of the following is the most likely diagnosis?

a Perthes disease

b Irritable hips

c Developmental dysplasia of the hips

d Slipped upper femoral epiphysis

e Septic arthritis

4 A premature infant, born at 27 weeks, was ventilated for the first 14 days and subsequently on CPAP for a further 21 days. A CXR is performed at three months of age. What is the likely appearance?

a 'White out' of the lungs

b Patchy bilateral ground-glass opacities with air bronchograms

c Hyperinflation with coarse linear densities and focal areas of emphysema

d Reduced lung volumes with bilateral reticulonodular opacities

e Normal volume lungs with no focal abnormality

5 A renal ultrasound on a five-year-old shows bilateral hyperechoic smoothly enlarged kidneys with a loss of corticomedullary differentiation and a few macroscopic (<1 cm) renal cysts. Which of the following is the most important additional investigation?

a Liver ultrasound

b Chest radiograph

c Micturating cystourethrogram

d Abdominal PET-CT

e Post-void bladder ultrasound

6 A 15-year-old child with Trisomy 21 presented to the Emergency Department with neck pain and loss of sensation over the occiput. He had fallen awkwardly on his head earlier during a game of touch rugby. What is most likely to be visible on plain radiographs of the neck?

a Sagittal cleft of the vertebral body

b Unilateral facet joint dislocation

c Abnormal odontoid peg formation

d Hypoplastic posterior arch of C1

e Atlantoaxial subluxation

7 A hip ultrasound performed on a one-month-old girl shows a shallow acetabulum and an alpha angle of 40 degrees. Which of the following is the most likely diagnosis?

a Perthes disease

   b Septic arthritis

   c Developmental dysplasia of the hip

   d Slipped upper femoral epiphysis

   e Irritable hip

8   An infant is born at 41 weeks following a traumatic delivery with passage of meconium. He quickly develops respiratory distress with grunting, tachypnoea and nasal flaring. A CXR is performed. What is the most likely appearance of the CXR?

   a Widespread ground-glass opacities

   b 'White out' of the lung

   c Widespread patchy consolidation and air trapping

   d Focal consolidation with air bronchograms

   e Small volume lungs with bilateral pleural effusions

9   An infant is born with an abdominal wall defect and exteriorised bowel loops. Which additional finding would suggest a diagnosis of gastroschisis rather than omphalocoele?

   a Herniated liver

   b Ascites

   c Bowel loops covered by peritoneum

   d Right paraumbilical abdominal wall defect

   e Bladder exstrophy

10 A one-year-old child is investigated for delayed speech development. He is found to have reduced hearing on the right side. There is no history of middle ear infections. The tympanogram shows a flattened and reduced response. On otoscopy there is abnormal discharge with granulation tissue in the upper quadrant of the auditory canal and an intact tympanic membrane. A diagnosis of congenital cholesteatoma is made. The patient has an MRI scan. What would you be looking for to confirm your diagnosis?

   a A soft-tissue erosion into the cochlear, which is hyper-dense on T1-weighted images and isodense on T2-weighted images relative to brain

   b A soft-tissue erosion into the cochlear, which is hyper-dense on T1-weighted images and hyper-dense on T2-weighted images relative to brain

   c A soft-tissue erosion into the cochlear, which is isodense on T1-weighted images and hyper-dense on T2-weighted images relative to brain

   d A soft-tissue erosion into the cochlear, which is isodense on T1-weighted images and hypo-dense on T2-weighted images relative to brain

   e A soft-tissue erosion into the cochlear, which is hyper-dense on T1-weighted images and hyper-dense on T2 images relative to brain

11 A 10-year-old boy presents with a painful lump on the left side of his head that has gradually increased in size. There is no definite history of trauma. Serum biochemistry reveals an eosinophilia and raised ESR. A skull radiograph shows a 6-cm round, punched out lesion in the left parietal bone with a bevelled edge and an overlying soft-tissue mass. Which of the following is the most likely diagnosis?

   a Osteomyelitis
   b Neuroblastoma metastases
   c Eosinophilic granuloma
   d Arachnoid granulation
   e Epidermoid cyst

12 A four-year-old child presents with recurrent urinary tract infections. They have had three culture-confirmed urinary tract infections with no evidence of pyelonephritis in any episode. What is the most appropriate investigation?

   a Ultrasound scan during an episode of infection
   b Ultrasound scan within six months
   c DMSA in four to six months
   d DMSA during acute infection
   e Micturating cysto-urethrogram at a time when symptom free

13 A two-year-old child presents with increasing abdominal girth. An ultrasound shows a 13-cm mass in the upper abdomen, arising on the right side and crossing the midline. A CT shows speckled calcification within it and a preliminary diagnosis of neuroblastoma is made. What is the most appropriate radionuclide study in this case?

   a I123 MIBG study with planar and SPECT images
   b In111 octreotide study planar and SPECT images
   c MDP Tc-99m bone scan whole body views
   d Tc-99m pertechnetate study with planar images of the whole abdomen at 24 and 48 hours
   e Whole body I123

14 An infant is diagnosed with Beckwith-Wiedemann syndrome and is therefore at increased risk of developing Wilms' tumour. How should they be followed up?

   a Abdominal ultrasound every three months
   b Annual abdominal ultrasound
   c Abdominal ultrasound at six months with further imaging only if the child becomes symptomatic
   d Annual abdominal CT
   e Abdominal CT every three months

15 A plain radiograph of the lower leg shows a lytic metaphyseal lesion within the tibia with a thinned cortex and fine internal trabeculations. There is no periosteal reaction. A bone scan is performed, which shows increased uptake around the periphery of the lesion with no uptake centrally. An MRI demonstrates multiple cysts of different signal intensity with a low signal rim and heterogeneous enhancement post-gadolinium. Which of the following is the most likely diagnosis?

a Fibrous dysplasia

b Aneurysmal bone cyst

c Enchondroma

d Bone island

e Chondrosarcoma

16 A 15-year-old girl with a history of recurrent lower respiratory tract infections during early childhood has a CXR to investigate a cough. The lungs are asymmetrical with a smaller, hyperlucent left lung with a small left hilum and evidence of air trapping during expiration. Which of the following is the most likely diagnosis?

a Congenital cystic adenomatoid malformation

b Congenital lobar emphysema

c Swyer-James syndrome

d Pulmonary artery atresia

e Intralobar pulmonary sequestration

17 A four-month-old child is brought to the Emergency Department with a reduced level of consciousness and has a CT brain scan. The child also has multiple healed fractures and a 'bucket handle' fracture of the left elbow. In this situation what is the most likely finding?

a Diffuse multiple foci of decreased density

b Epidural haemorrhage

c Occipital subdural haematoma

d Interhemispheric subdural haematoma

e Thalamic infarct

18 A previously well seven-year-old boy has a chest radiograph for a possible chest infection. The lungs are clear but the film is reported as showing a posterior mediastinal mass with an air-fluid level and hemivertebrae of T3 and T4. What is the most likely diagnosis?

a Intramural oesophageal tumour

b Morgagni diaphragmatic hernia

c Oesophageal duplication cyst

d Cystic hygroma

e Bronchogenic cyst

19 A three-year-old boy below the 0.25th centile for height has dystrophic nails and a yellowish discolouration of his teeth. Radiographs of both arms reveal generalised increased density of the long bones with thickened cortices and multiple healing fractures of varying ages. Which of the following is the most likely diagnosis?

a Osteopetrosis

b Nail-patella syndrome

c Pyknodysostosis

d Thanatophoric dwarfism

e Morquio syndrome

20 A three-month-old boy is brought into the Emergency Department with a dusky complexion. On CXR there is interstitial oedema with a prominent right atrial border but an absent left ventricular silhouette. What is the most likely diagnosis?

a Hypoplastic left heart syndrome

b Pulmonary atresia

c Patent ductus arteriosus

d Tetralogy of Fallot

e Tricuspid atresia

21 A 12-year-old girl with cystic fibrosis has a CT abdomen for recurrent bouts of colicky right lower quadrant abdominal pain. The positive findings include partial small bowel obstruction, diffuse colonic thickening, mural striation and mesenteric soft-tissue infiltration. What is the most likely diagnosis?

a Intussusception

b Distal intestinal obstruction syndrome

c Meconium ileus

d Crohn's disease

e Appendicitis

22 A nine-year-old girl falls from a height. She presents with ankle pain and swelling. The AP view of the ankle demonstrates a distal tibial fracture line running obliquely through the epiphysis and extending horizontally to the periphery of the physis. What is the Salter-Harris classification of this fracture?

a I

b II

c III

d IV

e V

23 The CXR of a neonate with a VSD and patent ductus arteriosus reveals a dilated right atrium and ventricle, absent aortic knuckle, and no oesophageal impression. Which of the following is the most likely diagnosis?

a Coarctation of aorta

b Aortic atresia

c Cor triatriatum

d Interruption of aortic arch

e Polysplenia syndrome

24 A three-month-old boy undergoes a renal tract ultrasound. This demonstrates a thick-walled bladder with trabeculations and bilateral hydroureteronephrosis. Which of the following is the most likely diagnosis?

a Pelvi-ureteric junction obstruction

b Megacystis-microcolon-intestinal hypoperistalsis syndrome

c Posterior urethral valve

d Vesico-ureteric junction obstruction

e Prune belly syndrome

25 An eight-month-old child presents with a rapid onset of lethargy and irritability. The child is hard to examine due to excessive crying. The child has a fever and diarrhoea but no purpuric rash. The paediatricians diagnose meningitis on a lumbar puncture. A week later the child is still septic, lethargic and is now showing signs of raised intracranial pressure. An enhanced CT brain is performed showing a hypodense lentiform zone with ring enhancement adjacent to the skull in the right parieto-temporal region. What complication is present?

a Subdural haematoma

b Extradural haematoma

c Cerebral aneurysm

d Epidural abscess

e Subdural empyema

26 A child is seen in the paediatric clinic and investigated for short stature and abnormal facies. As part of the investigation, he has plain radiographs of the thoracic and lumbar spine and lower limbs. These show generalised osteopenia. There is shortening of the long bones with widening of the metaphyses and diaphyses. In the spine there is kyphosis at the thoracolumbar junction with beaking of the anterior vertebral bodies. What is the most likely diagnosis?

a Gaucher's disease

b Achondroplasia

c Mucopolysaccharidosis

d Thanatophoric dysplasia

e Niemann-Pick disease

27 A father of a two-month-old boy is concerned that his son has been getting progressively blue, which becomes more apparent when he cries. On examination he is cyanosed with a pansystolic murmur. A CXR reveals a moderately enlarged heart. What is the likely diagnosis?

   a Tetralogy of Fallot

   b Corrected transposition of great arteries

   c Pulmonary atresia

   d Tricuspid atresia

   e Patent ductus arteriosus

28 An eight-year-old girl has never been continent of urine and complains of intermittent dribbling of urine, particularly when she is upright. Which of the following is the most likely diagnosis?

   a Complete ureteric duplication with infrasphincteric insertion of the upper moiety ureter

   b Complete ureteric duplication with suprasphincteric insertion of the upper moiety ureter

   c Partial ureteric duplication

   d Pseudoureterocoele

   e Congenital urethral diverticulum

29 A seven-year-old girl presented with lethargy and headache two weeks after a viral infection. On examination she was irritable and febrile. She became increasingly drowsy and soon after admission had a generalised seizure. An MRI brain was performed which showed high signal lesions at the junction between the deep cortical grey matter and subcortical white matter on T2-weighted images. There was surrounding vasogenic oedema. Which of the following is the most likely diagnosis?

   a Acute inflammatory demyelinating polyradiculoneuropathy

   b Viral encephalitis

   c Acute disseminated encephalomyelitis

   d Primary CNS lymphoma

   e Glioblastoma multiforme

30 A 12-month-old child presents with irritability and swelling of the wrists and ankles. She has had a prolonged period of exclusive breastfeeding. On examination she has softening of the cranial vault and bowed legs. A radiograph of the right wrist is performed. Which of the following is the most likely finding?

   a 'Ground-glass' osteoporosis with cortical thinning

   b Bands of increased density in the metaphyses

   c Cupping and fraying of the metaphyses with coarse trabeculation d Narrowed epiphyseal plates

e Lamellar periosteal reaction with multiple osteolytic areas within the metaphyses

31 A one-year-old boy presents with a six-day history of fever. On examination he has bilateral cervical lymphadenopathy, injected fissured lips, a strawberry tongue and bilateral non-purulent conjunctivitis. Which of the following should be performed in the acute setting?

a Neck ultrasound

b Slit-lamp examination of the eyes

c Echocardiogram

d Lumbar puncture

e Abdominal ultrasound

32 A neonate with obstructive jaundice undergoes a technetium labelled diiso-propyl iminodiacetic acid (DISIDA) nuclear scintiscan. What findings would confirm the diagnosis of biliary atresia?

a Good hepatic activity within five minutes and no visualisation of bowel at six hours or 24 hours

b Good hepatic activity within five minutes, no visualisation of bowel at six hours but good visualisation of bowel at 24 hours

c Good hepatic activity at one hour with no visualisation of bowel at six hours or 24 hours

d Absent hepatic activity at six hours and 24 hours

e Good hepatic activity at one hour, no visualisation of bowel at six hours but good visualisation of bowel at 24 hours

33 A two-year-old girl, who is failing to thrive, presents with bilateral facial swelling that has increased in size recently. On palpation the swellings are firm and non-tender. The child undergoes an ultrasound. The parotid glands are seen to contain multiple anechoic areas without associated posterior enhancement. What is the most likely diagnosis?

a Mumps

b HIV parotitis

c Lymphadenitis

d Warthin's tumour

e Branchial cleft cyst

34 A 10-month-old child is admitted to intensive care and ventilated following a significant head injury. An unenhanced CT brain is performed. Which of the following findings would be consistent with severe hypoxic brain injury?

    a Decreased grey and white matter density, decreased grey/white matter differentiation and increased density of the basal ganglia, thalami and cerebellum

    b Increased grey and white matter density, decreased grey/white matter differentiation and decreased density of the basal ganglia, thalami and cerebellum

    c Increased grey matter density and decreased white matter density

    d Decreased grey matter density, increased white matter density and decreased density of the basal ganglia, thalami and cerebellum

    e Increased grey and white matter density, increased grey/white matter differentiation and decreased density of the basal ganglia, thalami and cerebellum

35 A 12-year-old boy develops progressive shortness of breath on exercise and coughing at night. He has had two chest infections in the last year but his CXR is normal. What is the most likely diagnosis?

    a Cystic fibrosis

    b Asthma

    c Bronchiectasis

    d Congenital lobar emphysema

    e Tracheo-oesophageal fistula

36 A one-year-old boy presenting with abdominal pain has an abdominal ultrasound that confirms the diagnosis of intussusception. Which of the following ultrasound features is a good predictor of reducibility?

    a Absence of blood flow within the intussusceptum on colour Doppler

    b Fluid seen within the intussusception

    c Blood flow within the intussusceptum on colour Doppler

    d Presence of the 'target' sign

    e Small bowel obstruction

37 An eight-year-old boy with haemophilia A has repeated episodes of right knee pain and swelling. A radiograph of the right knee shows a joint effusion. What bony abnormalities might be seen?

    a Squared patella with widening of the intercondylar notch

    b Loss of joint space with subchondral sclerosis

    c Multiple erosions within the tibial plateau

    d Juxta-articular osteoporosis

    e Widened and irregular epiphyseal plate

38 A three-year-old girl with a chronic cough and recurrent chest infections is found to have atelectasis, mucous plugging, cystic bronchiectasis, and air trapping on CXR. What is the likely diagnosis?

a Congenital lobar emphysema

b Whooping cough

c Cystic fibrosis

d Asthma

e Cystic adenomatoid malformation

39 A neonate born at term is reviewed on the post-natal ward for not tolerating feeds. Every feed is regurgitated and on examination he is drooling. There is no evidence of respiratory distress. Attempts to pass a feeding NG tube are unsuccessful. What is the most likely diagnosis?

a Tracheoesophageal fistula without oesophageal atresia

b Oesophageal atresia and proximal and distal tracheoesophageal fistulae

c Oesophageal atresia without tracheoesophageal fistula

d Oesophageal atresia and proximal tracheoesophageal fistula

e Oesophageal atresia and distal tracheoesophageal fistula

40 A 10-year-old child is diagnosed with non-Hodgkin's lymphoma (NHL). He is found to have two single extranodal tumours on opposite sides of the diaphragm. What stage of disease does he have?

a I

b II

c III

d IV

e V

41 A tall eight-year-old with lax ligaments falls from her bicycle and undergoes plain radiographs of the right wrist and forearm, which show a mid-shaft fracture of the radius. The bone density of the radius and ulna is reduced with generalised osteoporosis and the carpal bones are abnormal with enlargement of the epiphyseal centres and epiphyseal calcification. Which of the following is the most likely diagnosis?

a Marfan syndrome

b Ehlers-Danlos syndrome

c Homocystinuria

d Rickets

e Scurvy

42 A neonate with persistent non-bilious vomiting has an abdominal radiograph that shows a 'double bubble' in the left upper quadrant and no gas distal to this in the abdomen. What is the most likely diagnosis?

a Choledochal cyst

b Duodenal duplication

c Duodenal atresia

d Duodenal diverticulum

e Peritoneal bands

43 An 11-month-old girl recently recovers from a viral chest infection but now develops shortness of breath and wheezing. Her CXR shows peribronchial thickening, some hyperinflation, and small parenchymal opacities. What is the most likely diagnosis?

a Asthma

b Bronchitis

c Reactive airways disease

d Cystic fibrosis

e Bronchopulmonary dysplasia

44 A girl who was born with Tetralogy of Fallot presented to the Emergency Department with fever and drowsiness. A CT scan was performed, which showed a ring-enhancing low-density lesion with surrounding oedema within the frontal lobe. What is the most likely diagnosis?

a Astrocytoma

b Metastasis

c Lymphoma

d Frontal lobe abscess

e Craniopharyngioma

45 A plain radiograph is performed on a four-year-old with progressive deformity of the right hand. This shows multiple radiolucent expansile lesions within the metacarpals and phalanges, some of which contain punctate calcifications. Which of the following is the most likely diagnosis?

a Chondroblastoma

b Chondromyxoid fibroma

c Langerhans cell histiocytosis

d Enchondromatosis

e Aneurysmal bone cyst

46 A 12-year-old girl with known osteosarcoma of the proximal femur presents with acute shortness of breath. What is the most likely finding on CXR?

a Bilateral hilar lymphadenopathy

b Pneumothorax

c Coarsened bronchovascular markings with reticular opacities

d Bilateral lower lobe atelectasis

e Multiple cavitating nodules

47 A two-year-old presents with an abdominal mass. He is found to be hypertensive and to have high levels of vanillylmandelic acid in his urine. A CT scan shows a heterogeneous mass containing calcification arising from the left adrenal gland and extending across the midline. There is no evidence of metastatic disease on the CT. Appearances are suggestive of an adrenal neuroblastoma. What is the most appropriate staging?

a Stage I

b Stage II

c Stage III

d Stage IV

e Stage IVs

48 A nine-year-old girl is investigated for precocious puberty. On examination she is noted to have two large café au lait spots with irregular edges on the right side of her back and to have a mild leg length discrepancy with a shorter right leg. A plain radiograph of the right leg is performed. Which of the following is the most likely finding?

a Several 'ground-glass' medullary lesions within the proximal femur with endosteal scalloping

b Anterolateral bowing of the lower half of the tibia

c Absent fibula

d Pseudoarthrosis of the tibia

e Generalised osteoporosis of the femur, tibia and fibula

49 A two-year-old boy is brought into the Emergency Department by his mother because she is concerned he has aspirated a foreign body. No foreign body is seen on CXR. What other CXR features might suggest recent foreign body aspiration?

a Hyperlucency

b Consolidation

c Effusion

d Pneumothorax

e Bronchiectasis

50 An MRI brain of an infant born at term with evidence of normal development demonstrates myelination of the brainstem, cerebellum and both the
anterior and posterior limbs of the internal capsule. Neither the splenium
nor genu of the corpus callosum appear myelinated. What is the likely age
of the infant?

a 2 months

b 3 months

c 6 months

d 9 months

e 1 year

51 A 15-year-old girl, who is short for her age and has not entered puberty, falls
off her bicycle onto her right hand. A plain radiograph of her right hand
shows shortened third and fourth metacarpals and a Madelung's deformity.
What is the most likely underlying diagnosis?

a Down's syndrome

b Angelman syndrome

c 21q deletion

d William's syndrome

e Turner's syndrome

52 A neonate is born with an imperforate anus. Before he has a colostomy
formed he has an echocardiogram, which reveals a ventricular septal defect.
He is also noted to have lumbar hemivertebrae on plain radiograph of the
lumbar spine. Further imaging is planned to look for associated conditions.
What further abnormality might be found?

a Radial dysplasia

b Tarsal coalition

c Developmental dysplasia of the hip

d Aneurysmal bone cyst

e Pyknodystosis

53 A 15-year-old boy is found to have metastatic deposits in his lungs. Osteogenic
sarcoma has been excluded. What is the most likely primary tumour?

a Rhabdomyosarcoma

b Wilms' tumour

c Ewing's sarcoma

d Medulloblastoma

e Retinoblastoma

54 A 12-year-old girl has a CT brain following head trauma. There is no evidence of any haemorrhage or fracture, but neither the maxillary antra nor mastoid are pneumatised and there is thinning of the outer table of the skull. Which of the following is the most likely diagnosis?

a Sickle cell disease

b Hereditary spherocytosis

c Thalassaemia major

d Fibrous dysplasia

e Von Gierke's disease

55 A seven-year-old girl presents with dysphagia and recurrent chest infections. She undergoes a barium study of her oesophagus, which reveals a right-sided impression in the upper chest and a left-sided impression slightly lower down. What is the most likely explanation for these findings?

a Right arch with aberrant left subclavian

b Right arch without aberrant vessels

c Left arch with aberrant right subclavian

d Double aortic arch

e Innominate artery compression syndrome

56 A 12-year-old boy presents with a six-week history of a painful leg mass. He has a fever and leucocytosis. A plain radiograph of the leg demonstrates a poorly defined lytic lesion in the tibial diaphysis. There is a lamellar periosteal reaction and penetration into the soft tissues with preservation of the tissue planes. Which of the following is the most likely diagnosis?

a Osteomyelitis

b Eosinophilic granuloma

c Neuroblastoma

d Osteosarcoma

e Ewing's sarcoma

57 A four-month-old boy presents in congestive heart failure. An abdominal ultrasound reveals several hyperechoic lesions within the liver. These demonstrate peritumoral flow on colour Doppler. A contrast enhanced CT abdomen is performed to further categorise the lesions, which are shown to have early peripheral nodular enhancement with complete central opacification on delayed images. Which of the following is the most likely diagnosis?

a Cavernous haemangioma

b Hepatoblastoma

c Hepatic metastases

d Haemangioendothelioma

e Focal nodular hyperplasia

58 A 12-month-old boy presents with pyrexia and a history of not moving his left leg for two days. On examination he is irritable and cries when the leg is manipulated. He has recently had an upper respiratory tract infection. Septic arthritis is suspected. Which of the following would be appropriate initial imaging?

a Bone scan of the hip

b Ultrasound of the ankle

c Ultrasound of the hip

d Plain radiograph of the knee

e CT of the knee

59 An F2 doctor from the Emergency Department has just seen a child who has chronic sinusitic symptoms. She has asked you to review the CXR because she is concerned to see the cardiac apex and gastric bubble on the right. On closer inspection, you also notice that the aortic arch is on the right side and there is some bronchiectasis. What is the likely diagnosis?

a Situs solitus

b Situs solitus with dextrocardia

c Situs inversus

d Levoversion with abdominal situs inversus

e Asplenia syndrome

60 Following minor trauma a six-year-old child has cervical spine radiographs. No cervical spine injury is identified and a diagnosis is made of pseudosub-luxation. What are the likely radiographic findings?

a A line between the anterior margins of C1 and C3 spinous processes passing within 2 mm of the anterior margin of the C2 spinous process

b 5-mm distance between the odontoid and the anterior arch of the axis

c Anterior displacement of up to 5 mm of the C2 vertebral body on the C3 vertebral body on flexion views

d Increase in the anterior displacement of the C2 vertebral body on the C3 vertebral body on extension views and reduction on flexion views

e 7-mm distance between the odontoid and anterior arch of the axis

61 A 10-year-old boy presents with acute pain in the upper pole of the right testis. On examination there is a small, firm right paratesticular nodule, which has a bluish tinge. Ultrasound demonstrates a normal left testis and an enlarged right testis. There is no focal lesion seen within the right testis and it has normal Doppler flow within it. Adjacent to the right testis is a small hypoechoic mass with absent Doppler flow. Which of the following is the most likely diagnosis?

a Testicular torsion

b Torsion of the appendix testis

c Haematocele

d Seminoma

e Acute orchitis

62 A young girl is brought to the Emergency Department with abdominal pain, nausea and vomiting. The working diagnosis is gastroenteritis but a heart murmur is heard and so a CXR and abdominal radiograph are requested. These show a 'three sign' of the aorta and the outline of the lower poles of the kidneys cannot be traced. How can these findings be explained?

a Down's syndrome

b Trisomy 13

c Trisomy 18

d Turner's syndrome

e Noonan's syndrome

63 A 14-year-old girl was the front passenger in a road traffic accident in which the driver died at the scene. She sustained multiple injuries. Her pulse is 110, blood pressure is 100/80 mmHg and GCS is 5/15. Radiographs show comminuted fractures of the right femur and humerus. There is a right pneumothorax. She has an abdominal CT scan. Findings in keeping with hypoperfusion complex are:

a Increased enhancement of the adrenal glands and decreased enhancement of the spleen and bowel wall

b Small calibre aorta, distended vena cava and increased bowel wall enhancement

c Collapsed vena cava, large aorta, and increased bowel wall enhancement

d Increased enhancement of the spleen and bowel wall and reduced enhancement of the adrenal glands

e Collapsed vena cava, increased enhancement of the adrenal glands and decreased splenic enhancement

64 A 10-year-old girl with a round moon face, truncal obesity, purple abdominal striae and proximal muscle weakness undergoes an abdominal ultrasound. Which of the following is the most likely finding?

a Multiple cysts within the left kidney

b 3-cm round hyperechoic left suprarenal mass

c 9-cm heterogeneous left suprarenal mass containing calcification

d 6-cm mixed reflectivity left suprarenal mass with a central area of low reflectivity

e 10-cm hyperechoic mass arising from the midpole of the left kidney

65 A child with Trisomy 13 is found to have a ventricular septal defect. What cardiac abnormality might you expect to see on his CXR?

a Dextroposition

b Dextroversion

c Dextrocardia

d Hypoplastic left ventricle

e Absent right heart border

66 A left multicystic dysplastic kidney is diagnosed on an antenatal ultrasound. Which of the following are the most likely findings in the left kidney on a post-natal ultrasound at three weeks?

a A 2-cm solitary cortical cyst within the upper pole

b Multiple cysts of varying sizes, an absent renal pelvis and dysplastic renal parenchyma

c A small kidney with poor corticomedullary differentiation and medullary cysts

d Enlarged hyperechoic kidney with poor corticomedullary differentiation and several cortical cysts

e Atrophic kidney measuring 1.5 cm in length

67 An infant is brought to the Emergency Department with a cough and temperature. The CXR reveals a well-circumscribed, rounded mass lesion behind the heart with air bronchograms. Which of the following would be appropriate further imaging?

a Enhanced CT chest

b Lateral chest radiograph

c Ultrasound chest

d Repeat CXR in six weeks

e High resolution CT chest

68 A six-day-old term neonate with congenital heart disease shows signs of septic shock with abdominal distension, bilious nasogastric aspirates and bloody diarrhoea. There is no change with supportive management. Plain abdominal radiographs taken 24 hours apart show a persistent loop of dilated bowel, intramural gas and gas in the portal venous system. The most appropriate next step in management is:

a Upper GI contrast study

b Barium enema

c Ultrasound abdomen

d Laparotomy

e Rectal biopsy

69 An infant presents with recurrent vomiting after every feed. You are asked to perform an upper GI contrast study to rule out malrotation. What is the best position in which to place the infant to rule out malrotation?

a Left lateral

b Right lateal

c Supine

d Prone

e Left oblique

70 A neonate born at term develops respiratory distress within the first few hours after birth. He is noted to have a scaphoid abdomen. A CXR is performed that shows multiple cystic structures within the left hemithorax. Which of the following is the most likely diagnosis?

a Bochdalek hernia

b Morgagni hernia

c Bronchogenic cyst

d Congenital lobar emphysema

e Intralobar pulmonary sequestration

Paediatric radiology

1   A six-week-old boy with non-bilious vomiting has an abdominal ultrasound. Which of the following findings confirm the diagnosis of pyloric stenosis?
    a   Pyloric muscle wall thickness of 2 mm
    b   Pyloric canal length of 10 mm
    c   Rapid gastric emptying
    d   Pyloric transverse diameter of 20 mm
    e   Absent peristaltic wave

2   An 18-month-old child is being investigated for reduced visual acuity and strabismus. She undergoes an ultrasound of the orbit, which demonstrates a heterogeneous, hyperechoic cystic intra-ocular mass with retinal detachment. What is the most likely diagnosis?
    a   Retinoblastoma
    b   Persistent hyperplastic primary vitreous
    c   Retinal astrocytoma
    d   Rhabdomyosarcoma
    e   Varix of the orbit

3   An overweight 12-year-old boy presents with right hip pain and a limp. An AP radiograph of the pelvis shows widening of the right proximal femoral physis and minimal medial displacement of the right femoral head. Which of the following is the most appropriate imaging to perform next?
    a   CT pelvis and right hip
    b   Ultrasound right hip
    c   Frog leg lateral of pelvis
    d   Plain radiograph of hips
    e   MRI right hip

4 A 12-year-old boy presents to the Emergency Department having swallowed a pen lid. A CXR is performed and the pen lid is seen in the midline below the level of the carina. However, it is noted that there is elevation of the right hemidiaphragm and some midline shift to the right. There is also a curved tubular structure running parallel to the right heart. The patient is re-examined and he is well. What is the most likely diagnosis to explain these findings?

  a Right lower bronchial obstruction and lower lobe collapse
  b Scimitar syndrome
  c Total anomalous pulmonary venous return
  d Hypoplastic right heart syndrome
  e Acute lung syndrome

5 A 15-year-old boy presents with a lump on the left side of his neck, which has grown recently. It lies along the anterior border of the sternocleidomastoid muscle. On ultrasound the lump is seen to be well circumscribed, compressible, have internal structure but lack internal flow. The mass extends between the bifurcation of the internal and external carotid artery. Using the Bailey classification, into which category would this lesion fall?

  a I
  b II
  c III
  d IV
  e V

6 A 13-year-old boy has short stature with a webbed neck. He has a delayed bone age and an abdominal ultrasound shows bilateral renal duplication. What is the most likely diagnosis?

  a Di George syndrome
  b Turner's syndrome
  c Cri du Chat syndrome
  d Noonan's syndrome
  e Edward's syndrome

7 A seven-year-old boy presents with left hip pain and a limp. The anteroposterior and frog-leg lateral hip radiographs demonstrate a small left femoral epiphysis with a subchondral fracture on the anterolateral aspect of the epiphysis and a widened medial joint space. Which of the following is the most likely diagnosis?

  a Perthes disease
  b Slipped upper femoral epiphysis
  c Septic arthritis

    d Developmental dysplasia of the hips

    e Irritable left hip

8   A three-year-old girl with a cough and fever has a CXR. This shows a spherical mass in the posterior left lower lobe with slightly ill-defined borders and air bronchograms. Which of the following is the most likely diagnosis?

    a Aspergilloma

    b Round pneumonia

    c Pertussis

    d Bronchiolitis

    e Neuroblastoma metastasis

9   A series of 48 children with suspected rhabdomyosarcomas are evaluated by MRI and the results show that 28 patients' scans are reported as normal. There are 18 true positives and four false negatives. What is the positive predictive value of the test?

    a 9/10

    b 6/7

    c 9/11

    d 1/7

    e 1/10

10   A male neonate is found to have a wrinkled hypotonic abdominal wall and no palpable testes within the scrotum. What is the most important radiological investigation to perform in the first instance?

    a Abdominal radiograph

    b Renal tract ultrasound

    c Scrotal ultrasound

    d Chest radiograph

    e Micturating cystourethrogram

11   At the baby check a baby boy is found to have both a positive Barlow dislocation test and a positive Ortolani reduction test. Which of the following would be appropriate follow-up imaging?

    a Hip ultrasound at one week

    b Hip ultrasound at seven months

    c Hip ultrasound at one month

    d AP pelvic radiograph at one week

    e AP pelvic radiograph at one month

12 A CXR is performed as part of a septic screen on a lethargic two year old who does not have any specific chest signs. The lungs and pleural spaces appear clear, but a large anterior mediastinal mass is identified, the edge of which appears wavy. Which of the following is the likely cause?

   a Reactive lymphadenopathy
   b Normal thymus
   c Non-Hodgkin's lymphoma
   d Thymic hyperplasia
   e Hodgkin's lymphoma

13 A six-year-old child presents with sudden onset of difficulty in breathing with inspiratory stridor. The child is febrile and irritable. A lateral neck radiograph shows enlargement of the epiglottis and circumferential narrowing of the subglottic portion of the trachea. Which of the following is the most likely cause?

   a Aspiration
   b *Streptococcus* group A
   c Respiratory syncytial virus
   d Norwalk virus
   e *Haemophilus ducreyi*

14 A four-day-old boy born at term presents with bilious vomiting, abdominal distension and failure to pass meconium. An abdominal radiograph shows dilated loops of small bowel without air-fluid levels and a 'soap bubble' appearance within the right lower quadrant. What is the most likely diagnosis?

   a Necrotising enterocolitis
   b Meconium ileus
   c Small bowel atresia
   d Duodenal duplication cyst
   e Malrotation

15 Plain radiographs of the right foot are performed on an eight year old. On the frontal view, the talar line lies lateral to the first metatarsal and the calcaneal line lies lateral to the fifth metatarsal. On the lateral view, the talocalcaneal angle is reduced and there is a step-like configuration of the metatarsals. Which of the following is the most likely diagnosis?

   a Hindfoot valgus
   b Metatarsus adductus
   c Vertical talus
   d Pes cavus
   e Talipes equinovarus

16 A neonate born at term is admitted to the neonatal intensive care unit with respiratory distress and generalised hypotonia. A CXR is performed that does not show any focal abnormality, but the chest is noted to be bell-shaped. Which of the following is the likely underlying diagnosis?

   a Down's syndrome

   b Group B streptococcal pneumonia

   c Foetal alcohol syndrome

   d Congenital toxoplasmosis

   e Neuromuscular disease

17 Which of the following is used in the diagnosis of Meckel's diverticulum?

   a Tc-99m pertechnetate

   b Ga-67 citrate

   c I-123 metaiodobenzylguanidine

   d Tc-99m diethylenetriamine pentaacetic acid

   e Tc-99m dimercaptosuccinic acid

18 A four-year-old boy has a plain radiograph of the left wrist. This demonstrates fraying and irregularity of the radial and ulnar metaphysis and widening of the growth plates. Which of the following is the most likely diagnosis?

   a Scurvy

   b Osteomalacia

   c Rickets

   d Hypothyroidism

   e Haemophilia

19 A four-year-old boy presented with loss of visual acuity and a change in iris pigmentation. A CT of his brain and orbits showed a diffuse thickening of the left optic nerve. An MRI was then performed, which showed the abnormality to be isodense to the cortex and hypodense to the white matter on T1-weighted images, and hyperdense to the cortex and white matter on T2-weighted images. It was hypodense to orbital fat on all sequences. There was intense enhancement post-gadolinium. Which of the following is the most likely diagnosis?

   a Isolated meningioma

   b Neurofibromatosis type 1

   c Oligodendroglioma

   d Subdural haematoma

   e Previous cranial trauma

20 A three month old with feeding difficulties and intermittent respiratory distress has a CXR. This shows a well-defined homogeneous triangular mass adjacent to the posterior medial hemidiaphragm. A contrast-enhanced CT chest is performed and the mass seen on the CXR corresponds to a homogeneous well-circumscribed soft-tissue mass, which drains into the right heart via the IVC. Which of the following is the most likely diagnosis?

 a Congenital cystic adenomatoid malformation
 b Intralobar pulmonary sequestration
 c Extralobar pulmonary sequestration
 d Neuroblastoma
 e Morgagni diaphragmatic hernia

21 A 25-month-old child presents to their GP with a recently expanded lump on the side of the neck. The mass spans both the anterior and posterior triangles of the neck, is soft, non-tender and doughy to palpation. An ultrasound is performed which shows multiple fluid-filled cysts with thin walls. What is the most common genetic abnormality associated with this diagnosis?

 a Turner's syndrome
 b Alpert's syndrome
 c Klinefelter's syndrome
 d Crouzon syndrome
 e Patau's syndrome

22 A renal ultrasound of a one month old shows a grossly abnormal left kidney with the normal renal architecture replaced by cysts of varying sizes, separated by septae. A nuclear medicine scan shows a non-functioning right kidney. Which is the most likely diagnosis?

 a Autosomal recessive polycystic kidney disease
 b Multicystic dysplastic kidney
 c Multilocular cystic renal tumour
 d Hydronephrosis
 e Nephroblastomatosis

23 A nine-year-old girl presents with severe pain in the left leg following a trivial fall. A radiograph shows an abnormality within the proximal femur. There is a lucent intramedullary lesion with a thinned cortex and an apparent fragment of bone within the inferior part of the lesion. Which of the following is the most likely diagnosis?

 a Simple bone cyst
 b Osteosarcoma
 c Langerhans cell histiocytosis
 d Aneurysmal bone cyst
 e Ewing's sarcoma

24 A three-day-old infant presents with poor feeding and lethargy. He was born at term following prolonged rupture of membranes. A CXR shows bilateral patchy infiltrates and a left-sided pleural effusion. Which of the following is the most likely diagnosis?

a Respiratory distress syndrome

b Group B Streptococcal pneumonia

c Meconium aspiration

d Congenital listeriosis

e Staphylococcal pneumonia

25 You are asked to perform a cranial ultrasound scan on a neonate who was born with poor APGAR scores and made a poor inspiratory effort. On the ultrasound you find multiple irregular foci of calcification throughout the periventricular region, the thalamus and basal ganglia. What is the most likely diagnosis?

a Congenital *Cytomegalovirus* infection

b Tuberous sclerosis

c Congenital toxoplasmosis infection

d Grade IV acute haemorrhage

e Periventricular leukomalacia due to hypoxic injury

26 A neonate presents with progressive respiratory distress. Which of the following plain film findings is suggestive of a tracheo-oesophageal fistula without oesophageal atresia?

a Abdomen distended by bowel gas

b Gasless abdomen

c Nasogastric tube coiled within the pharynx

d Air distended proximal oesophagus

e Displaced trachea

27 A 12-year-old keen footballer presents with left knee pain. There is no history of a specific injury. On examination there is soft-tissue swelling overlying the left knee and generalised tenderness. Plain radiographs of the knee show fragmentation of the tibial tubercle and increased radiodensity of the infra-patellar fat pad. Which of the following is the most likely diagnosis?

a Osgood-Schlatter disease

b Osteomyelitis

c Salter Harris III fracture of the tibia

d Sinding-Larsen Johansson syndrome (jumper's knee)

e Osteochondritis dissecans

28 An infant born at 26 weeks requires intubation and ventilation for respiratory distress. A CXR is performed at eight hours of age. What is the likely appearance of the CXR?

a Left lower lobe consolidation and bilateral pleural effusions

b Hyperinflation with areas of air trapping

c Bilateral patchy ground-glass opacities with air bronchograms

d Bilateral basal atelectasis

e Bilateral patchy consolidation with no evidence of air bronchograms

29 A neonate is on intensive care with high-output cardiac failure. The cardiac ultrasound did not show any intracardiac or great vessel abnormalities. A cranial ultrasound is requested. What is the likely finding?

a Hydrocephalus

b Pseudotumour cerebri

c Primary neonatal brain tumour

d Vein of Galen malformation

e Intracranial haemorrhage

30 A neonate has a full thickness abdominal wall defect on the right side of the umbilical cord. There is no peritoneal covering of the bowel loops. Which of the following abnormalities is associated?

a Ventricular septal defect

b Intestinal atresia

c Imperforate anus

d Trisomy 21

e Beckwith-Wiedemann syndrome

31 A six-year-old with conductive deafness and blue sclerae has a skull radiograph that shows wormian bones and a thin calvarium. Which of the following is the most likely diagnosis?

a Ehlers-Danlos

b Homocystinuria

c Osteogenesis imperfecta

d Hurler's syndrome

32 An 11-year-old girl with recurrent sinusitis and a chronic productive cough has a CXR. This shows bronchial wall thickening and cystic spaces with air-fluid levels. What additional findings would be expected?

a The heart lying in the normal position with the stomach bubble on the right

b The heart and stomach bubble lying in the normal position

c The left ventricle lies on the right and the stomach bubble lies on the left

d The left ventricle lies on the right with the stomach bubble on the right

e The heart is of normal shape but is displaced to the right

33 An ultrasound of a four-year-old with an abdominal mass shows a mixed reflectivity, predominantly solid spherical mass arising from the left kidney. Further imaging in the form of a contrast-enhanced CT shows a well-circumscribed partly cystic mass arising from the left kidney. The mass enhances less than the residual renal parenchyma and does not contain any calcification. What is the most likely diagnosis?

a Neuroblastoma

b Nephrogenic carcinoma

c Nephroblastomatosis

d Wilms' tumour

e Multicystic kidney

34 A radiograph of the thoracolumbar spine shows rounded anterior beaking of the upper lumbar vertebrae. Which additional finding would suggest achondroplasia rather than Hurler's syndrome?

a Thoracolumbar kyphosis

b Posteriorly concave vertebral margin

c Vertebra plana

d Anteriorly concave vertebral margin

e Long slender pedicles

35 A five-year-old has a CT chest following surgery for a structural congenital heart abnormality. The CT shows a right atrial baffle and an anastomosis between the pulmonary artery and the right atrium. There are bilateral pleural effusions. Which of the following procedures has been performed?

a Fontan procedure

b Blalock-Taussig shunt

c Aorticopulmonary window shunt

d Glenn shunt

e Norwood procedure

36 A seven-month-old presents with spasmodic abdominal pain, vomiting and the passage of bloodstained stool. A plain abdominal radiograph shows a soft-tissue mass in the right upper quadrant. What is the most likely diagnosis?

a Appendicitis

b Haemolytic uraemic syndrome

c Volvulus

d Intussusception

e Inflammatory bowel disease

37 A three-year-old presents with polyuria and polydipsia. Serum and urine biochemistry confirm the diagnosis of diabetes insipidus. On examination there is bilateral exophthalmos. A CT brain demonstrates multiple lytic skull lesions with overlying soft-tissue nodules. Which of the following is the most likely diagnosis?

a Hand-Schüller-Christian disease

b Letterer-Siwe disease

c Eosinophilic granuloma

d Neuroblastoma metastases

e Lymphoma

38 A CXR performed for cough in a 10-year-old does not show any abnormality of the lungs. It is reported as having a posterior indentation of the mid-oesophagus. Which of the following is the most likely cause of this appearance?

a Right aortic arch without aberrant vessels

b Right aortic arch with aberrant left subclavian artery

c Double aortic arch

d Left aortic arch with aberrant right subclavian artery

e Left aortic arch without aberrant vessels

39 A five-day-old presents with bilious vomiting. Which of the following findings on barium meal is most commonly associated with the diagnosis of malrotation?

a Duodenojejunal junction over the right pedicle

b Duodenojejunal junction to the left of the spine but low

c Duodenojejunal junction low and in the midline

d Normal position of the duodenum

e Duodenal redundancy to the right of the spine

40 A 12-year-old girl attended the Accident and Emergency Department following a fall from a bicycle. On examination she had some neck tenderness and was noted to have a short neck and a low hairline. Plain cervical spine radiographs were performed. No fracture was identified, but there was apparent fusion of the C2 and C3 vertebral bodies. Which of the following is the most likely diagnosis?

a Turner's syndrome

b Klippel-Feil syndrome

c Sprengel's deformity

d Cleidocranial dysplasia

e Previous fracture at C2/C3

41 A neonate presents with poor feeding. On examination he is found to be cyanotic, with symptoms of congestive heart failure and a systolic murmur. A CXR shows extreme right atrial enlargement and a hypoplastic aorta and pulmonary trunk. Which of the following is the most likely diagnosis?

a Ebstein's anomaly

b Eisenmenger's syndrome

c Transposition of the great arteries

d Patent ductus arteriosus

e Tricuspid atresia

42 A six-week-old infant with a confirmed urinary tract infection presents seriously unwell with septicaemia. Which of the following is the most appropriate investigation according to current NICE guidelines?

a DMSA during the acute infection

b DMSA four to six months after the acute infection

c MCUG with antibiotic cover during infection

d Ultrasound renal tract within six weeks

e MAG 3 renogram to exclude urinary tract obstruction

43 A 13-year-old presenting with abdominal pain is found to have an enlarged liver on examination. An ultrasound shows a solitary well-defined echogenic mass containing a low-reflectivity central scar. A contrast-enhanced CT abdomen is performed. The mass is transiently high attenuation in the arterial phase and low attenuation on portal venous phase. The central scar does not enhance. Which of the following is the most likely diagnosis?

a Hepatoblastoma

b Hepatic metastases

c Fibrolamellar hepatocellular carcinoma

d Undifferentiated embryonal sarcoma

e Haemangioma

44 A 14-year-old keen hurdler presents with left hip pain and tenderness. A plain radiograph of the pelvis shows irregularity of the left anterior inferior iliac spine and an avulsed crescent of bone lateral to this. Which of the following is the most likely underlying cause of this?

a Avulsion of the hamstrings

b Avulsion of the iliopsoas muscle

c Avulsion of the rectus femoris muscle

d Avulsion of the sartorius muscle

e Avulsion of the gluteus medius muscle

45 A five-month-old boy is admitted with difficulty feeding and episodes of unconsciousness. On examination he is cyanosed with a systolic murmur in the pulmonary region. A CXR shows an enlarged right ventricle and pulmonary oligaemia. An echocardiogram is performed. What findings would be expected?

a Large VSD, overriding aorta, right ventricular outflow tract obstruction and right ventricular hypertrophy

b Aorta originating from the right ventricle, pulmonary artery originating from the left ventricle and VSD

c Left atrial dilatation and mitral valve atresia

d Tricuspid atresia and right atrial dilatation

e Pericardial defect

46 A three-day-old baby boy born at 26 weeks develops abdominal distension, bilious vomiting and respiratory distress. Which of the following abdominal radiograph features indicate the greatest degree of severity?

a Portal venous gas

b Pneumatosis intestinalis

c Pneumoperitoneum

d Ascites

e Bowel wall thickening

47 A child has a suspected hip effusion and undergoes ultrasound assessment of the hip. The distance from the joint capsule to the bony femoral neck is measured. If there is no hip effusion, the greatest distance this could be is:

a 1 mm

b 4 mm

c 0.5 mm

d 3 mm

e 1 mm

48 A neonate is found to be in congestive heart failure and has a loud murmur. On CXR there is cardiomegaly with a wide mediastinum. What other abnormality might be seen on the CXR?

a Inferior rib notching

b Superior rib notching

c Forked ribs

d Ribbon ribs

e Wide ribs

49 Which of the following is associated with an increased risk of testicular cancer?

    a No testes within the scrotum in a two-week-old infant born at 26 weeks

    b Congenital monorchia

    c One testis within the scrotum and one between the internal and external inguinal ring in a newborn infant born at 31 weeks

    d Unilateral undescended testis post-orchidopexy in a nine month old

    e Bilateral retractile testes

50 A developmentally normal male child falls and injures his elbow. A plain radiograph of the elbow shows no evidence of a fracture. There is ossification at the radial head, medial epicondyle and capitellum, but not at the lateral epicondyle, olecranon or trochlea. What is the most likely age of the child?

    a 1 year

    b 5 years

    c 7 years

    d 10 years

    e 11 years

51 A seven-month-old child who is crying uncontrollably and vomiting is brought to hospital. On examination he is drowsy with a bulging fontanelle. The child undergoes a CT brain scan that shows a mildly hyperdense mass that enhances homogeneously above the level of background brain. The mass is sitting at the trigone of the left lateral ventricle and is large with a smooth lobulated border with no invasion. There are small foci of calcification within the mass. The left ventricle is dilated. What is the most likely diagnosis?

    a Choroid plexus carcinoma

    b Choroid plexus cyst

    c Choroid plexus papilloma

    d Astrocytoma

    e Glioblastoma multiforme

52 A child presents with chronic cough, shortness of breath, excess sputum production, recurrent chest infections, and haemoptysis. His CXR shows bronchial wall thickening. What other features would you expect to see to confirm your diagnosis?

    a Dilated cystic spaces with air-fluid levels

    b Consolidation

    c Pulmonary infiltrates

    d Soft-tissue mass

    e Pleural effusion

53 A micturating cystourethrogram performed on a child showed reflux into a tortuous ureter with a moderately dilated pelvicalyceal system, blunted forniceal angles and distinct papillary impressions. These findings represent what grade of reflux?

a Grade I vesicoureteric reflux

b Grade II vesicoureteric reflux

c Grade III vesicoureteric reflux

d Grade IV vesicoureteric reflux

e Grade V vesicoureteric reflux

54 A six-year-old is investigated for malaise, weight loss and shortness of breath. A CXR shows multiple, well-defined spherical opacities of varying sizes throughout both lungs. Which of the following is the most likely underlying diagnosis?

a Testicular carcinoma

b Medulloblastoma

c Retinoblastoma

d Rhabdomyosarcoma

e Brainstem glioma

55 A teenage boy suffers from thoracic pain aggravated by exertion. On examination he is found to have a thoracic kyphosis. He is thought to have Scheuermann's disease. Radiographs of the thoracic and lumbar spine are performed. Which of the following would be the most likely findings?

a Multiple vertebral fusion abnormalities

b Loss of anterior vertebral height and Schmorl's nodes

c Loss of posterior vertebral height

d Calcification of the anterior spinal ligament

e Multiple vertebral segmentation abnormalities

56 A full-term male infant was started on phototherapy for presumed physiological jaundice on day three. After two days of phototherapy the bilirubin levels had declined sufficiently for him to be discharged home. He was re-referred by the GP on day 16 and serum liver function tests confirmed obstructive jaundice. Ultrasound showed an enlarged and echogenic liver. What further feature on ultrasound would suggest biliary atresia rather than neonatal hepatitis?

a 'Triangular cord' sign in porta hepatis

b Small gallbladder (1 cm)

c Non-visualisation of the gallbladder

d Decreased visualisation of the peripheral portal veins

e Normal-calibre intrahepatic bile ducts

57 A three-month-old infant has an axial non-enhanced CT brain following a fall. There is a low-density subdural haematoma on one side and a high-density subdural haematoma on the contralateral side. Which of the following is the most likely diagnosis?

a Bleeding diathesis

b Haemorrhagic meningitis

c Accidental trauma

d Non-accidental injury

e Arteriovenous malformation

58 A three-year-old boy is taken to an optician following problems reading. The optician finds the child has a loss of visual acuity and visual fields; he also did not think the boy looked well. He referred the child to the hospital. The paediatrician found the boy to be thin, hyperactive and unusually alert for his age. A CT brain was performed, which showed a mass in the suprasellar region that appeared to be extending into the optic chiasm. This had mixed enhancement with some cystic areas and calcifications. What is the most likely diagnosis?

a Hypothalamic glioma

b Hypothalamic hamartoma

c Craniopharyngioma

d Astrocytoma

e Pituitary adenoma

59 A neonate has a CXR for respiratory distress following a precipitous normal vaginal delivery at term. This shows mild cardiomegaly and mild hyperexpansion but no focal lung abnormality. Which of the following is the most likely underlying diagnosis?

a Respiratory distress syndrome

b Transient tachypnoea of the newborn

c Meconium aspiration

d Group B Streptococcal pneumonia

e Pulmonary haemorrhage

60 A 10-year-old girl presents with a long history of right hip pain. A plain radiograph shows a lucent lesion in the greater trochanter. It has sclerotic margins and contains central irregular calcifications and is associated with a thick periosteal reaction. Which of the following is the most likely diagnosis?

a Enchondroma

b Aneurysmal bone cyst

c Giant cell tumour

d Chondroblastoma

e Chondromyxoid fibroma

61 An abdominal ultrasound performed on a neonate demonstrates multiple calculi within a thin-walled gallbladder. Which of the following is the most likely underlying diagnosis?

   a Hereditary spherocytosis
   b Congenital *Cytomegalovirus*
   c Congenital rubella
   d Hypothyroidism
   e Toxoplasmosis

62 A radiograph of the femur in a 10-year-old shows an ill-defined mixed sclerotic/lytic metaphyseal lesion in the distal femur. There is cortical disruption with a sunburst periosteal reaction and an associated soft-tissue mass containing speckled calcification. Which of the following is the most likely diagnosis?

   a Ewing's sarcoma
   b Osteosarcoma
   c Osteoid osteoma
   d Osteoblastoma
   e Osteochondroma

63 A 12-year-old girl has developed a chesty cough and temperature. Her Emergency Department CXR shows some interstitial infiltrates and multifocal lobar consolidation. Which of the following is the most likely pathogen?

   a Adenovirus
   b *Chlamydia trachomatis*
   c *Bordetella pertussis*
   d RSV
   e *Mycoplasma pneumoniae*

64 A three-year-old girl presents to the paediatricians with headaches and intermittent ataxia. She has an MRI that shows a medulloblastoma. When you review the images what pattern of signal characteristics would you expect to see in the tumour?

   a Hyperintense on T1-weighted images, variable on T2-weighted images and hypointense rim post gadolinium
   b Hyperintense on both T1- and T2-weighted images without enhancement post gadolinium
   c Hypointense on both T1- and T2-weighted images, heterogeneous enhancement post gadolinium
   d Hypointense on T1-weighted images, variable on T2-weighted images, homogeneous enhancement with a hypointense rim post gadolinium
   e Hypointense on T1-weighted images, hyperintense on T2-weighted images, homogeneous enhancement with a hyperintense rim post gadolinium

65 A four-year-old boy presents with a three-week history of intermittent pyrexia. On examination he is miserable and febrile with a widespread salmon-coloured rash, bilaterally enlarged lymph nodes and hepatosplenomegaly. Which of the following is the most likely diagnosis?

a Kawasaki disease

b Stevens-Johnson syndrome

c Still's disease

d Non-Hodgkin's lymphoma

e Henoch-Schönlein purpura

66 A four-year-old girl presents with a three-day history of bloody diarrhoea. On examination she is pale and irritable with dry mucous membranes and a tachycardia. Blood tests reveal a microangiopathic haemolytic anaemia, thrombocytopaenia and acute renal failure. A renal ultrasound demonstrates bilateral slightly enlarged kidneys with hyperechoic cortices. What is the most likely diagnosis?

a Idiopathic thrombocytopaenic purpura

b Gram-negative sepsis

c Haemolytic uraemic syndrome

d Acute lymphoid leukaemia

e Acute glomerulonephritis

67 A CXR of an acyanotic infant shows a straight left heart border and absence of the SVC. What is the likely diagnosis?

a ASD

b VSD

c PDA

d Pulmonary artery stenosis

e Aortic coarctation

68 On a chest radiograph of a child there is noted to be expansion and widening of a number of ribs at the neck. There is increased uptake on bone scintigraphy. What is the most likely diagnosis?

a Fracture due to accidental injury

b Ewing's sarcoma

c Rickets

d Fracture due to non-accidental injury

e Fracture due to Osteogenesis imperfecta

69 A five-year-old girl presented with a history of chronic constipation and faecal soiling. She was otherwise well. On examination there was a palpable retroanal mass. An MRI pelvis showed a spherical, well-defined lesion posterior to the rectum that communicated with the rectum. The lesion was predominantly high signal on T2-weighted images, containing a few foci of low signal, and low signal on T1-weighted images. What is the most likely diagnosis?

   a Rectal duplication cyst
   b Perianal abscess
   c Rectal prolapse
   d Solitary rectal ulcer syndrome
   e Rectal carcinoma

70 A 10-year-old boy is found to have an incidental murmur. His CXR demonstrates a dilated subclavian artery, a dilated descending thoracic aorta, and rib notching. What is the likely diagnosis?

   a ASD
   b VSD
   c PDA
   d Pulmonary artery stenosis
   e Aortic coarctation

Paediatric radiology

PAPER 3

1   A two year old presents with weight loss and fatigue. On examination he has a palpable abdominal mass and bluish nodules on the skin. He undergoes a CT of the abdomen. What are the most likely radiological findings?

   a   Enlarged liver containing multiple low-attenuation lesions
   b   Heterogeneous suprarenal mass containing calcification displacing the left kidney
   c   Well-circumscribed heterogeneous mass arising from the left kidney with a beak of renal tissue extending partially around the mass
   d   Well-circumscribed multi-septated cystic mass replacing the lower pole of the left kidney
   e   Solitary heterogeneous lesion within the right lobe of the liver

2   The paediatric team sees a neonate with respiratory distress, bradycardia and poor swallowing. Following imaging investigation the child was found to have a small posterior fossa and dysgenesis of the hindbrain. The fourth ventricle and hindbrain are displaced caudally and the tonsils and vermis are herniating through the foramen magnum. What further CNS abnormalities may be present?

   a   A funnel-shaped posterior fossa
   b   Klippel-Feil deformity
   c   Basilar impression
   d   Herniation of the cerebellar tonsils
   e   Lumbar myelomeningocele

3 A neonate born at term by emergency Caesarean section for foetal distress is admitted to the neonatal unit. She is below the 0.25th centile and has dysmorphic features and clenched fists with overlapping second and third fingers. Chest radiograph shows a hypoplastic sternum and thin ribs and clavicles. Which of the following is the most likely diagnosis?

a Trisomy 13

b Trisomy 21

c Trisomy 18

d Turner's syndrome

e Cleidocranial dysplasia

4 A full-term infant born by ventouse delivery required resuscitation immediately after birth following a difficult labour. He was admitted onto the neonatal unit for observation and examination the following day revealed a palpable mass in the left lumbar region. Further tests revealed an elevated serum creatinine and haematuria. Ultrasound showed an enlarged left kidney with loss of corticomedullary differentiation. What is the most likely diagnosis?

a Autosomal recessive polycystic kidney disease

b Renal vein thrombosis

c Wilms' tumour

d Glomerulonephritis

e Medullary sponge kidney

5 The CXR of a tachypnoeic term neonate delivered by Caesarean section shows linear densities radiating from the hila, thick fissures and small pleural effusions. What is the most likely diagnosis?

a Transient tachypnoea of the newborn

b Hyaline membrane disease

c Meconium aspiration

d Bronchopulmonary dysplasia

e Pulmonary haemorrhage

6 You are approached by a paediatric registrar who has an externally performed cranial ultrasound report. The ultrasound was performed in a district general hospital prior to the child being transferred to your hospital's neonatal intensive care unit. The report concludes the child has a Grade 3 haemorrhage. What does this mean?

a Intraventricular haemorrhage with ventricular dilatation, 20% mortality

b Intraventricular haemorrhage with ventricular dilatation, 50% mortality

c Intraventricular haemorrhage without ventricular dilatation, 20% mortality

d Intraparenchymal haemorrhage, 70% mortality

e Intraventricular haemorrhage without ventricular dilatation, 10% mortality

7 A seven-year-old girl is above the 99th centile for height with long limbs. She wears glasses to correct her myopia. She undergoes a plain radiograph of the thoracic and lumbar spine. Which of the following findings would suggest a diagnosis of Marfan's syndrome rather than homocystinuria?

a Biconcave vertebrae

b Scoliosis

c Osteoporosis of vertebrae

d Posterior scalloping of vertebral bodies

e Segmentation abnormality

8 A premature infant was born at 32 weeks' gestation requiring intubation at birth and a nasogastric tube to be inserted. A CXR was performed to check the endotracheal tube position. On the CXR you see the nasogastric tube is doubled up within the neck and no air in the gut. What is the likely diagnosis?

a Oesophageal atresia with distal tracheo-oesophageal fistula

b Pyloric stenosis

c Oesophageal atresia without tracheo-oesophageal fistula

d Laryngeal web

e Duodenal atresia

9 A previously well 15-year-old girl presents with a three-hour history of abdominal pain. On examination she has low-grade pyrexia and is diffusely tender over the right lower quadrant. An abdominal ultrasound shows an unremarkable upper abdomen. Within the right lower quadrant there are enlarged mesenteric lymph nodes, prominent pericaecal fat and a focal collection of fluid. What is the most likely diagnosis?

a Meckel's diverticulitis

b Crohn's disease

c Pelvic inflammatory disease

d Appendicitis

e Infectious enteritis

10 A hip ultrasound is performed on a three-month-old infant with suspected developmental dysplasia of the hips. The alpha angle is measured. Which of the following would be the expected alpha angle if the hip were dislocated?

a 77 degrees

b 60 degrees

c 55 degrees

d 45 degrees

e 41 degrees

11 A seven-year-old boy with developmental delay is being investigated for myoclonic seizures, which appear to be reducing in frequency. On examination he has a facial angiofibroma. A CT brain is performed, which shows multiple areas of cortical abnormality with a hypodense centre, broadened gyri and curved linear calcifications. Which other intracranial abnormality may be seen?

a Giant cell astrocytoma

b Hydrocephalus

c Arteriovenous malformations

d Neuroblastoma

e Venous angiomas

12 A four-year-old girl is referred by her GP with a six-month history of persistent cough and wheeze despite being treated for several chest infections. She has a CXR, which reveals a cystic mediastinal mass, with widening of the carina and mild narrowing of the proximal aspect of both left and right main bronchi. The lung volumes are normal. What is the most likely diagnosis?

a Lymphoma

b Hiatus hernia

c Tracheo-oesophageal fistula

d Pericardiac tumour

e Bronchogenic cyst

13 A nine-year-old boy presents with colicky right upper quadrant pain and weight loss. He has a long history of intermittent obstructive jaundice and an intermittent palpable mass in the right upper quadrant. He undergoes an abdominal ultrasound. Which of the following are the most likely radiological findings?

a Thickened gallbladder wall with intramural gas and no evidence of gallstones

b Thickened and striated gallbladder wall containing multiple calculi

c Dilated common bile duct and brightly echogenic portal triads

d Complex collection surrounding the gallbladder

e Fusiform cyst beneath the porta hepatis, separate from the gallbladder

14 A 12-year-old obese boy presents with hip pain. It is thought that his capital epiphysis has slipped in relation to the femoral neck. A frontal radiograph is taken and a line is drawn along the superior edge of the femoral neck. In relation to the capital epiphysis the line is most likely to be:

a Superior and lateral

b Superior and medial

c Inferior and lateral

d Inferior and medial

e Crossing it

15 A neonate presents with feeding difficulties. On examination he is moderately cyanosed, becoming more so when crying, with evidence of congestive heart failure and a systolic murmur. The CXR shows an enlarged heart with a widened mediastinum and pulmonary plethora. Which of the following is the most likely diagnosis?

a Tetralogy of Fallot

b Tricuspid atresia

c Truncus arteriosus

d Patent ductus arteriosus

e Hypoplastic left heart

16 A six-year-old girl is investigated for having pubic and axillary hair. She undergoes an abdominal ultrasound as part of her work-up. This shows a 2-cm well-circumscribed mass arising from the left adrenal gland. It is hypoechoic to the kidney and does not contain any calcification. Which of the following is the most likely diagnosis?

a Phaeochromocytoma

b Neuroblastoma

c Adrenal haemorrhage

d Adrenocortical carcinoma

e Adrenal metastasis

17 A six-year-old girl falls and suffers a hyperextension injury of the elbow. A plain radiograph of the elbow shows elevation of the anterior and posterior fat pads. What is the most likely underlying injury?

a Avulsion of the medial epicondyle

b Fracture between the lateral condyle and trochlea

c Fracture through the capitellum

d Supracondylar fracture

e Transverse radial neck fracture

18 A mother brings her two-week-old baby to the GP surgery complaining that she is looking blue. The GP immediately refers the mother and baby to the paediatrician who examines the child and requests a CXR, which reveals right heart enlargement, an absent pulmonary trunk, and an ascending aorta with convexity to the right. What is the most likely diagnosis?

a Tetralogy of Fallot

b Pulmonary ductus arteriosus

c VSD

d Coarctation of aorta

e Transposition of great arteries

19 A patient with known Dandy-Walker malformation presents with seizures and is investigated with a CT scan of the brain. This demonstrates the large posterior fossa cyst expected in Dandy-Walker malformation, but also a high and enlarged third ventricle with parallel lateral ventricles. The anterior horns of the ventricles are small in comparison to the posterior horns. What other abnormality is represented on this scan?

a Prominent cavum vergae

b Hydrocephalus

c Holoprosencephaly

d Arachnoid cyst in the midline

e Agenesis of the corpus callosum

20 A five-month-old boy is treated for a proven urinary tract infection. He does not respond well to suitable antibiotics within 48 hours and becomes septic. Which of the following would be appropriate imaging follow-up?

a Ultrasound during the acute infection, DMSA four to six months after the acute infection and MCUG

b Ultrasound during the acute infection, DMSA four to six months after the acute infection, no MCUG

c Ultrasound within six weeks of the acute infection, DMSA four to six months after the acute infection, no MCUG

d Ultrasound within six weeks of the acute infection, no DMSA or MCUG

e Ultrasound and DMSA within six weeks of the acute infection

21 A 12-year-old boy presents with a three-month history of a painful knee, which clicks and locks. A PA radiograph of the knee shows a linear lucency separating a fragment of bone from the lateral aspect of the medial femoral condyle. MR shows the fragment to be of intermediate signal on all sequences. On T2-weighted imaging a rim of high signal separates this from the condyle. Which of the following is the most likely diagnosis?

a Spontaneous osteonecrosis

b Osteochondritis dissecans

c Blount disease

d Acute osteochondral fracture

e Osteogenesis imperfecta

22 A five-year-old girl complains of shortness of breath and on CXR is found to have an enlarged cardiac silhouette with discrete calcific densities. Ultrasound reveals a pericardial complex cystic mass containing calcific foci and a pericardial effusion. What are the calcific foci most likely to be?

a Bone

b Teeth

c Stones

d Foreign bodies

e Calcified pericardial cyst

23 A 10-year-old boy presents with a history of severe left-sided testicular pain lasting for 48 hours. On examination the left testis is swollen and exquisitely tender. The urinalysis is negative. He undergoes a scrotal ultrasound. Which of the following are the most likely radiological findings?

a Enlarged hyperechoic left testis with increased peritesticular flow and absent parenchymal flow

b Small atrophied left testis with absent peritesticular and parenchymal flow

c Normal-sized hypoechoic left testis with absent peritesticular and parenchymal flow

d Enlarged hypoechoic left testis with normal parenchymal flow

e Normal-sized hyperechoic left testis with increased peritesticular and parenchymal flow

24 A five-year-old girl is systemically unwell with left leg pain and a limp. On examination she is exquisitely tender over the left femur. *Staphylococcus aureus* is grown from her blood cultures. A plain radiograph of the left leg confirms the diagnosis of osteomyelitis. Where is the abnormality likely to be?

a Femoral metaphysis

b Femoral epiphysis

c Femoral diaphysis

d Distal femoral physis

e Multicentric involvement

25 A two-year-old boy presents with a one-week history of fever, vomiting and conjunctivitis. On examination he is found to have a red tongue, a rash on both elbows and bilateral non-purulent conjunctivitis. Which of the following is the most likely diagnosis?

a Takayasu's arteritis

b Polyarteritis nodosa

c Kawasaki syndrome

d Stevens-Johnson syndrome

e Henoch-Schönlein purpura

26 A two-year-old child is under investigation for delayed walking and wide-based gait. Their speech is difficult to understand. There is a history of recurrent chest infections. A CT brain is performed, which demonstrates cerebellar cortical atrophy and dilatation of the fourth ventricle. There is also a cerebral infarct. What is the most likely diagnosis?

   a Friedreich's ataxia

   b Ataxia telangiectasia

   c Multiple sclerosis

   d Wolman disease

   e Niemann-Pick disease

27 An abdominal radiograph on a two-year-old child shows a paucity of bowel gas. An abdominal ultrasound is then performed which shows a 5 cm × 2 cm mass in the right upper quadrant. In the longitudinal plane, this has a 'pseudokidney' appearance with a central echogenic focus and in the transverse plane it has the appearance of a 'bull's-eye'. What is the most likely diagnosis?

   a Ischaemic colitis

   b Intussusception

   c Volvulus

   d Necrotising enterocolitis

   e Appendicitis

28 A skull radiograph of a one-year-old infant demonstrates a diastatic fracture. The paediatricians suspect non-accidental injury. There are no neurological signs on examination. What should the next investigation be?

   a CT head with intravenous contrast

   b CT head without intravenous contrast

   c MRI brain

   d Radioisotope scintigraphy

   e Transfontanellar cranial ultrasound

29 A two-year-old with previous urinary tract infections is investigated by ultrasound and DMSA. The ultrasound shows possible duplex systems but normal-sized kidneys and no obvious scarring. How will the DMSA study aid the investigation?

   a Differential function can be measured

   b Obstruction can be demonstrated on dynamic images

   c Reflux can be assessed without the need for invasive tests

   d GFR can be performed based on the post DMSA blood results

   e Horseshoe kidney can be excluded

30 A five-year-old girl presents with colicky abdominal pain and a purpuric rash on her legs and the extensor surface of her arms. Urinalysis reveals haematuria and proteinuria. An abdominal ultrasound shows enlarged slightly hyperechoic kidneys and areas of bowel wall thickening in the terminal ileum. What is the most likely diagnosis?
   a Haemolytic uraemia syndrome
   b Henoch-Schönlein purpura
   c Crohn's disease
   d Eosinophilic gastroenteritis
   e Coeliac disease

31 A six-year-old child presents with a two-month history of anterior thigh pain and a limp. Radiographs of the hips demonstrate femoral head fragmentation, subchondral fracture and femoral neck cysts. Radionucleotide bone scan demonstrates increased tracer uptake in the femoral head. What is the most likely cause?
   a Developmental dysplasia of the hip
   b Late-phase Perthes disease
   c Early-phase Perthes disease
   d Moderate slipped capital femoral epiphysis
   e Severe slipped capital femoral epiphysis

32 A 16-month-old girl presented with an enlarging head circumference and bulging occiput. She was noted to have poor fine motor control. An MRI of the head was performed, which showed a large uniformly low signal cystic area in the posterior fossa on T1-weighted images and an elevated tentorium cerebelli. On axial images the cerebellar hemispheres appeared widely spaced. What is the most likely diagnosis?
   a Dandy-Walker malformation
   b Large arachnoid cyst
   c Cystic cerebellar astrocytoma
   d Epidermoid cyst
   e Haemangioblastoma

33 A two-year-old boy is brought in with a sudden onset of cough. On CXR there is a radio-opaque midline opacity and atelectasis. Which of the following additional features are you most likely to see?
   a Consolidation
   b Cardiomegaly
   c Pneumothorax
   d Pulmonary infiltrates
   e Air trapping and hyperinflation

34 A nine-year-old undergoes a Tc-99m pertechnetate scan for possible Meckel's diverticulum. Which of the following would give a false negative result?

a Urinary obstruction

b Inflammatory bowel disease

c Malrotation of the ileum

d Haemangioma

e Intussusception

35 A 12-year-old boy presents with long-standing left knee pain with no history of trauma. A plain radiograph shows a lucent lesion within the metaphysis of the proximal tibia. This has a well-defined sclerotic margin and contains trabeculations. There is no associated periosteal reaction. Which of the following is the most likely diagnosis?

a Enchondroma

b Chondromyxoid fibroma

c Simple bone cyst

d Non-ossifying fibroma

e Fibrous dysplasia

36 An 11-year-old boy presents with abdominal pain, nausea and vomiting and has an inhaler for a chronic cough. His CXR reveals gas-filled loops of bowel in the centre of his chest. What is the likely diagnosis?

a Bochdalek hernia

b Morgagni hernia

c Septum transversum defect

d Hiatal hernia

e Eventration

37 A 10-year-old boy presents with a mass in the posterior triangle of the neck, night sweats and significant weight loss. The mass is biopsied under ultrasound guidance and found to be Hodgkin's lymphoma. A staging CT shows abnormal lymph nodes within the right axilla and left cervical chain. Which of the following would be the appropriate staging?

a Stage 1A

b Stage 2A

c Stage 2B

d Stage 3A

e Stage 3B

38 A 15-year-old girl complaining of long-standing right-sided chest pain has a CXR. This shows a right-sided pleural effusion and an abnormality of the sixth right anterior rib. There is a 4-cm ill-defined lytic lesion within the rib associated with a very large inhomogeneous soft-tissue mass. Which of the following is the most likely diagnosis?

a Fibrous dysplasia

b Enchondroma

c Ewing's sarcoma

d Haematopoiesis

e Aneurysmal bone cyst

39 A six-year-old child presented with loss of vision, nausea and vomiting. On examination there was papilloedema and an ataxic gait. A brain MRI was performed, which did not show any abnormality on T1-weighted images, but revealed a well-circumscribed hyperintense lesion with a rim of low signal, containing multiple cysts on T2-weighted images. Which of the following is the most likely diagnosis?

a Schwannoma

b Pilocytic astrocytoma

c Primitive neuroectodermal tumour (PNET)

d Medulloblastoma

e Ependymoma

40 The newborn daughter of a diabetic mother is noted to have nasal flaring and expiratory grunting. The CXR shows complete lung white out. What is the likely diagnosis?

a Respiratory distress syndrome

b Neonatal pneumonia

c Unilateral pulmonary agenesis

d Cystic fibrosis

e Persistent foetal circulation syndrome

41 A three-month-old girl undergoes a renal ultrasound for a urinary tract infection. This demonstrates a horseshoe kidney. Her parents mention that she was born with very puffy hands and feet, which has now resolved. Which of the following is the most likely underlying diagnosis?

a VACTERL (syndrome of vertebral, anal, cardiac, tracheo-oesophageal fistula/oesophageal atresia, renal and limb abnormalities)

b Turner's syndrome

c Prader-Willi syndrome

d Noonan's syndrome

e Edward's syndrome

42 A 15-year-old boy presents with a two-month history of dull thoracic back pain that is worse at night. On examination there is a scoliosis concave to the right. A radiograph of the thoraco-lumbar spine confirms the scoliosis and shows a lucent lesion originating in the spinous process of T8 extending into the T8 vertebral body. Which of the following is the most likely diagnosis?

a Osteoblastoma

b Osteochondroma

c Osteoid osteoma

d Haemangioma

e Fibrous dysplasia

43 A four-year-old girl presents with a fractured radius. The history given is inconsistent with the injury and non-accidental injury is suspected. A skeletal survey is carried out. No further fractures are demonstrated. Which would be the next most appropriate investigation?

a MRI brain

b Scintigraphy

c None

d Ultrasound abdomen

e Repeat skeletal survey in one to two months

44 A four-month-old boy presents with cough and difficulty feeding. On examination he is in respiratory distress with nasal flaring and subchondral recession and there is widespread wheeze. A CXR shows hyperexpansion and prominent hila with no focal parenchymal abnormality. Which of the following is the most likely diagnosis?

a Respiratory syncytial virus bronchiolitis

b Streptococcal pneumonia

c Varicella pneumonitis

d *Haemophilus* pneumonia

e Croup

45 An otherwise well three-year-old child of Caribbean origin has lower limb bowing bilaterally. Radiographs demonstrate tibia vara. There is beaking and irregularity of the tibial proximal medial metaphysis. What is the most likely diagnosis?

a Rickets

b Osteogenisis imperfecta

c Osgood-Schlatter disease

d Physiological bowing

e Blount disease

46 A six-year-old girl presented with jaundice and malaise. Examination showed evidence of portal hypertension and a dark ring around the iris of both eyes. An ultrasound demonstrated a small nodular liver with an irregular capsule but no focal lesions. Further imaging in the form of a CT abdomen was performed and the liver was found to be of normal attenuation. Which of the following is the most likely diagnosis?

a Cystic fibrosis

b Galactosaemia

c Wilson's disease

d Haemochromatosis

e Alpha-1 antitrypsin deficiency

47 A CXR of a newborn is shown to have an indistinct right heart border with opacification in this area. A few days later the CXR shows a well-defined lucency in the right hemithorax with displacement of the mediastinum to the left, widened rib interspaces, and an intact right hemidiaphragm. What is the most likely diagnosis?

a Venolobar syndrome

b Sequestration

c Congenital lobar emphysema

d Cystic adenomatoid malformation

e Lymphangiectasia

48 A 14-year-old girl is referred to the orthopaedic clinic with scoliosis. AP radiographs of the spine are taken. Two lines are drawn and the Cobb angle is measured between them to confirm the diagnosis. Where should the lines be drawn to correctly measure the Cobb angle?

a From the centre of the apical vertebra to the centre of the superior end vertebra and from the centre of the apical vertebra to the centre of the inferior end vertebra

b Tangential to the superior end plate of the apical vertebra and tangential to the inferior endplate of the apical vertebra

c Tangential to the inferior end plate of the superior end vertebra and tangential to the superior end plate of the inferior end vertebra

d Tangential to the superior end plate of the superior end vertebra and tangential to the inferior end plate of the inferior end vertebra

e From the centre of the apical vertebra to the superior end plate of the superior end vertebra and from the centre of the apical vertebra to the inferior end plate of inferior end vertebra

49 A five-year-old girl presented with acute severe left upper quadrant pain. On examination she was found to have a massively enlarged spleen. Blood tests revealed low haemoglobin, low platelets and high reticulocytes. An ultrasound of the abdomen was performed that confirmed an enlarged spleen and showed multiple hypoechoic lesions at the periphery of the spleen. Which of the following is the most likely diagnosis?

a Acute splenic sequestration crisis

b Autosplenectomy

c Idiopathic thrombocytopaenic purpura

d Thalassaemia

e Acute lymphoid leukaemia

50 A nine-year-old girl presents with a two-month history of right knee swelling and morning stiffness with no definite history of trauma. On examination she is afebrile and the knee is swollen and tender with a reduced range of movement. She is thought to have juvenile rheumatoid arthritis. A knee radiograph is performed. Which of the following are the likely findings?

a Soft-tissue swelling and transverse metaphyseal bands

b Osteosclerosis and small epiphyses

c Soft tissue swelling, juxta-articular osteopenia and periosteal reaction

d Retarded bone growth and transverse metaphyseal bands

e Soft-tissue swelling and osteosclerosis

51 An MRI brain was performed on a toddler who had failed to attain gross motor skills after initially achieving them on time. It was also noted that the child's head circumference was increasing faster than expected. The child's medical history and birth record were unremarkable. The MRI showed communicating hydrocephalus. What is the most likely underlying cause?

a Medulloblastoma

b Subdural haematoma

c Meningitis

d Venous obstruction

e Repetitive subarachnoid microhaemorrhage

52 A young boy with tracheal stenosis undergoes a CT of his chest. He is found to have a tracheal bronchus. What findings would you expect to see?

a Right upper lobe apical segmental bronchus originates from the trachea rather than the right upper lobe bronchus

b Left upper lobe apical segment originates from the trachea rather than the left upper lobe bronchus

c Right lower lobe apical segment bronchus originates from the trachea rather than the right lower lobe bronchus

d Left lower lobe apical segment bronchus originates from the trachea rather than the left lower lobe bronchus

e Right upper lobe anterior segmental bronchus originates from the trachea rather than the right upper lobe bronchus

53 A 10 month old with known neurofibromatosis type I has a plain radiograph of the tibia and fibula. Which of the following is the most likely finding?

a Anterolateral bowing of the tibia

b Elongated tibia in relation to the fibula

c Multiple lytic lesions within the medulla of the tibia

d Expanded medullary cavity of the tibia

e Posterior bowing of the fibula

54 Radiographs of both legs are performed on a neonate. They demonstrate diffuse demineralisation, multiple fractures with pseudoarthrosis and bowing deformity. There is exuberant callus formation. The baby is noted to have blue sclerae. What is the likely diagnosis?

a Non-accidental injury

b Osteogenesis imperfecta

c Osteomalacia

d Pyknodystosis

e Rickets

55 A three-year-old girl is brought into hospital with vomiting, having swallowed household cleaning fluid. Her CXR at 10 hours is normal. How should this be interpreted?

a She is likely to have aspirated but the findings have not yet appeared on CXR

b She is likely to have aspirated but the findings have resolved

c She is unlikely to have aspirated

d The CXR is most likely to be inadequate

e She can be discharged home

56 A three-year-old boy presents with an acute onset of generalised abdominal pain. On examination he is jaundiced with tender hepatomegaly and ascites and is diagnosed as being in acute hepatic failure. A contrast-enhanced CT scan reveals an enlarged liver with increased enhancement of the caudate lobe and patchy enhancement of the other hepatic segments. Non-enhancing thrombus is seen within the hepatic veins. Ascites and gallbladder wall oedema are present. Which of the following is the most likely diagnosis?

a Hepatocellular carcinoma

b Hepatoblastoma

c Budd-Chiari syndrome

d Hepatic veno-occlusive disease

e Wilson's disease

57 A 14-year-old boy presented with history of aching leg pain for a few months that was more severe at night and relieved by non-steroidal anti-inflammatory drugs. A lateral radiograph of his leg showed a <1 cm lucent nidus surrounded by dense sclerosis within the diaphysis of the tibia and an osteoid osteoma is suspected. A CT is planned for further evaluation. What are the expected findings on the CT scan?

a A well-demarcated low-attenuation lesion a few millimetres in size, surrounded by an area of high attenuation

b A localised low-attenuation lesion, which does not enhance with contrast with surrounding high attenuation and a small channel to the surrounding soft tissues

c Well-demarcated low-attenuation area of 2.5 cm in size, surrounded by an area of high attenuation

d A high-attenuation lesion with no area of low attenuation

e A linear high-attenuation lesion

58 A CT chest is performed on a six year old. An incidental soft-tissue mass is seen in the middle mediastinum. Which of the following is it most likely to represent?

a Neurogenic tumour

b Great vessel aneurysm

c Thymoma

d Lateral meningocele

e Teratoma

59 A six-year-old boy attends for a scrotal ultrasound following the discovery of a seemingly painless lump in his left testis. As he is undressed for the ultrasound he is noted to have bilateral gynaecomastia. The ultrasound reveals a normal-looking right testis and a well-defined hypoechoic mass within the left testis. Which of the following is the most likely diagnosis?

a Gonadoblastoma

b Seminoma

c Yolk sac carcinoma

d Orchitis

e Leydig cell tumour

60 A 16-year-old girl is having a third CT scan of her chest, which reveals dilated and beaded bronchi, bronchial wall thickening, and peripheral bronchial mucous plugging. There is also hyperinflation and hilar enlargement, which has progressed since the previous scan. What is the most likely diagnosis?

a Bronchiectasis

b Cystic fibrosis

c Swyer-James syndrome

d Juvenile rheumatoid arthritis

e Systemic lupus erythematosus

61 A three-week-old boy has an abdominal ultrasound, which shows a hyper-peristaltic stomach with a thickened and elongated pylorus measuring 5 mm in thickness and 25 mm in length. Which of the following is the most likely diagnosis?

a Pylorospasm

b Pyloric stenosis

c Gastric volvulus

d Gastro-oesophageal reflux

e Microgastria

62 A two year old with pneumonia is not improving with antibiotics. CXR shows hyperinflation and patchy infiltrates. What is the likely diagnosis?

a *Chlamydia*

b *Streptococcus pneumoniae*

c *Pneumocystis carinii*

d RSV

e Adenovirus

63 A one month old with bilious vomiting has an abdominal radiograph that shows a dilated stomach and duodenum with only a trace of gas distally. Which of the following is the most likely diagnosis?

a Duodenal duplication cyst

b Intussusception

c Midgut malrotation

d Gastric volvulus

e Duodenal atresia

64 A seven-year-old boy presents with visual field defects. He is felt to be small for his age, taking into account the heights of his parents. A plain skull radio-graph is performed, which shows marked destruction of the sella containing curvilinear calcifications. What is the most likely diagnosis?

a Epidermoid

b Rathke's cleft cyst

c Pituitary adenoma

d Teratoma

e Craniopharyngioma

65 A CXR is taken of a child two days after surfactant replacement therapy for hyaline membrane disease. The findings include left-sided cardiac enlarge-ment, an enlarged aorta, and pulmonary oedema. How can these findings be explained?

a ASD

b VSD

c PDA

d Pulmonary artery stenosis

e Aortic coarctation

66 A three-day-old neonate born at 34 weeks' gestation shows signs of septic shock with abdominal distension and bilious nasogastric aspirates. Plain abdominal radiograph shows dilated loops of bowel and intramural gas. Which of the following is the most likely diagnosis?

a Hirschsprung disease

b Midgut volvulus

c Necrotising enterocolitis

d Intussusception

e Duplication cyst

67 A 15-year-old boy has a small, deformed right chest wall. The CXR demonstrates that the soft tissues over the right hemithorax are thinned. On CT there is an absence of the right-sided pectoral muscles. What is the most likely diagnosis?

a Askin tumour

b Poland syndrome

c Pectus excavatum

d Pectus carinatum

e Muscular dystrophy

68 A 14-day-old boy is admitted with prolonged jaundice and poor feeding. On examination he is hypotonic with cool, mottled skin, abdominal distension and an umbilical hernia. Serum biochemistry reveals a low T4 and an elevated TSH. Which of the following is the most likely ultrasound appearance?

a No thyroid tissue seen

b Ectopic thyroid tissue seen in the suprahyoid position

c Enlarged echogenic thyroid

d Solitary low reflectivity nodule within the thyroid

e Multiple low reflectivity nodules within an enlarged thyroid

69 A baby has a chest radiograph that shows 11 pairs of ribs and a hypersegmented manubrium. Which of the following is the most likely diagnosis?

a Cleidocranial dysplasia

b Campomelic dysplasia

c No further underlying abnormality

d Down's syndrome

e VACTERL syndrome

70 A six-year-old girl presents with a history of weight loss, malaise and intermittent jaundice. An abdominal ultrasound reveals a heterogeneous, low reflectivity soft-tissue mass with high Doppler flow in the porta hepatis and both intra-hepatic and extra-hepatic duct dilatation. Which of the following is the most likely diagnosis?

a Gallbladder carcinoma

b Cholangiocarcinoma

c Caroli's disease

d Rhabdomyosarcoma of the biliary tract

e Choledochal cyst

Neuroradiology, head and neck and ENT radiology

PAPER 1

1 An orthopantomogram (OPG) was requested following trauma. No fractures are visible on the film, but there is loss of the lamina dura and a well-defined expansile lytic lesion affecting the ramus of the mandible. This lesion has a narrow zone of transition and no associated soft-tissue mass. The bones are diffusely osteopaenic. What is the most appropriate investigation?

   a CT scan
   b Biopsy of the mass
   c ESR
   d PTH level
   e Calcium level

2 A five-month-old baby girl was being investigated for blindness. On CT both her globes were elongated with a cone-shaped deformity affecting the posterior globe, which involved the optic nerve. The defect passed inferiorly and communicated with vitreous. The girl had cardiac abnormalities and choanal atresia. What is the eye abnormality?

   a Coloboma
   b Congenital glaucoma
   c Rubella retinitis
   d Trauma
   e Orbital haematoma

3   A six-month-old child has bilateral leukocoria. On CT there were bilateral solid smooth lobulated hyperdense lesions with nodular calcification within both orbits. The tumours were in the posterolateral region and were indistinguishable from the wall of the globe. The globes were both of normal size. What other abnormality should be looked for on CT?

   a   Cortical tubers
   b   Subependymal heterotopia
   c   Pineoblastoma
   d   Persistent hyperplastic primary vitreous
   e   Coat's disease

4   A CT head on a 60-year-old male demonstrated bilateral small calcific densities overlying the junction of the retina and optic nerve. The intraconal portion of the optic nerve appeared normal. No other abnormalities were seen on CT. What is the most likely diagnosis?

   a   Retinoblastoma
   b   Drusen
   c   Coat's disease
   d   Bilateral optic gliomas
   e   Choroidal osteoma

5   A newborn child is noted to have leukocoria. A CT was performed. What feature makes persistent hyperplastic primary vitreous more likely than retinoblastoma?

   a   A calcified intra-orbital mass
   b   Microphthalmia
   c   A diffuse infiltrating mass
   d   Moderately high signal on T1
   e   Bony destruction

6   A 45-year-old male complained of worsening vision. On cross-sectional imaging the left optic nerve appeared thickened. What feature makes optic glioma more likely than optic nerve sheath meningioma?

   a   A unilateral mass
   b   Hyperostosis affecting the optic canal
   c   Diffuse homogeneous enhancement
   d   Calcification
   e   Kinking and buckling of the optic nerve

7   A 55-year-old gentleman was investigated for sudden onset visual loss affecting the right temporal region. Ultrasound of the globe demonstrated right-sided retinal detachment with an associated well-defined flat echogenic mass was seen. An uveal melanoma was suspected and a MRI scan performed. What are the likely signal characteristics of the lesion?

a High signal on both T1- and T2-weighted imaging

b High signal on T1-weighted imaging and intermediate on T2

c High signal on T1-weighted imaging and intermediate on T2

d High signal on T1-weighted imaging and intermediate on T2

e Low signal on both T1- and T2-weighted imaging

8 A seven-year-old was referred from the maxillofacial surgeons for assessment of facial asymmetry. X-rays revealed expansion of the right maxilla and frontal bone with a featureless 'ground-glass' appearance. He was also known to have multiple café au lait spots. What other feature occurs commonly with this condition?

a Osteosarcoma

b Precocious puberty

c En plaque meningioma

d Dentigerous cysts

e Brown tumours

9 A 17-year-old male patient with recurrent left-sided epistaxis and associated mucopurulent discharge was investigated urgently in ENT outpatients. He underwent a CT scan which revealed a unilateral, low-attenuation mass filling the left maxillary sinus with extension into an expanded nasal cavity and middle meatus. A subsequent MRI also showed the mass, which appeared bright on T2-weighted images and displayed peripheral enhancement following IV gadolinium. What is the most likely diagnosis?

a Juvenile angiofibroma

b Mucocele of the maxillary sinus

c Nasopharyngeal carcinoma

d Antrochoanal polyp

e Inverted papilloma

10 A five-year-old boy presented with hearing loss. An intact, dry tympanic membrane was visualised and audiology confirmed a conductive hearing loss. A CT was performed which revealed a lesion medial to and eroding the ossicular chain which fills the oval window niche and does not enhance following contrast. An MRI confirmed the lesion was low intensity on T1 and high signal intensity on T2-weighted images. What is the most likely diagnosis?

a Acquired cholesteatoma

b Glomus tympanicum

c Cholesterol granuloma

d High jugular bulb

e Congenital cholesteatoma

11 A 15-year-old girl complained of a six-month history of left-sided unilateral tinnitus. A pulsatile mass was visible in the ipsilateral middle ear. A high-resolution CT scan of the temporal bone showed an absent foramen spinosum with the internal carotid artery following an aberrant course laterally in the middle ear on this side. A carotid angiogram revealed a vascular structure arising from the aberrant carotid artery terminating in the middle meningeal artery. What is the most likely diagnosis?

a Persistent stapedial artery

b Glomus jugulare tumour

c High jugular bulb

d Middle ear paraganglioma

e Glomus tympanicum

12 A 65-year-old man attended the ENT outpatients complaining of a one-year history of unilateral tinnitus and vertigo. Audiology confirmed a unilateral sensorineural hearing loss on the affected side. An MRI scan demonstrated a mass that was thought to be an acoustic neuroma. What signal characteristics are most likely?

a Hyperintense on T1-weighted images

b Enhancement following gadolinium

c No enhancement following gadolinium

d Hypointense on T2-weighted images

e Isointense to grey matter on T2-weighted images

13 A patient with post-nasal drip and a 'persistent foul taste in the back of the mouth' was diagnosed as having a Tornwaldt's cyst. What was the likely appearance on imaging?

a Low signal intensity on T1-weighted images

b High signal intensity on T2-weighted images

c Low signal intensity on post gadolinium T1-weighted images

d Low signal intensity on T2-weighted images

e Very low attenuation on CT

14 A patient presents to the ophthalmologist with proptosis and bossing of the forehead. A CT scan shows complete opacification of the frontal sinus with bony expansion and remodelling. On MRI there is opacification of the frontal sinus with peripheral rim enhancement. What is the most likely diagnosis?

a Mucous retention cyst

b Frontal sinus mucocele

c Inverted papilloma

d Sinusitis

e Frontal sinus squamous cell carcinoma

15 An elderly diabetic patient presented to his GP with severe right ear pain out of keeping with the visible findings of an erythematous external auditory canal with some granulation tissue. A CT scan was performed and an abnormal soft-tissue mass was visualised in the eternal auditory canal. He was subsequently diagnosed with malignant otitis externa. Which of the following is the most appropriate?

a On MRI the granulation tissue would be expected to be low intensity on both T1- and T2-weighted images

b CT is the imaging modality of choice to assess skull base involvement

c The radiological appearances are usually contemporaneous with the clinical findings

d SPECT is ineffective in monitoring for disease progression and post-therapeutic recurrence

e Sclerosis of the mastoid and temporal bones is a characteristic feature of malignant otitis externa on CT

16 A 65-year-old smoker presents with hoarseness and investigations demonstrate a laryngeal carcinoma. A lymph node metastasis is identified in a cervical node lying anteriorly to sternocleidomastoid and above the hyoid bone. What anatomical classification is appropriate?

a Level I

b Level II

c Level III

d Level IV

e Level V

17 A 48-year-old man presents with a hard mass in the parotid gland. CT and MRI were performed and as a result of the radiological appearances a differential of mucoepidermoid carcinoma and adenoid cystic carcinoma was postulated. What characteristic radiological feature do they both exhibit?

a Ground-glass appearance on CT

b Hyperintense signal on both T1- and T2-weighted images

c Signet ring enhancement post contrast

d Honeycombing on CT

e Perineural extension

18 A 20-year-old man presented via the Emergency Department following a suspected punch directed low on the maxillary alveolar rim in a downward direction. Examination findings included facial oedema and mobility of the hard palate. Facial view X-rays revealed a fracture line extending from the nasal septum to the lateral pyriform rims, running horizontally above the teeth apices, crossing below the zygomaticomaxillary junction and traversing the pterygomaxillary junction to interrupt the pterygoid plates. What is the most likely diagnosis?

a Le Fort I

b Le Fort II

c Le Fort III

d Orbital blow out fracture

e Tripod fracture

19 A six-month-old child was admitted with lethargy, fever and dysphagia. A lateral neck plain film demonstrated thickening of the retropharyngeal soft tissue with smooth bowing of the anterior border. On CT there was extensive prevertebral soft-tissue swelling with fat streaking and a 2-cm peripherally enhancing low-density mass medial to the carotid artery. What is the most likely pathogen?

a *Haemophilus influenzae*

b *Staphylococcus aureus*

c *Pseudomonas aeruginosa*

d *Escherichia coli*

e Herpes simplex virus

20 A 55-year-old female presents with a right-sided facial weakness, hyperacusis, loss of lacrimation and taste. What pathology is most likely to cause this pattern of clinical findings?

a Facial nerve schwannoma

b Acoustic neuroma

c Brain stem glioma

d Parotid malignancy

e Malignant otitis media

21 A 60-year-old lady presented complaining of a hoarse voice and signs of a vocal cord palsy associated with lower cranial nerve palsies affecting cranial nerves IX, X and XI. CT demonstrated a large extra axial soft-tissue mass with calcification and a dural tail entering the jugular foramen. What further imaging features would you expect?

a En plaque spread along the skull base

b Permeative erosion of jugular foramen

c Smooth expansion

d Enhancement with contrast

e Thickening of the dura

22 A young man presents to the ENT Department with a painless palpable soft-tissue swelling in the right perialveolar region. Contrast-enhanced CT revealed an inhomogeneous contrast-enhancing mass in the mandible. On bony windows the mass was a multilocular cyst with a thin sclerotic margin and a narrow zone of transition. The patient had gingival disease. Which is the most likely diagnosis?

a Giant cell granuloma

b Pleomorphic adenoma

c Oropharyngeal carcinoma

d Lymphoma

e Nasopharyngeal angiofibroma

23 A 55-year-old man with known squamous cell carcinoma of the larynx was noted to have some enlarged level II nodes on CT and an USS has been arranged. What feature on USS would make you most suspicious that they were enlarged due to infiltration with metastatic carcinoma?

a Orientated with long axis in axial plane

b Orientated with long axis orientated along cranio-caudal axis

c Round shape

d Reduced vascularity on Doppler imaging

e Prominent fatty hilum

24 A 16-year-old girl with gradual onset of a swelling below her chin presents to the ENT surgeons. MR revealed a well-defined cystic lesion in the sublingual space with no septations or wall thickening. It was bright on T2-weighted imaging and low signal on T1-weighted imaging. What is the most likely diagnosis?

a Ranula

b Second branchial cleft cyst

c Thyroglossal duct cyst

d Cystic hygroma

e Pleomorphic adenoma

25 A seven-day-old infant presented with poor feeding and increased sweating. On examination he had an enlarged head, prominent forehead veins and a cranial bruit. A cranial USS revealed dilated lateral ventricles and increased vascularity posterior to the third ventricle. What is the most likely diagnosis?

a Sagittal sinus thrombosis

b Vein of Galen malformation

c Giant MCA aneurysm

d Dural fistula

e Sturge-Weber syndrome

26 A nine-year-old girl presented with nystagmus, ataxia and diplopia to outward gaze. On CT there was a mass within the optic chiasm, which extended into the left optic nerve. The mass had poor patchy enhancement. A further eccentrically enhancing lesion was identified in the left occipital lobe. The most likely underlying condition is

a Tuberous sclerosis

b Neurofibromatosis type 1

c Neurofibromatosis type 2

d Von Hippel-Lindau syndrome

e Sturge-Weber syndrome

27 A middle-aged male had a CT following prolonged seizures which showed a rounded cystic lesion in the cerebellum with an avidly enhancing mural nodule. Other imaging demonstrated bilateral renal cell carcinoma. At what other site is he at risk of developing further cystic lesions?

a Lateral ventricles

b Insular cortex

c Corpus callosum

d Spinal cord

e Pons

28 An eight-year-old girl is admitted following a fall from a horse and complains of neck pain. A CT of the cervical spine demonstrates no evidence of fractures/dislocations. Incidentally, a lucent line is seen across the peg with sclerosis of the margins. The anterior arch appears hypertrophied. With which syndrome is this condition associated?

a Hurler's

b Morquio

c Down's

d Achondroplasia

e Turner's

29   A newborn baby was noted to have a thoracolumbar myelomeningocele and
     upper limb spasticity. An MRI scan revealed a small posterior fossa, low-lying
     tonsils, an elongated fourth ventricle, tectal beaking and partial agenesis of
     the corpus callosum. What is the most likely diagnosis?
     a   Dandy-Walker syndrome
     b   Chiari I malformation
     c   Chiari II malformation
     d   Chiari III malformation
     e   Septo-optic dysplasia

30   A 15-month-old boy was investigated for developmental delay. On clin-
     ical examination he was found to have a cleft palate. On CT he had a large
     posterior fossa, agenesis of the vermis with a large cystic dilatation of the
     fourth ventricle and agenesis of the corpus callosum. What is the most likely
     diagnosis?
     a   Chiari I malformation
     b   Schizencephaly
     c   Dandy-Walker malformation
     d   Septo-optic dysplasia
     e   Vein of Galen aneurysm

31   An 11 year old was investigated for widespread cutaneous lesions. Imaging
     revealed ribbon ribs, tibial bowing and a hypoplastic sphenoidal ala on the left.
     An MRI of the spine was also performed which showed a mid-thoracic lesion
     along with some bone remodelling. What is this lesion most likely to be?
     a   Ependymoma
     b   Astrocytoma
     c   Neurofibroma
     d   Lipoma
     e   Dermoid cyst

32   A 32 year old was imaged following sudden onset right hemiplegia. A CT
     showed subtle atrophy of the left occipital lobe and unusual gyral calcification.
     MRI demonstrated prominent pial and deep medullary veins in the region
     with a prominent left choroid plexus. What is the underlying aetiology?
     a   Tuberous sclerosis
     b   Ataxia telangiectasia
     c   Meningiomatosis
     d   von Hippel-Lindau syndrome
     e   Sturge-Weber syndrome

33 A 12 year old undergoing chemotherapy for acute myeloid leukaemia developed seizures. CT revealed multiple punctate areas of calcification scattered throughout the brain, with little enhancement and no mass effect. Ventricular size was normal. Comparison was made with a CT from two years previously which revealed no abnormality. What is the most likely diagnosis?

a Mineralising angiopathy

b *Cytomegalovirus* infection

c Fahr's disease

d Toxoplasmosis

e Carbon monoxide poisoning

34 A 22-year-old male presents to his GP with a history of a headache four weeks ago, which he describes as the worst headache of his life. He did not seek medical advice at the time as he was on holiday. The GP suspects he has had a subarachnoid haemorrhage. Which investigation would best determine if he did have a subarachnoid haemorrhage?

a CT cerebral angiogram

b Lumbar puncture

c Axial STIR MRI images

d Coronal FLAIR MRI images

e Axial T2*-weighted MRI images

35 A 25-year-old fitness instructor presented to the Emergency Department with a two-week history of left-sided nystagmus, past pointing and vertigo. CT revealed low-density changes affecting the left superior part of the cerebellum, the left vermis and tectum. What vascular territory is involved?

a Right vertebral artery

b Left posterior inferior cerebellar artery

c Left anterior inferior cerebellar artery

d Right superior cerebellar artery

e Left superior cerebellar artery

36 A five-year-old child was admitted with diarrhoea associated with *Escherichia coli* infection, having stopped feeding at home. She was started on antibiotics but started complaining of a headache and then became drowsy. On CT there was high density within the right transverse sinus. The rest of the brain appeared normal and there was no hydrocephalus. What is the most likely cause for this?

a Frontal sinusitis

b Head injury

c Iatrogenic

d Dehydration

e Mastoiditis

37 A 64-year-old lady is being consented for a diagnostic cerebral angiogram for a suspected MCA aneurysm. She asks about the risk of stroke. What is the risk due to the angiogram?

a 4.7%

b 0.2%

c 1.3%

d 10%

e 3.5%

38 A 32-year-old woman had a stormy post-natal period complicated by post-partum haemorrhage (PPH). On the fifth post-partum day she developed nausea and vomiting followed by generalised tonic clonic seizures. A diagnosis of cerebral venous sinus thrombosis with likely infarction was made. Which of the following is an unlikely feature on the MRI?

a Empty delta sign

b High signal in the cerebral venous sinuses on T2-weighted images

c Bilateral thalamic infarcts

d Basal ganglia haemorrhage

e Insular ribbon sign

39 A 55-year-old man is undergoing a coiling for a right PICA aneurysm. Where is likely to be the preferred arterial puncture site

a Left radial artery

b Left brachial artery

c Left common carotid artery

d Right common femoral artery

e Right common carotid artery

40 A 55-year-old woman who is hypothyroid with a large goitre undergoes a thyroid ultrasound, which demonstrates a diffusely enlarged thyroid with increased vascularity. She then undergoes a technetium-99m pertechnetate study. What findings would you expect to see?

a Homogeneous diffuse increase uptake

b Heterogeneous diffuse increase uptake

c Diffuse low uptake with a small nodule with increased uptake

d Diffuse low uptake

e Normal uptake

41 A 45-year-old female fell down a flight of stairs under the influence of alcohol and presented to the Emergency Department with a deteriorating GCS. A non-contrast CT revealed a 13-mm deep left temporoparietal lenticular haematoma. What is the most likely source of the bleed?

   a Middle meningeal artery

   b Internal cerebral veins

   c Bridging cortical veins

   d Choroidal arteries

   e Vein of Labbe

42 A 46-year-old motorcyclist was involved in a high-speed RTA. On arrival of the paramedics, the GCS was recorded as 4/15 and the patient was intubated at the site of injury. An emergency non-contrast CT showed multiple subtle petechial haemorrhages characteristic of diffuse axonal injury. What is the most likely site of the petechial haemorrhage?

   a Insular ribbon

   b Watershed areas

   c Periventricular white matter

   d Grey-white matter junction

   e Cerebellum

43 A 22-year-old female rear-seat passenger suffered a high-speed road traffic accident and presented to the Emergency Department with several left temporal facial injuries. Following stabilisation of her bony injuries she was discharged. A week later she developed painful left orbital swelling and third nerve palsy. A post-contrast CT was unremarkable barring some fullness of the left orbital apex and mild enlargement of the left superior ophthalmic vein. A catheter angiogram revealed early opacification of the left superior ophthalmic vein and a vascular blush posteriorly. What is the most likely diagnosis?

   a Dural fistula

   b Traumatic ICA aneurysm

   c Caroticocavernous fistula

   d Carotid dissection

   e Cavernous angioma

44 Regarding *Cryptococcus neoformans* in human immunodeficiency virus. Which of the following statements is correct?

   a *Cryptococcus neoformans* is the most common fungal infection in AIDS

   b It is found in bird excrement and spreads by direct invasion

   c Results in abscess formation in the basal ganglion

   d Results in a florid meningitic response

   e Results in effacement of the perivascular spaces

45 Regarding *tuberculosis* in the HIV population. Which of the following statements is correct?

a *Tuberculosis* abscess are the most common presentation

b Typically results from direct spread from adjacent structures

c Tuberculomas occur in the posterior fossa

d The typical imaging feature of a tuberculoma is a target lesion

e Hydrocephalus is typically obstructive in nature

46 A patient with known tuberous sclerosis had a routine follow-up CT. A 3 × 2-cm partly calcified heterogeneously enhancing lesion was seen at the level of the foramen of Monro. What is the most likely pathology?

a Colloid cyst

b Subependymal giant cell astrocytoma

c Intraventricular

d Meningioma

e Germinoma

47 A seven-year-old boy presented with sudden onset gait problems and subtle uncoordination on the finger nose test. CT demonstrated a low density cystic solid lesion with subtle calcification centred on the vermis. Thick heterogeneous enhancement was seen within the solid area along with obstructive hydrocephalus. What is the most likely diagnosis?

a Pilocytic astrocytoma

b Medulloblastoma

c Haemangioblastoma

d Ependymoma

e Brainstem glioma

48 A 62-year-old female presented to the Emergency Department with gradual onset weakness in the right upper and lower limbs. CT demonstrated multiple rounded hyperdense lesions with marked vasogenic oedema which showed prominent enhancement following IV contrast. Assuming the lesions are metastases, what is the most likely primary?

a Bladder

b Renal cell carcinoma

c Colon

d Adenocarcinoma of the lung

e Uterus

49 A five-year-old boy was admitted with nausea and increased somnolence. Obstructive hydrocephalus was seen on CT with a posterior fossa tumour. What typical features make medulloblastoma more likely than ependymoma?

a Arising form the floor of the fourth ventricle

b Extension through the foramina of Luschka

c Calcification on CT

d Arising from the vermis

e Small cystic area within the mass

50 A 50-year-old female was investigated for chronic headaches. A CT demonstrated a well-defined hyperdense parasagittal lesion with calcification that avidly enhanced with contrast. The superior sagittal sinus was invaded and thrombus was present. What other feature on CT would you look for to help clinch the diagnosis?

a Dural tail

b Bony destruction

c Vasogenic oedema

d Ventricular distortion

e Corpus callosal involvement

51 A 47-year-old male was investigated for progressive left-sided weakness. On CT of his head there was loss of grey-white matter differentiation with thickening of the cortex and minor effacement of the sulci affecting the right frontal and temporal lobes. On MRI there was generalised high signal on T2 in this region. On FLAIR there was diffuse enlargement of the right frontal and temporal lobes cortex with vasogenic oedema in the surrounding white matter. What is the most likely diagnosis?

a Oligodendroglioma

b Gliomatosis cerebri

c Metastasis

d Glioblastoma multiforme

e Heterotopia

52 A 25-year-old male had an MRI for chronic headaches. On MR there was a cystic mass with an enhancing nodule in the left Sylvian fissure. The mass had an enhancing dural tail and exhibited only minor vasogenic oedema. What is the most likely diagnosis?

a Meningioma

b Pleomorphic xanthoastrocytoma

c Anaplastic astrocytoma

d Metastasis

e Lymphoma

53 A 43-year-old male underwent an MRI to evaluate hearing loss. In the right cerebellopontine angle there was a well-defined mass which was low signal on T1W, high signal on T2W and low on FLAIR. The signal intensity was similar to CSF. There was scalloping of the bony margins. What would you expect the signal characteristics to be on diffusion weighted imaging?

a Low signal

b Similar signal to fat

c Bright signal

d Intermediate signal

e Similar signal to the ADC map

54 A 55-year-old chronic alcoholic was admitted following an extended period of heavy drinking. He was noted to be very confused, confabulating and suffering from delusions. On examination he was ataxic and had ophthalmoplegia. What features on MRI would you look for in order to make the diagnosis?

a Cerebellar atrophy

b High signal perpendicular to the lateral ventricle

c High signal within the periaqueductal region

d High signal within the vermis

e High signal within the lentiform nucleus

55 A 35 year old presents with progressive personality changes and increasing withdrawal. CT brain demonstrated cerebral atrophy affecting the frontal lobes and anterior temporal lobe with associated compensatory enlargement of the frontal horns of the lateral ventricles. The rest of the brain was normal. What is the likely diagnosis?

a Alzheimer's disease

b Parkinson's disease

c Progressive supranuclear palsy

d Fabry's disease

e Pick's disease

56 A 39-year-old man was being investigated for progressive involuntary movement. On CT he was found to have caudate atrophy with compensatory enlargement of the anterior horns of the lateral ventricles. What would one expect to see on MRI imaging?

a Eye of the tiger sign

b High signal in the caudate and putamen on T2-weighted MR images

c High signal in the thalamus on T2-weighted MR images

d Loss of the pars compacta

e High signal in the pons on T2-weighted MR images

57 A 63-year-old male undergoing a CT for unwitnessed fall had marked widening of the cerebellar sulcal spaces suggestive of cerebellar atrophy. Which of the following is unlikely to be a cause?

a Phenytoin

b Alcohol

c Ataxia telangiectasia

d Tuberous sclerosis

e Bronchial carcinoma

58 A 17-year-old boy was being investigated for partial complex seizures refractory to drug treatment and was being considered for a lobectomy. An interictal FDG-PET scan demonstrated reduced signal in the right temporal lobe. What would be the next appropriate step in management?

a Continue with medical management

b Perform an ictal FDG-PET scan

c Right temporal lobe resection

d Left temporal lobe resection

e Radiotherapy

59 A 45-year-old male patient attempted suicide by taking all of his prescription tablets. Eighteen hours later he was found unconscious at home. He was stabilised and a CT head was performed the next morning. He is found to have wedge-like low densities affecting the occipito-parietal and mid-frontal regions. What tablets is he most likely to have taken?

a Antiepileptics

b Antihypertensives

c Antibiotics

d Antipsychotics

e Antiflammatories

60 You are teaching an F1 about interpreting the difference between vasogenic and cytotoxic oedema. Which is a feature of cytotoxic oedema?

a Sharply demarcated border

b Demonstrates restricted diffusion on DWI

c Oedema involving the cortex

d Oedema extending across the corpus callosum

e Associated with ischaemia

61 On plain film X-ray of the lumbar spine a dense single vertebra is seen (ivory vertebra). The vertebra is not expanded and the trabeculae are not thickened. There is no evidence of disc space narrowing, periosteal reaction or soft-tissue mass. What is the most likely diagnosis?

a Low-grade infection

b Paget's disease

c Sclerotic metastasis

d Lymphoma

e Haemangioma

62 A four-year-old child had a skeletal survey, which revealed central beaking of the vertebral body. What is the most likely diagnosis?

a Hurler's syndrome

b Morquio syndrome

c Achondroplasia

d Down's syndrome

e Congenital hypothyroidism

63 A 22-year-old gymnast was admitted with signs of right L4 radiculopathy. An MR was performed which revealed disc pathology. What is the most likely site of abnormality on the MR?

a Right L5/S1 paracentral disc bulge

b Left L5/S1 central disc bulge

c Right L4/L5 paracentral disc bulge

d Left L4/L5 paracentral disc bulge

e Right L4/L5 lateral disc bulge

64 An 86-year-old woman complains of chronic neck pain. She has had multiple admissions for fractures and is on a bisphosphonate. A skull X-ray is taken. On the lateral film the odontoid peg is seen at the level of McGregor's line. What is this condition?

a Platybasia

b Craniocaudal disassociation

c Basilar invagination

d Basilar impression

e Normal finding

65 A 60-year-old woman was admitted with severe back pain. She had a past medical history of breast cancer and was on tamoxifen. She underwent an MRI scan for further assessment. What feature makes an osteoporotic fracture more likely than metastatic disease?

a Multiple levels affected

b A focal paraspinal mass

c Normal pedicles

d Convex posterior border of the vertebral body

e An epidural mass

66   A 39-year-old male who was being investigated for neck pain was noted on CT to have posterior vertebral scalloping of the C4-7 vertebra. On MRI the cord was expanded at this level by a well-defined tumour, which was high signal on T2 and low on T1. There was intense homogeneous enhancement with contrast. What is the most likely diagnosis?

   a Meningioma

   b Astrocytoma

   c Ependymoma

   d Lipoma

   e Intramedullary haematoma

67   A 60-year-old woman was admitted with immobility and was found to have a raised ESR. The remainder of her blood tests were normal. On T1-weighted MR there was some nodularity along the nerve roots with nodular contrast enhancement along the cauda equina. What is the most likely diagnosis?

   a Drop metastasis from ependymoma

   b Metastatic breast cancer

   c Sarcoid

   d Dural sepsis

   e Meningioma

68   A 46-year-old male complained of lower back pain and faecal incompetence. On plain film there was a large expansile lytic destructive mass in the sacrum with moderate internal calcification. It was heterogeneous and of low signal on T1 and high on T2. The mass enhanced with contrast. The patient had no other medical history. What is the most likely diagnosis?

   a Metastasis

   b Plasmacytoma

   c Insufficiency fracture

   d Teratoma

   e Chordoma

69   A 55-year-old female with progressive lower limb weakness was being investigated by a neurologist. On spinal MR there was a well-defined 1-cm intramedullary spinal mass at D6 level, which was high signal on both T1 and T2. A low-signal rim was present on T2-weighted imaging. On T2* there was blooming. No high signal was seen in the cord. What is the most likely diagnosis?

   a Ependymoma

   b Pilocytic astrocytoma

   c Spinal cord cavernous angioma

   d AVM

   e Metastasis

70 A six-month-old baby underwent a chest X-ray for a persistent cough and was found to have absent clavicles and supernumerary ribs. On pelvic X-ray there was a widened symphysis pubis. What feature would you expect to see on the plain skull X-ray?

a Thickened skull vault

b Hair on end

c Scaphocephaly

d Wormian bones

e Enlarged maxillary sinuses

Neuroradiology, head and neck and ENT radiology

PAPER 2

1   A 30-year-old male had an OPG and multiple well-defined unilocular and multilocular lytic lesions were visible. These lesions involved the body and angle of the mandible and were associated with unerupted molars. What is the most likely diagnosis?
    a Dentigerous cyst
    b Osteomyelitis
    c Gorlin's disease
    d Fibrous dysplasia
    e Metastatic disease

2   An OPG was performed on a 15-year-old following an alleged assault. The plain film revealed generalised expansion of the mandible with a ground-glass appearance to the bone and multiple multiloculated cystic lesions affecting both bodies of the mandible. What is the likely diagnosis?
    a Gorlin's disease
    b Cherubism
    c Paget's disease
    d Metastases from Wilms' tumour
    e Hyperparathyroidism

3   A 55-year-old female was admitted with a worsening headache. On imaging the right optic nerve appeared thickened with linear plaque-like calcification and optic canal hyperostosis. What pattern of enhancement is most likely?
    a Patchy enhancement of the optic canal
    b No enhancement
    c Generalised tram track enhancement
    d Peripheral enhancement
    e Avid enhancement with flow voids

4   A 67-year-old woman was admitted with right-sided diplopia and proptosis. She was known to have metastatic breast cancer and was on Herceptin. On CT there was gross bony destruction of the right greater wing of sphenoid with soft-tissue filling the superior orbital fissure. The inferior orbital fissure and optic canal were not affected. What nerves may be affected?

  a III, IV, V1, V2 and VI

  b II, III, IV, V1, V2 and VI

  c III, IV, V1 and VI

  d III, IV, V1, V2 and VI

  e III, V1, V2 and VI

5   A 45-year-old woman with known multiple sclerosis complained to her GP that she had visual loss. On examination she was found to have upper right-sided quadrantanopia. Where is she likely to have a new plaque?

  a Right optic nerve

  b Optic chiasm

  c Left lateral geniculate nucleus

  d Right optic tracts

  e Left optic radiation

6   A five-year-old boy was noted by his parent to be bumping into things on his left. On examination he was found to have a soft-tissue mass affecting his left retina. On CT there was a poorly enhancing mass causing irregularity of the orbit and surrounding conal fat haziness. This mass was most likely to be a secondary from which tumour?

  a Neuroblastoma

  b Wilms'

  c Sarcoma

  d Leukaemia

  e Medulloblastoma

7   A 25-year-old male was admitted with a painful partial right Horner's syndrome. A contrast CT was performed. In which area of the scan would you expect to find the pathology?

  a Right intraconal region

  b Left occipital cortex

  c Left vertebral artery

  d Right carotid artery

  e Left carotid artery

8 A 54-year-old underwent a CT of the paranasal sinuses for functional endoscopic sinus surgery (FESS) planning. The right frontal sinus appeared significantly larger than the left and was opacified. At the base there was a dense lesion, which appeared to contain compact cortical bone and protruded into the sinus cavity. On MRI the lesion appeared as a signal void. What is the most likely diagnosis?

    a Ivory osteoma

    b Fibrous dysplasia

    c Meningioma

    d Ossifying fibroma

    e Foreign body

9 A newborn baby boy developed respiratory distress post delivery. He was intubated and did well but as soon as he was extubated he again developed respiratory distress. CT demonstrated bilateral air/fluid levels within the nasal cavities and narrowing of the posterior choanae with bowing of the posterior maxilla. What is the most likely diagnosis?

    a Polyp disease

    b Unilateral choanal atresia

    c Sudden infant death syndrome

    d Encephalocele

    e Bilateral choanal atresia

10 A 37-year-old woman was being investigated for pulsatile tinnitus and was found on otoscopy to have a blue mass deep to the tympanic membrane. On CT there was a small left-sided soft-tissue mass abutting the left cochlear promontory. This enhanced brightly with contrast. What is the most likely diagnosis?

    a Glomus tympanicum

    b Glomus jugulare

    c Left aberrant internal carotid artery

    d Cholesteatoma

    e Carotid artery aneurysm

11 A patient is due to have an operation on their parotid gland and the ENT surgeon is concerned he cannot identify the facial nerve on the patient's pre-op CT or MRI scans. Which structure that lies medial to the nerve can be used as a landmark?

    a Facial artery

    b Facial vein

    c Retromandibular vein

    d Wharton's duct

    e Terminal segment of hypoglossal nerve

12 A two-year-old boy presented with a discharging mass on the bridge of the nose, which did not heal despite a prolonged course of broad-spectrum antibiotic therapy. Prior to biopsy, imaging was performed. An MRI scan confirmed a cystic lesion, which was of heterogeneous increased signal on T1W and T2 imaging. The density of the lesion on CT was that of fat. What is the most likely diagnosis?

    a Encephalocele

    b Dermoid cyst

    c Nasal glioma

    d Sebaceous cyst

    e Potts puffy tumour

13 A 33-year-old male presented with a history of gradually worsening unilateral nasal obstruction and epistaxis. Endoscopy revealed a polypoidal mass filling the left nasal cavity. CT scan showed a soft-tissue mass arising from the lateral nasal wall with associated bone destruction of the medial wall of the maxillary sinus and heterogeneous enhancement post administration of contrast. An MRI scan confirmed intermediate signal intensity on both T1 and T2W images with avid enhancement post administration of gadolinium. What is the most likely diagnosis?

    a Mucocele of ethmoidal sinus

    b Inverted papilloma

    c Mucous retention cyst

    d Nasopharyngeal carcinoma

    e Nasal polyp

14 A 40-year-old man who presented with progressive right-sided facial pain and paraesthesia underwent a CT scan. This revealed a bilobed mass arising from Meckel's cave and ultimately a trigeminal nerve schwannoma was diagnosed. What signal characteristics would be most characteristic on MRI?

    a Isointense to grey matter on T2-weighted images

    b Hyperintense on T1-weighted images

    c Hypointense on T2-weighted images

    d Does not enhance following IV gadolinium on T1-weighted images

    e Isointense to grey matter on T1-weighted images

15 A patient presents with acute onset headache, right-sided otorrhoea and associated abducent nerve palsy. CT revealed opacification of the petrous apex on the symptomatic side and cavernous sinus enhancement. On MRI there was a low signal mass within the petrous apex, which demonstrated bright peripheral enhancement with contrast. The mass was hyperintense on T2W. What syndrome is this patient suffering from?

a Gradenigo's syndrome

b Korsakoff's syndrome

c Chilaiditi's syndrome

d Riley-Day syndrome

e Gerstmann's syndrome

16 A 16-year-old male presented with epistaxis following contact sports. CT revealed a large mass in the nasopharynx extending into the pterygopalatine and infratemporal fossa. Following contrast, there was significant enhancement and erosion of the medial pterygoid plate was seen. What treatment would be an appropriate next step in his management?

a Conservative management

b Medical management

c Embolisation

d Direct intratumoral alcohol injection

e Surgical excision

17 A seven-year-old presented with a midline neck swelling following a respiratory tract infection. On examination this moved with swallowing and an ultrasound revealed a hypoechoic nonvascular lesion. MRI confirmed an infrahyoid location and demonstrated a high signal on T2. What percentage of these lesions is likely to undergo malignant change?

a <1%

b 2%

c 7%

d 12%

e 25%

18 An 18-year-old man presents to the maxillofacial team suffering from a blow to the mid maxillary region. Examination findings included marked facial oedema, bilateral subconjunctival haemorrhages, and epistaxis. Plain facial views reveal a fracture segment that has a pyramidal shape and extends from the nasal bridge below the nasofrontal suture through the frontal processes of the maxilla, inferolaterally through the lacrimal bones and inferior orbital floor and into the orbital foramen. Inferiorly the fracture extended through the anterior wall of the maxillary sinus. The zygoma and pterygoid plates were both fractured. What type of fracture is this?

a Le Fort I fracture

b Le Fort II fracture

c Le Fort III fracture

d Orbital blow out fracture

e Tripod fracture

19 A 30-year-old man presents with bilateral external ear masses. Otoscopic examination reveals these lesions to be a build up of layers of flaky skin. Further history elucidates chronic sinusitis and bronchiectasis. What is the most likely diagnosis?

a Keratosis obturans

b Van der Hoeve syndrome

c Malignant otitis externa

d Surfer's ear

e Cholesteatoma

20 A 10-year-old girl presented with a unilateral enlarged orbit. Facial X-rays revealed opacification of the maxillary sinus with no air/fluid level. CT demonstrated depression of the right orbital floor with enlargement of the orbit and lateral displacement of the lateral wall of the nasal fossa. The middle turbinate was large but morphologically normal. What is the most likely diagnosis?

a Sinus hypoplasia

b Maxillary dentigerous cyst

c Primordial dentigerous cyst

d Acute sinusitis

e Ameloblastoma

21 The report on a child's neck X-ray reads, 'There is loss of the normal subglottic angle resulting in a wine bottle-shaped appearance on AP projection. On the lateral film there is an ill-defined haziness of the soft-tissue/air interface between the glottic and subglottic regions.' What is the most likely diagnosis?

a Croup

b Supraglottitis

c Congenital tracheal stenosis

d Subglottic haemangioma

e Laryngomalacia

22 You are considering the utility of CT in detecting acoustic neuromas and read a study evaluating its use in 200 people of whom 10 actually had the condition. The study reports that CT was reported as abnormal in seven patients and there were 188 true negatives. What is the sensitivity of CT for detection of acoustic neuroma in this study?

a 2.5%

b 29%

c 50%

d 70%

e 99%

23 This question relates to the descent of the thyroid gland during development. At which of the following anatomical sites are you least likely to find maldescended thyroid tissue?

a Within foramen lacerum

b Within foramen caecum

c Anterior to the thyroid cartilage

d Within the hyoid bone

e Anterior to the hyoid bone

24 A four-year-old girl who weighs 16 kg presented in status epilepticus and a lesion was visible in her posterior fossa on an unenhanced CT scan. A post-contrast scan is being planned for further assessment. How much 300 mg/mL iohexol non-ionic contrast would be appropriate?

a 4 mL

b 8 mL

c 16 mL

d 32 mL

e 48 mL

25 A nine-year-old boy underwent an MRI while being investigated for cognitive difficulties. Prominent occipital horns and a high-riding third ventricle were seen. Sagittal sections revealed a radial orientation of the gyri. What is the most likely diagnosis?

a Joubert syndrome

b Septo-optic dysplasia

c Corpus callosum agenesis

d Holoprosencephaly

e Porencephaly

26 A six-month-old male baby underwent neurological work-up. An MRI showed a wide CSF communication between the left lateral ventricle and the cortical subarachnoid space. A similar smaller communication was seen on the right without pouching along the lateral border of the right lateral ventricle. What is the most likely diagnosis?

a Schizencephaly

b Hydranencephaly

c Megalencephaly

d Lobar holoprosencephaly

e Arrhinencephaly

27 A five year old with seizures and cognitive impairment had an MRI scan. This revealed features highly suggestive of heterotopia. What are the likely findings on the MRI?

a CSF lined cleft extending from the ependymal surface to cortical pia

b Shallow Sylvian fissures and agyric cortex

c Bilateral nodular subependymal grey matter

d Squared appearance of the frontal horns and an absent septum pellucidum

e Poor brain sulcation with intraparenchymal calcification

28 A six-year-old female was investigated for a neurogenic bladder and persistent leg pain. Clinical examination revealed a hairy patch overlying the lumbosacral region. An MRI showed a bony cleft within the spinal canal and two hemicords from T11 to L1. What is the most likely diagnosis?

a Diastematomyelia

b Sirenomelia

c Myelocystocele

d Dorsal enteric sinus

e Syringohydromyelia

29 A healthcare worker noted that a three-month-old child had an unusual-shaped head. She was seen by the paediatrician who requested a CT head. This demonstrated bony fusion of the sagittal suture. The metopic and coronal sutures were open. What is the most likely diagnosis?

a Brachycephaly

b Clover leaf skull

c Plagiocephaly

d Trigonocephaly

e Scaphocephaly

30 A five-month-old child was being investigated for a nasopharyngeal mass. He had a cleft palate but otherwise appeared morphologically normal. On CT there was a bony defect in the roof of the sphenoid sinus and a soft tissue and CSF density mass extended into the nasopharynx. What is the diagnosis?

a Mucocele

b Transsphenoidal meningocele

c Transsphenoidal encephalocele

d Leptomeningeal cyst

e Dermoid cyst

31 A 19-year-old boy was admitted with new onset seizures. On T2-weighted MRI there was high signal within the atrophied left hippocampus. What other feature is likely to be associated with this condition?

a Enlargement of the occipital horn of the lateral ventricle

b Generalised cerebral atrophy

c Ipsilateral atrophy of the mammillary body

d Atrophy of the amygdala

e Heterotopia

32 A 76-year-old was scanned 14 hours post onset of left-sided weakness and facial droop. Which of the following would you not expect to find on the CT scan?

a Hyperdense MCA sign

b Loss of grey/white matter differentiation

c Obscuration of the lentiform nucleus

d Mass effect with midline shift

e Insular ribbon sign

33 A 55-year-old lady was repeatedly imaged following surgical evacuation of a large right-sided extra-axial bleed sustained in a high-speed RTA. On her latest CT there was widespread cerebral oedema, with effacement of the right suprasellar cistern and medial displacement of the uncus and parahippocampus. Enlargement of the right CP angle cistern was also seen. What territory is she currently at most risk of infarcting?

a Right ACA territory

b Right MCA territory

c Right PCA territory

d Left MCA territory

e Left PCA territory

34 A 22-year-old male developed a post-coital headache and was admitted via the Emergency Department with a CT which demonstrated diffuse subarachnoid blood in the suprasellar cistern. CT cerebral angiogram and conventional cerebral catheter angiogram performed six weeks after the event were both negative. What is the most likely cause?

a Anterior communicating artery aneurysm

b Middle cerebral artery aneurysm

c Carotid dissection

d Venous bleed

e Subdural bleed

35 A 45-year-old woman was admitted with a GCS of 12. There was no history available. On CT there was bilateral parasagittal haemorrhage affecting the posterior frontal lobe and parietal lobes. The lateral ventricles were dilated and the basal cisterns partially effaced. The rest of the brain parenchyma was normal. What is the most likely diagnosis?

a Hydrocephalus

b Sagittal sinus thrombosis

c Hypertensive angiopathy

d Amyloid angiopathy

e Haemorrhage from metastatic disease

36 A 10-year-old child of oriental origin was being investigated for right-sided hemiplegia. MRI revealed a left MCA territory infarct. Multiple flow voids were seen within the basal ganglia and the left supraclinoid ICA appeared small in calibre on the MRA. Multiple collaterals were present in the basal cisterns and the vertebro-basilar circulation appeared normal. What do the intracranial features indicate?

a ICA dissection

b Polyarteritis nodosa

c Sarcoidosis

d Moyamoya disease

e Kawasaki's disease

37 A 66-year-old presented with symptoms of dizziness, ataxia and nausea. CT showed a low-density non-enhancing area along the right anterolateral aspect of the cerebellum. The ipsilateral cerebellar vermis and tonsil also appeared involved. A diagnosis of cerebellar infarction was made. What territory is involved?

a Superior cerebellar artery

b Posterior inferior cerebellar artery

c Anterior inferior cerebellar artery

d Basilar artery

e Right vertebral artery

38 A patient has a dual phase subtraction study for investigation of hyperparathyroidism and a focus of uptake is seen on the Tc-99m-mibi scan with a corresponding area of increased uptake on the I123 study in the region of upper pole of the right lobe of the gland. What is the most likely cause for this finding?

a Functioning parathyroid adenoma

b Papillary thyroid tumour

c Multinodular goitre with prominent nodule

d Solitary functioning thyroid nodule

e Submandibular salivary gland

39 A 22-year-old male was catapulted from his motorbike. He was admitted unconscious and lateral cervical spine X-ray demonstrated a small triangular fragment of bone antero-inferior to the anterior margin of C4 with widening of the spinous processes at C4–C5. What was likely to have been the mechanism of injury?

a Vertical compression

b Flexion with rotation

c Hyperextension

d Hyperflexion

e Lateral flexion/shearing

40 A six-month-old child was brought to the Emergency Department by his parents following a fit. The attending doctor discovered multiple bruises to his chest and pelvis and suspected non-accidental injury. A skeletal survey revealed multiple fractures and a head CT revealed a subdural haematoma. An MR was performed and demonstrated high signal on T1 and low signal on T2. How long is it likely the injury was sustained?

a Less than 24 hours (oxyhaemoglobin)

b 1–3 days (deoxyhaemoglobin)

c 3–7 days (intracellular methaemoglobin)

d 7–14 days (extracellular methaemoglobin)

e Greater than 14 days (haemosiderin)

41 Following a high-speed RTA a 45-year-old male had a multitrauma scan. A fracture was seen running across the right petrous temporal bone extending from the squamous portion laterally to the mesotympanum medially. Opacification of the mastoid air cells was evident. What is the patient most at risk of?

a Sensorineural deafness

b Ossicular dislocation

c Irreversible facial paralysis

d CSF rhinorrhea

e Recurrent mastoiditis

42 A female is referred from a thyroid clinic with suspected Graves' disease with an elevated T3 and low TSH. She is a tachycardic at 90 bpm but has a regular pulse and has minor eye symptoms. She is booked for a technetium-99m pertechnetate scan prior to any therapy. If the diagnosis is correct, what is the scan likely to show?

a Normal uptake

b Diffuse avid uptake in a uniform pattern

c Patchy appearance with areas of intense uptake

d Uniform reduced uptake throughout the gland

e A technetium scan is contraindicated due to the risk of thyroid storm

43 A 42-year-old woman with a proceeding history of flu-like symptoms presented with a day history of increasing confusion followed by three generalised seizures. Initial CT revealed no abnormality while an MRI showed high signal on T2 in the medial right temporal and right insula region. No enhancement with gadolinium and little mass effect were seen. She remained in intensive care and a repeat MRI a week later showed extensive high signal in the temporal lobes and frontal lobes with multiple low-signal foci on T2 GRE. There was no ventricular dilatation. What is the most likely diagnosis?

a Toxoplasmosis

b Herpes encephalitis

c Low-grade glioma

d Paraneoplastic syndrome

e *Cytomegalovirus* infection

44 A 40-year-old man with headaches was assessed with a CT which showed a thin-walled uniformly enhancing lesion with marked vasogenic oedema in the right temporal lobe adjacent to the petrous ridge. On MRI the lesion appeared iso-hypointense on T1 and hyperintense on T2-weighted images. On DWI there was high signal and low signal on the ADC map. What is the most likely diagnosis?

a Glioblastoma multiforme

b Cerebral abscess

c Arachnoid cyst

d Metastasis

e Chronic haematoma

45 A 38-year-old immunocompromised male presented with increasing head-aches and worsening memory. CT showed three discrete hyperdense lesions in the corpus callosum and centrum semiovale. Partial enhancement with eccentric necrotic areas was seen. What is the most likely diagnosis?

  a Cryptococcosis

  b Primary CNS lymphoma

  c Toxoplasmosis

  d Herpes encephalitis

  e *Tuberculosis*

46 A 32 year old had a CT head following a road traffic accident. Note was made of an incidental finding of a low-density lesion in the right cerebellopontine angle. There was no enhancement following IV iodinated contrast. On MRI the lesion was low on T1 and bright on T2-weighted images. DWI demon-strated signal similar to CSF in this region with no apparent signal loss on the ADC map. What is the most likely diagnosis?

  a Arachnoid cyst

  b Epidermoid

  c Dermoid

  d Acoustic neuroma

  e Choroid plexus cyst

47 A 32-year-old male presented with recent onset headaches and seizures. CT showed a rounded extra-axial mass in the interpeduncular cistern with peri-pheral calcification. Low-density homogeneous foci were also seen within the basal cisterns. No enhancement was visible post contrast. On MRI the lesion appeared bright on T1 and T2 with a low signal rim. On proton dens-ity (PD) images it was of homogeneously high signal. What is the most likely diagnosis?

  a Lipoma

  b Rathke's cleft cyst

  c Epidermoid

  d Arachnoid cyst

  e Craniopharyngioma

48 A 12-year-old male was scanned following visual complaints. An MRI showed a suprasellar lesion, which was high signal on T1- and T2-weighted images. Multiple areas of low signal were also seen within it and the dorsum sellae was partially eroded. Given the patient's age and radiological features, what is the most likely diagnosis?

  a Lipoma

  b Craniopharyngioma

  c Rathke's cleft cyst

d Arachnoid cyst

e Pituitary macroadenoma

49 A six-year-old boy was investigated for precocious puberty. On sagittal T1-weighted MRI there was a homogeneous 1-cm, well-defined soft-tissue mass between the pituitary stalk and the mammillary bodies. The mass did not enhance with contrast. What is the most likely diagnosis?

a Craniopharyngioma

b Pituitary adenoma

c Eosinophilic granuloma

d Hypothalamic hamartoma

e Chiasmatic glioma

50 A 13-year-old boy was being investigated for progressive confusion, lethargy and increased thirst. CT was performed which demonstrated a well-defined, smooth-walled homogeneous hyperdense lesion in the pineal region. At which other site does this tumour most often occur?

a Posterior fossa

b Spinal cord

c Suprasellar cistern

d Lateral ventricle

e Frontal lobe

51 A 35-year-old woman is three months post partum. She had a normal vaginal delivery with an epidural as anaesthetic. Since her child's birth she has complained of a postural headache but otherwise feels well and is not depressed. On MRI brain she was noted to have generalised thickening of the dura, which enhanced uniformly and small bilateral subdural collections. No parenchymal or bony abnormality was visible and there was no hydrocephalus. What is the most likely diagnosis?

a Dural metastasis

b En plaque meningioma

c Intracranial hypotension

d Meningitis

e Sarcoid

52 A 25-year-old woman had an MRI and CT for investigation of headaches. She appeared morphologically normal and had normal blood tests. She was found to have a well-defined mass, which was homogeneously high signal on both T1- and T2-weighted MRI in the midline suprasellar region deviating the pituitary posteriorly. On CT there was again a well-defined homogenously low-defined mass within the suprasellar region with no enhancement. The rest of the pituitary appeared normal. What is the likely diagnosis?

a Rathke's cleft cysts

b Craniopharyngiomas

c Pituitary adenoma

d Metastasis

e Hypothalamic glioma

53 A 40-year-old female was being investigated for a familial movement disorder. On CT of her brain there was caudate atrophy with compensatory enlargement of the frontal horns of the lateral ventricles. How is this condition inherited?

a X-linked recessive

b X-linked dominant

c Autosomal dominant

d Autosomal recessive

e Not inherited

54 A 15-year-old girl with a neurocutaneous disorder had an MRI which showed vermian and interhemispheric atrophy with compensatory enlargement of the IVth ventricle. There were also multiple small cortical wedge infarcts. What cutaneous abnormalities is she most likely to have?

a Café au lait spots

b Axillary freckles

c Telangiectasia

d Port wine stain

e Adenoma sebaceum

55 A 22-year-old Australian gap year student started to develop unusual behaviour, dystonia and dysarthria while travelling around Europe. On MRI she was found to have high signal in the caudate and putamen. There were no mass lesions, hydrocephalus or extra axial blood. What is the most likely diagnosis?

a Wilson's disease

b Ataxic telangiectasia

c Leigh's disease

d Carbon monoxide poisoning

e HIV

56 A 39-year-old man had a CT of his head, on which a fat density was seen in the most superior parts of the frontal horns of the lateral ventricles. No other abnormalities were visible. What is the most likely reason for these findings?

a Ruptured dermoid cyst

b Intraventricular epidermoid

c Germinal teratoma

d Intraventricular lipoma

e Metastasis

57 A 35-year-old woman is being investigated for demyelinating disease. What is the best sequence to demonstrate plaques in the posterior fossa?

a Axial T2

b Coronal FLAIR

c Axial proton density

d Axial FLAIR

e Coronal T1

58 A five-year-old boy was noted to have multiple well-defined lucent areas with no sclerotic margin and a narrow zone of transition on his skull X-ray. A contrast-enhanced CT was then performed, which demonstrated an enhancing soft-tissue mass within the abnormal areas of the skull vault. What is the most likely diagnosis?

a Dermoid

b Metastasis

c Encephalocele

d Eosinophilic granuloma

e Prominent venous lakes

59 A 30-year-old West African woman was being investigated for a right Bell's palsy and diabetes insipidus. She was known to have an abnormal CXR. On MRI she was found to have diffuse meningeal enhancement with some modularity. What would be your next investigation?

a Repeat CXR

b CT brain

c Meningeal biopsy

d Staging CT

e Full blood count

60 A middle-aged male presented with increasing paraesthesia in the right leg. An X-ray of his lumbar spine and views of his leg were unremarkable. An MRI was performed which showed a lesion displacing the thecal sac away from the bony spinal canal. Which of the following would you not include in the differential diagnosis?

a Prolapsed disc

b Epidural metastases

c Neurofibroma

d Ependymoma

e Meningioma

61 A six-year-old child presented with gait problems and neurologic deficit. An MRI of the brain and whole spine was performed. There was a diffuse abnormality in the upper thoracic cord extending over approximately five vertebral levels. The lesion appeared intramedullary in location and was hypo-isointense on T1 and hyperintense on T2-weighted images with enhancement on T1 following IV Gadolinium. A syrinx was seen more superiorly. What is the most likely diagnosis?

a Ependymoma

b Transverse myelitis

c Astrocytoma

d Metastases

e Haemangioblastoma

62 A 26-year-old male with haemophilia developed sudden onset cauda equina syndrome and an emergency MRI of the lumbar spine was performed. A large fusiform posterior extradural mass extending from L1 to L5 was present. It was hypointense on T2-weighted images. What is the most likely diagnosis?

a Epidural abscess

b Metastasis

c Arachnoid cyst

d Neurofibroma

e Haematoma

63 A 70-year-old male was seen in outpatients with left T12 nerve root pain. CT demonstrated generalised expansion of the whole of the T12 vertebra with coarsening of the trabeculae. On T1-weighted imaging there was effacement of the fat around the left T12 nerve root. What is the cause for these symptoms?

a Fibrous dysplasia

b Metastastatic disease

c Paget's disease

d Haemangioma

e Langerhans cell histiocytosis

64 A middle-aged woman had a three-year history of change in sensation in her lower legs. On MRI of her whole spine there was diffuse cord expansion in the thoracic region with cystic areas. The abnormality was isointense on T1 and hyperintense on T2 with multiple flow voids and peripheral enhancement. Bilateral renal masses were just visible on the edge of the MR images. What is the most likely diagnosis?

a Renal cyst with astrocytoma

b Von Hippel-Lindau syndrome with haemangioblastoma and renal cell carcinomas

c Neurofibromatosis with renal cysts and spinal neurofibromas

d Metastatic breast cancer

e Arteriovenous malformation with myelolipomas

65 Regarding *Cytomegalovirus* (CMV) in human immunodeficiency virus, which of the following statements is correct?

a CMV infections are the result of primary infection

b CMV infections most commonly affect the nervous system

c It rarely occurs with other opportunistic infections

d CMV infections can cause a brachial plexus neuropathy

e Causes periventricular calcification

66 A newborn girl was found at birth to have a hairy naevus overlying the sacral region and an imperforate anus. She underwent an ultrasound of her spine. The conus was found to lie at L4 and the filum terminale measured 4 mm in diameter. What is the most likely diagnosis?

a Caudal regression syndrome

b Tethered cord

c Diastematomyelia

d VACTRL

e Spinal bifida occulta

67 A 35-year-old female was being investigated for bilateral lower limb neurology. On plain film X-ray she was found to have bilateral pars defect with a 50% spondylolisthesis. MR was performed which did not demonstrate any neural foraminal narrowing or nerve root impingement. What investigation would you suggest was performed next?

a Axial T2-weighted brain

b Coronal FLAIR brain

c Nerve conduction studies

d Psychiatric opinion

e Flexion extension views of lumbar spine

68 An 18-year-old boy was involved in a road traffic accident. He had multiple injuries and one month after his accident he still had a right T1 nerve root palsy. MRI of the brachial plexus was normal. A further MRI study of his cervicothoracic spine was performed which showed an absent right T1 nerve root. No conjoint roots were seen at C7 or T2. There was a small, well-defined area of CSF signal at the right T1 neural exit foramina. What is the most likely diagnosis?

a Lateral myelomeningocele

b Traumatic nerve root avulsion

c Tarlov cyst

d Neurogenic cyst

e Synovial cyst from the facet joint

69 A 55-year-old woman was being investigated for right lower limb weakness. On MRI there was a well-defined high signal cystic area in the right S1 lateral recess. There was expansion of the right S1 neural canal with bone scalloping. Nerve roots are visualised along the wall of the cyst. What is the most likely diagnosis?

a Tarlov cyst

b Myelomeningocele

c Schwannoma of right S1 nerve root

d Pilocytic astrocytoma

e Haematoma

70 Regarding carotid artery Doppler, what features help differentiate the external carotid artery from the internal carotid artery?

a There are no branches arising from the external carotid artery

b Usually larger than the internal carotid artery

c The external carotid artery is orientated posterolaterally towards the mastoid process

d Low resistance flow pattern is seen

e Early diastolic flow reversal

Neuroradiology, head and neck and ENT radiology

PAPER 3

1   A 30-year-old woman saw her GP with increasing toothache. She was referred to the local hospital for a formal OPG. This demonstrated a mixed lytic and sclerotic mass centred on the apex of the right lower canine. What is the likely diagnosis?
   a Odontogenic cyst
   b Apical cyst
   c Cementoma
   d Brown tumour
   e Metastasis

2   A multilocular cystic lesion with expansile scalloped margins is seen lying adjacent to the right lower first molar on an OPG of a 30-year-old woman. The cyst has thin septated margins and the root of the molar is absorbed. What is the likely diagnosis?
   a Brown tumour
   b Metastasis
   c Dentigerous cyst
   d Apical cyst
   e Ameloblastoma

3   A 65-year-old known arteriopath was admitted via the emergency eye clinic with new onset right-sided homonymous hemianopia (hemianopsia). What part of the optic pathway is most likely to be affected?
   a Left optic tract
   b Right primary visual cortex
   c Right optic radiation
   d Optic chiasm
   e Left optic nerve

4 A 42-year-old female is seen in the emergency eye clinic with a left-sided proptosis and chemosis. What features on imaging make thyroid eye disease more likely than pseudotumour?

a Intraconal fat haziness

b Enhancement of the fat

c Thickening and enhancement of Tenon's capsule (fascia bulbi)

d Lacrimal gland enlargement

e Swelling limited to the muscle bellies of the recti muscles

5 A 44-year-old hyperthyroid woman develops chemosis, proptosis and lid lag affecting the right eye. She underwent a CT. Which orbital muscle is the most commonly affected?

a Lateral rectus

b Superior rectus

c Medial rectus

d Inferior oblique

e Inferior rectus

6 A 34-year-old male with known Burkitt's lymphoma has a new right-sided proptosis. Where is the most likely site of the lymphomatous deposit?

a Rectus muscles

b Bony destruction of the sphenoid wing

c Intraconal

d Intraorbital

e Lacrimal gland

7 A 76-year-old man with deranged liver enzymes underwent an MRI for investigation of a possible cerebrovascular event. On T1-weighted MR he was noted to have an incidental 0.5-cm high-signal lesion in his right choroid. Apart from age-related small-vessel changes within the periventricular white matter the rest of the MRI was within normal limits. What is the most likely diagnosis?

a Haemorrhagic cysts

b Choroidal lipomas

c Kayser-Fleischer rings

d Melanoma

e Foreign body

8 A patient with suspected Alzheimer's presents with memory impairment, personality change and mild but definite cogwheel rigidity. The referrer is keen to start Alzheimer's therapy soon due to the high clinical suspicion and success rate of early therapy. Out of the following options, which is the best investigation to ensure therapy will not exacerbate a Parkinsonian crisis?

a CT scan

b DaTSCAN

c Tc-99m HMPAO brain scan

d MRI scan

e PET-CT with FDG

9 An 18-month-old child with Turner's syndrome presented to the paediatric outpatient department following the sudden appearance of a large fluctuant mass in the posterior triangle of the neck. An MRI study revealed a multi-loculated mass posterior to sternocleidomastoid on the left side, which was hypointense on T1-weighted imaging and of increased signal intensity on a T2-weighted sequence. CT scan showed the lesion to be hypodense. What is the most likely diagnosis?

a Branchial cleft cyst

b Cystic hygroma

c Ranula

d Thyroglossal duct cyst

e Leiomyoma

10 A 24-year-old patient presented with a painless lump in the right submandibular region, which had been present for three years and had been gradually increasing in size, now measuring 1.5 cm. A FNA revealed features suggestive of a submandibular pleomorphic adenoma. What are the most likely imaging characteristics?

a Isointense to muscle on T1W MRI

b Hypointense to muscle on T2W

c Poor enhancement post gadolinium

d A smooth margin

e Areas of calcification on CT

11 A 14-year-old female exhibited painless facial asymmetry, which had been progressing since birth and for which she had undergone multiple surgical procedures with reconstruction. CT findings revealed expansion of the medullary cavity of the left maxillary bone with a 'ground-glass' appearance. The skull base was also imaged and the neural foramina were not involved. The lesion was hypointense on both T1- and T2-weighted images. What is the most likely diagnosis?

a Paget's disease

b Noonan's syndrome

c Ossifying fibroma

d Fibrous dysplasia

e Osteogenesis imperfecta

12 The posterior triangle of the neck is divided anatomically into the supraclavicular and occipital triangles by which structure?

    a Posterior belly of digastric

    b Inferior belly of omohyoid

    c Vagus nerve

    d Anterior scalene

    e Clavicular head of sternocleidomastoid

13 A 68-year-old male with no previous psychiatric history was referred with declining memory and confusion. A CT showed patchy low density in the deep white matter with marked generalised atrophy and multiple small well-defined areas of low density, which lacked mass effect. He was then referred for a radionuclide HMPAO scan which demonstrated reduced perfusion to the superior parieto-temporal cortices bilaterally. What is the most likely diagnosis?

    a Frontotemporal dementia with concurrent vascular disease

    b Alzheimer's disease/DLB (dementia of the Lewy body type) probably secondary to vascular pathology

    c A mixed pattern of Alzheimer's/DLB type and vascular dementia

    d Drug-induced Parkinson's disease

    e Mesial temporal sclerosis

14 A 42-year-old smoker presented with right arm weakness and left-sided ptosis with a constricted left pupil. A contrast-enhanced CT of his neck was performed. What is the most likely appearance of the carotid arteries?

    a Normal appearance on left

    b Luminal narrowing on left

    c Double lumen sign on right

    d Double lumen sign on left

    e Luminal narrowing on right

15 A 66-year-old man with a history of chronic schizophrenia, for which he receives medication, presents to the neurologists with recent onset tremor and apathy. A DaTSCAN shows bilateral 'comma-shaped' tracer uptake in the striatal pathways. CT shows ill-defined low density in the periventricular deep white matter with a mild degree of atrophy. What is the most appropriate preliminary diagnosis at this stage?

    a Idiopathic Parkinson's disease

    b Vascular dementia

    c Drug-induced Parkinsonian syndrome

    d Early-onset Alzheimer's disease

    e Depression

16 A 59-year-old lady is being investigated for hypercalcaemia after being referred with general malaise, weight loss and bone pain. A whole body bone scan demonstrates markedly increased and diffuse tracer uptake in the appendicular skeleton with increased bone to soft tissue ratio and absent renal uptake. Plain films show speckled soft-tissue calcification. An ultrasound of the neck shows a small low-reflectivity lesion posterior to the right lobe of the thyroid. What is the likely explanation for the bone scan appearances?

a Hyperparathyroidism secondary to parathyroid adenoma
b Widespread metastases with metastatic deposits in nodes in the neck
c Renal osteodystrophy
d Myeloproliferative disease
e Hyperthyroidism with a multinodular goitre

17 A 55-year-old woman is being treated for hyperthyroidism using I131. How soon after it is ingested should imaging be performed?

a Within 30 minutes
b 1–2 hours
c 6 hours
d 24 hours
e One week

18 A 28-year-old man presents to Accident and Emergency following trauma to the nasal bridge and upper maxilla. Examination revealed the maxilla to be displaced posteriorly causing an anterior bite. Facial views reveal a fracture line extending across the nasofrontal and frontomaxillary sutures. On CT the fracture passes through the medial wall of the orbit, through the nasolac-rimal groove and ethmoid bones and along the floor and lateral orbital wall to the zygomaticofrontal junction and the zygomatic arch. A branch of the fracture extends through ethmoid, vomer, pterygoid plates and to the base of the sphenoid. What type of fracture is this?

a Le Fort I fracture
b Le Fort II fracture
c Le Fort III fracture
d Orbital blow out fracture
e Tripod fracture

19 A 23-year-old man presents to the Emergency Department following a fight, is assessed and diagnosed with a right-sided tripod fracture. No other facial fractures are apparent. How many of McGrigor's lines are disrupted?

a None
b 1
c 2
d 3
e 4

20 A 58-year-old man presented with a two-year history of a painless palpable swelling in the region of his left parotid. On examination the mass was mobile and superficial to his facial nerve. Imaging with MR revealed a septated well-defined mass in the parotid tail. On T1-weighted sequences it was of low signal relative to the parotid gland and enhanced with contrast. On T2-weighted imaging the mass was of heterogeneously high signal. What is the most likely diagnosis?

a Warthin's tumour

b Siladenitis

c Lipoma

d Mucoepidermoid carcinoma

e Sjögren's syndrome

21 A 60-year-old woman presents with a painless mastoid swelling. Investigations reveal a mixed hearing loss. CT shows a coarsening of the trabeculae with cortical expansion and thickening. What is the most likely diagnosis?

a Paget's disease

b Osteomyelitis of skull base

c Ossifying fibroma

d Polyostotic fibrous dysplasia

e Monostotic fibrous dysplasia

22 A 35-year-old pregnant female with a family history of deafness presented with accelerated hearing loss. Otological examination was unremarkable and audiological assessment confirmed a mixed hearing loss primarily affecting the higher frequencies. A working diagnosis of cochlear otosclerosis was postulated. What classical finding would you expect to see on CT?

a A ring of low density around the cochlea

b Hypersclerosis of a poorly pneumatised mastoid

c Ossification of the oval window

d Hypodense opacity of the mesotympanum without bony erosion

e Ossicular destruction and bony scalloping

23 A 40-year-old male presents to his GP with a gradual onset of increasing dizziness. Investigations in the ENT clinic reveal a sensorineural hearing loss and gradual hemifacial spasm. Imaging studies revealed a lesion in the cerebellopontine cistern with low T1 and high T2 signal similar to that of the CSF. It was of high signal on FLAIR sequences. What is the most likely diagnosis?

a Epidermoid

b Arachnoid cyst

c Cystic meningioma

    d Acoustic neuroma

    e CPA aneurysm

24 A 40-year-old patient has unilateral pulsatile tinnitus. Audiometry reveals a conductive hearing loss on that side, otoscopy shows a vascular retrotympanic mass lying behind the inferior tympanic membrane and CT reveals a tubular mass crossing the middle ear cavity from posterior to anterior with no associated bone changes, although there is an enlarged inferior tympanic canaliculus. What is the most likely diagnosis?

    a Aberrant internal carotid artery

    b Dehiscent jugular bulb

    c Glomus tympanicum

    d Glomus jugulotympanicum

    e Cholesterol granuloma

25 A one-month-old hypotonic baby was morphologically abnormal. He had a cleft lip and hypotelorism. A CT demonstrated fused thalami, a large monoventricle, agenesis of the corpus callosum, absence of the falx cerebri and interhemispheric fissure. What further structure is most likely to be absent?

    a Pituitary

    b Septum pellucidum

    c Septum vergae

    d Olfactory nerves

    e Optic nerves

26 A 14-year-old boy with recurrent fits since birth undergoes an MRI. On T2-weighted images there is gyriform, low-signal intensity changes with associated atrophy affecting the left occipital lobe. On T1-weighted contrast enhanced images there is enhancement of the leptomeninges. What other feature is likely on MRI?

    a Right V1 venous angiomatous lesion

    b Left V2 venous angiomatous lesion

    c Left occipital skull vault thinning

    d Ipsilateral enlargement of the choroid plexus

    e Cavernoma

27 A 15-month-old child was being investigated for chronic fits. On T1- and T2-weighted MRI a grey matter cleft extends from the surface of the right temporal horn of the lateral ventricle to the parietal lobe cortex. CSF signal is seen within this cleft. The corpus callosum is present but the septum pellucidum is absent. What is the diagnosis?

a Open-lipped schizencephaly

b Lobar holoprosencephaly

c Porencephaly cyst

d Closed-lipped schizencephaly

e Burr hole track

28 A 26-month-old child had a skull X-ray as a part of skeletal survey for suspected non-accidental injury. Multiple intrasutural ossicles were seen. Which of the following should be considered?

a Scurvy

b Achondroplasia

c Turner's syndrome

d Down's syndrome

e Hurler's syndrome

29 A premature baby girl born at 28 weeks' gestation was intubated for respiratory distress. On day three a cranial USS showed right periventricular flare and hydrocephalus. A month later, on a repeat cranial USS, there was diffuse cystic changes in the right periventricular region with dilatation of the right lateral horn. What is the most likely diagnosis?

a Periventricular leukomalacia

b Porencephalic cyst

c Intraventricular haemorrhage

d Encephalitis

e Meningitis

30 A 23-year-old woman was undergoing an anomaly scan at 16 weeks' gestation. Her maternal alpha fetoprotein level was very high. An obstetric USS demonstrated the banana sign and the lemon sign. What is the most likely cause?

a Schizencephaly

b Holoprosencephaly

c Meningitis

d Neural tube defect

e Septo-optic dysplasia

31 A 38-year-old male with a known left parietal AVM presented with ataxia and progressive hearing loss. A CT (pre and post contrast) did not reveal any new abnormality apart from the known AVM. On the MRI T1- and T2-weighted

images showed cerebellar atrophy and FLAIR sequences revealed a hypointense rim along the cerebellar margins and the brainstem. What is the most likely diagnosis?

a Meningitis

b Chronic subarachnoid haemorrhage

c Leptomeningeal metastases

d Subdural abscess

e Meningiomatosis

32 A 55-year-old male was brought in unconscious following a house fire. He was intubated and had a CT head, which was unremarkable. Three days later he did not regain consciousness and an MRI head was performed. This showed low signal intensity on T1-weighted images and high signal on T2-weighted and FLAIR images within the medial portions of the globus pallidus bilaterally. What is the most likely diagnosis?

a Hypoxic ischaemic encephalopathy

b Carbon monoxide poisoning

c Central pontine myelinolysis

d Venous infarction

e Wilson's disease

33 A 55-year-old female was admitted with a short history of headache and drowsiness. She was found to be hypertensive with a BP of 220/140. On ophthalmoscopy she was found to have grade IV papilloedema. PRES (posterior reversible encephalopathy syndrome) was suspected clinically. What features would be expected on CT?

a Periventricular low-density white matter changes perpendicular to the lateral ventricles

b Low-density white matter changes within the occipital lobes

c Intraparenchymal haemorrhage affecting the basal ganglia

d Low-density changes affecting the cerebellar white and grey matter

e Diffuse bilateral asymmetrical perivenous low-density changes

34 A 53-year-old patient underwent investigation for an incidental neck lump. CT demonstrated a 1-cm lesion at the carotid bifurcation, which was a homogenous lesion with avid post-contrast enhancement. A typical salt and pepper appearance was seen on MRI. What is the most likely diagnosis?

a Schwannoma

b Carotid body tumour

c Branchial cyst

d Glomus tumour

e Neurofibroma

35 A 35-year-old woman presented with headaches and left-sided weakness. CT showed hyperdense venous sinuses. On MRI there was high signal within the superior sagittal, straight and right transverse venous sinuses. What further complication is she at most risk of?

   a Bilateral thalamic infarcts

   b Bacterial abscess

   c Right middle cerebral artery infarct

   d Basal meningitis

   e Right cerebellar infarction

36 A 40-year-old man was making a good recovery following drainage of post-traumatic large-volume extra-axial bleeds. He suddenly deteriorated 24 hours following surgery and a repeat CT did not demonstrate re-accumulation of the bleeds. Bilateral tentorial hygromas were seen. MR showed inferior displacement of the midbrain and crowding of the suprasellar cistern. Following contrast there was strong enhancement of the dura. What is the most likely diagnosis?

   a Meningitis

   b Subarachnoid haemorrhage

   c Cerebral hypotension

   d Diffuse cerebral oedema

   e Venous sinus thrombosis

37 A 42-year-old female presented with intractable facial pain. A diagnosis of trigeminal neuralgia was considered and an MRI was performed. On high resolution CISS sequences, vascular contact with the root entry zone was evident. Which vessel is most likely involved?

   a Superior cerebellar artery

   b Posterior inferior cerebellar artery

   c Anterior inferior cerebellar artery

   d Basilar artery

   e Vertebral artery

38 A young male presented with symptoms of neck pain and ipsilateral headache following a weekend of rock climbing. Signs of ipsilateral Horner's syndrome were also elicited. Following an MRI, a diagnosis of carotid artery dissection was made. Which segment of the carotid artery is most likely to be involved?

   a Cervical segment

   b Petrous segment

   c Lacerum segment

   d Cavernous segment

   e Supraclinoid segment

39 A 56-year-old man was investigated for intermittent arm claudication and gait problems. A recent Doppler scan performed as part of an insurance check up had shown no disease in the carotids but did show flow reversal in the left vertebral artery. An angiogram was performed which revealed occlusive disease in the left subclavian artery origin with flow reversal in the ipsilateral vertebral artery on delayed images. What is the most appropriate treatment?

a Open endarterectomy

b Endovascular endarterectomy

c Surgical bypass with vein graft

d Balloon angioplasty

e Endovascular stent placement

40 A 25-year-old homosexual man went to a GUM clinic with penile warts. He reported having unprotected sex with multiple casual partners. An HIV test was positive and his CD4 count was 300. He complained of painless swelling of his parotid glands and a MRI was performed. What would you expect to see?

a Diffuse generalised enlargement of the parotid glands

b Multiple normal-sized lymph nodes

c Diffuse heterogeneous low signal with increase vascularity

d Multiple bilateral small cysts within both parotid glands

e Diffusely enlarged glands with microcalcification.

41 A 14-year-old girl presented after her parents became aware that her walking was slower than usual and she kept tripping over. On examination she had an ataxic gait and bilateral reduction in toe proprioception. MRI brain and spinal cord were performed and showed atrophy of the cervical spinal cord without evidence of cerebellar atrophy. Which of the following is the most likely diagnosis?

a Ataxia telangiectasia

b Guillain-Barré syndrome

c Multiple sclerosis

d Friedreich's ataxia

e Joubert syndrome

42 A 15-month-old child was placed under the care of social services for sus-
    pected child abuse. She had had a CT scan aged six months, which was
    normal. A repeat CT scan demonstrated a defect in the right temporal bone
    with indistinct scalloped margins and a prominent CSF space lying adja-
    cent to it. There was right temporal encephalomalacia. What is the likely
    diagnosis?

    a Dermoid cyst
    b Lacunar skull
    c New fracture
    d Leptomeningeal cyst
    e Accessory suture

43 A five-month-old baby girl was admitted fitting. On non-contrast CT head
    a crescent-shaped extra-axial mixed-density collection was seen. No history
    was forthcoming from the parents. What other pathology would most help
    you to clinch the diagnosis?

    a Subconjunctival haemorrhage
    b Metaphyseal corner fracture of the tibia
    c Diffuse periosteal reaction of the tibia
    d Anterior rib fractures
    e Bruising to the forehead

44 A three-month-old baby presents with intractable crying and respiratory dis-
    tress. The patient has a facial CT scan, which shows a bony septum extending
    across the posterior choanae. Which of the following additional features are
    likely to be seen?

    a 5-mm-wide posterior choanae
    b Outward bowing of the posterior maxilla
    c Thickening of the vomer
    d Absence of the vomer
    e 1-cm-wide posterior choanae

45 A 46-year-old HIV-positive female with a CD4 count of 40cells/cu mm
    was admitted with a month's history of progressive confusion. A MRI was
    performed which demonstrated bilateral, asymmetrical patchy white mat-
    ter changes with no mass effect or enhancement. What is the most likely
    diagnosis?

    a Progressive multifocal leukoencephalopathy
    b Toxoplasmosis
    c Lymphoma
    d HIV encephalopathy
    e CMV

46 A 27-year-old HIV positive man was admitted with increasing confusion and lethargy. He had a CD4 count of 150 but had no history of an AIDS-defining illness. Cross-sectional imaging of the head was performed. What features make a diagnosis of toxoplasmosis more likely than lymphoma?

    a Corpus callosum involved

    b Haemorrhage on CT

    c Basal ganglia lesions

    d Single lesion

    e Subependymal spread

47 A four-year-old boy was being investigated for short stature and diabetes insipidus. On CT there was a rounded cystic solid mass with some peripheral calcification in the suprasellar cistern with peripheral enhancement after administration of iodinated contrast. What is the most likely diagnosis?

    a Pituitary adenoma

    b Germinoma

    c Optic chiasm glioma

    d Craniopharyngioma

    e Rathke's cleft cyst

48 A 35-year-old male was investigated for worsening progressive headache. On CT there was a 5 × 6-cm cystic solid mass with heavy nodular calcification affecting the left frontal lobe. The tumour extended to the cortical surface with associated erosion of the calvarium. There was peripheral enhancement following administration of contrast. What is the likely diagnosis?

    a Mucinous adenocarcinoma

    b Oligodendroglioma

    c Meningioma

    d Post-radiation changes

    e Glioblastoma multiforme

49 A six-year-old female child complained of a worsening headache and vomiting. On CT there was hydrocephalus and a lobulated soft-tissue mass in the trigone of the right lateral ventricle, which enhanced brightly with contrast. What is the cause for the hydrocephalus?

    a Overproduction of CSF

    b Obstruction at the foramen of Monro

    c Reduced absorption

    d Obstructing hydrocephalus

    e Obstruction at the foramen of Luschka

50 A 45-year-old male was being investigated for reduced hearing on the left. The left internal auditory canal was expanded by a soft-tissue mass, which extended into the left cerebellopontine angle. There was minor calcification and the mass showed strongly enhanced following IV contrast. What is the most likely diagnosis?

   a Meningioma

   b Acoustic neuroma

   c Epidermoid

   d Metastasis

   e Arachnoid cyst

51 A 56-year-old man was being investigated for a right seventh nerve palsy. On CT there was a lobulated heterogeneous hypodense mass extending across from the prepontine cistern to the right cerebellopontine angle mass causing compression of the right side of the pons. The mass was slightly hyperdense relative to CSF. What is the most common signal characteristics of this mass on MRI?

   a High signal on T1 and low signal on T2

   b Low signal on T1 and low signal on T2

   c Low signal on T1 and high signal on T2

   d High signal on T1 and high signal on T2

   e Intermediate signal on T1 and T2

52 A 32-year-old Caucasian female was scanned following worsening weakness of the lower limbs. Several discrete oval and round lesions were identified in the periventricular white matter perpendicular to the ventricles on MRI. A sample of CSF confirmed the diagnosis made on MRI. Which of the following is not a usual feature of this condition?

   a Cortical lesions

   b Haemorrhage

   c Ring enhancement

   d Corpus callosal involvement

   e Periventricular extension

53 A middle-aged alcoholic man was admitted with a reduced level of consciousness and quadriplegia. He had been discharged a few days earlier when he was noted to have a low sodium. On the most recent admission he had a CT, which appeared normal. A MRI, however, demonstrated a butterfly-shaped area of high signal in the pons on T2 and FLAIR images. Similar lesions were also seen in the thalami. What is the most likely diagnosis?

   a Brainstem glioma

   b Central pontine myelinolysis

   c Multiple sclerosis

d Gliomatosis cerebri

e Venous infarction

54 A 22 year old with widespread cutaneous lesions, axillary freckling and multiple café au lait spots is known to have a neurocutaneous syndrome. What abnormality would you be most likely see on CT?

a Optic nerve glioma

b Acoustic schwannoma

c Haemangioblastoma

d Subependymal astrocytoma

e Subependymal nodules

55 A 43-year-old male underwent an MRI for evaluation of hearing loss. In the right cerebellopontine angle there was a well-defined mass, which was low signal on T1, high signal on T2 and low signal on FLAIR with an intensity similar to CSF. There was scalloping of the bony margins. What would you expect the signal characteristics to be on diffusion weighted imaging?

a Low signal

b Similar signal to fat

c High signal

d Intermediate signal

e Similar signal to the ADC map

56 You are called to perform a cranial ultrasound on a neonate who has been critically ill after birth with low APGAR scores. The baby has not progressed as expected and is lethargic and less responsive than hoped. On the ultrasound, in the coronal view, a line of hyper-reflective dots is seen under the lateral ventricles. Which of the following is the most likely diagnosis?

a Tuberous sclerosis

b Congenital toxoplasmosis infection

c Periventricular infarcts

d Rubella

e Congenital *Cytomegalovirus* infection

57 A six-year-old girl with a repaired myelomeningocele at birth and hydrocephalus had an MRI scan to check the position of her V-P shunt. Sagittal T1 and T2 images demonstrated a small posterior fossa with tectal beaking and a cervicomedullary kink. What finding in the cervical spine would account for any recent onset of neurological symptoms?

a Cervical astrocytoma

b Syringomyelia

c Epidural abscess

d Neurofibroma

e Vertebral collapse

58 An MRI of the thoracolumbar spine in a 26 year old showed multilevel anterior vertebral scalloping. Which of the following conditions is likely to be a cause?

  a Neurofibromatosis type 1
  b Ehlers-Danlos syndrome
  c Marfan's syndrome
  d Down's syndrome
  e Morquio syndrome

59 A 29-year-old heroin addict presented with sudden onset left-sided leg pain. An X-ray of the lumbar spine was performed followed by an MRI, which confirmed the clinical suspicion of infective spondylitis. What features would you expect on the MRI?

  a Narrowing of the disc space with high signal in the adjacent vertebral bodies on T1-weighted images
  b Narrowing of the disc space with high signal in the adjacent vertebral bodies on T2-weighted images
  c Widening of the disc space with high signal in the adjacent vertebral bodies on T1-weighted images
  d Widening of the disc space with high signal in the adjacent vertebral bodies on T2-weighted images
  e None of the above

60 A 20-year-old man had progressive upper and lower limb weakness, worse in the lower limbs. On MR there was widening of the spinal canal with posterior vertebral scalloping between D3 and D7. On T1- and T2-weighted imaging a well-defined high-intensity mass was present anterior to the spinal cord with atrophy of the cord at this level. The CSF space was slightly expanded immediately superior to the mass. No high signal was present in the cord on T2. What is the most likely diagnosis?

  a Epidural abscess
  b Epidural haematoma
  c Neuroma
  d Neurogenic cyst
  e Meningioma

61 A 54-year-old female was scanned following insidious onset of bilateral leg weakness. MRI of the thoracolumbar spine revealed gibbus deformity centred at T10. Destructive changes were seen involving both anterior and posterior elements above and below this level with loss of vertebral body and intervertebral disc height. An epidural abscess was seen tracking down to L1 level. What is the most likely diagnosis?

  a Brucellosis
  b *Tuberculosis*

c Pyogenic spondylitis

d *Actinomycosis*

e Herpes simplex virus

62 Following surgery for a herniated L4/L5 disc a 66-year-old obese patient had little symptomatic relief. An MRI scan performed in the second post-operative week revealed extradural soft-tissue material within the spinal canal, which demonstrated little enhancement following contrast. Nerve root enhancement was striking. What is the most likely diagnosis?

a Arachnoiditis

b Epidural haematoma

c Residual disc material

d Epidural fibrosis

e Neuritis

63 A 46 year old undergoing a CT of the abdomen and pelvis for small bowel pathology was noted to have an abnormal-looking T10 vertebral body. This demonstrated some expansion with internal lucencies and areas of coarse trabeculation; the posterior elements were spared. An X-ray of the spine demonstrated vertical striations at this level. What is the most likely diagnosis?

a Haemangioma

b Osteoid osteoma

c Giant cell tumour

d Osteoblastoma

e ABC

64 A 35-year-old woman with a known spondylolysis and 50% spondylolisthesis presented with new onset lower limb weakness. She had an episode of vertigo six months previously, which had resolved. MRI of the spine demonstrated the spondylolisthesis and bilateral pars defects, but no cause for the symptoms was found. On flexion extension films the spondylolisthesis was found to be stable. What would be the next investigation you would suggest to the clinician?

a Lumbar puncture

b CT brain

c MRI brain

d Nerve conduction studies

e Repeat the MR in six months

65 A 12-year-old with a webbed neck, low hairline and a decreased range of neck movement underwent a CT of the cervicothoracic spine for surgical planning. Clinically, a diagnosis of Klippel-Feil syndrome had been made. Which of the following would not be an expected feature on the scan?

a Fusion of two or more vertebrae

b Raised and rotated scapula

c Paravertebral ossification

d Omovertebral bar

e Spinal stenosis

66 A 38-year-old male had a long history of back stiffness and restricted movement. Spinal X-rays followed by a CT of the thoracolumbar spine revealed flowing calcifications and ossifications along the right anterolateral aspect of the T7–T11 vertebral bodies. Disc spaces appeared preserved. What is the most likely diagnosis?

a Ankylosing spondylitis

b Diffuse idiopathic skeletal hyperostosis

c Reiter's disease

d Psoriatic arthritis

e Primary osteoarthritis

67 A 60-year-old man was being investigated for progressive bilateral leg weakness. An MR lumbar spine was performed on which multiple tortuous tubes with signal voids on the posterior aspect of the cauda equine were visible on both T1- and T2-weighted images. Subtle bumps were seen along the surface of the cord. The conus was expanded with high signal within it on T2. What is the likely diagnosis?

a Epidural haematoma

b Epidural abscess

c Cavernoma

d Spinal dural arteriovenous fistula

e Spinal cord arteriovenous malformation

68 A 55-year-old woman complained of left retro-orbital pain and double vision. On examination she was found to have left III, IV and VI nerve palsies. She has no past medical history and is otherwise well. Imaging demonstrated abnormalities in the ipsilateral cavernous sinus and superior orbital fissure. What is the most likely diagnosis?

a Moyamoya

b Ramsay Hunt syndrome

c Herpes simples encephalitis

d Tolosa-Hunt syndrome

e Sarcoidosis

69 An unwell 60-year-old man who is being treated for a large diverticular abscess was witnessed to have a grand mal seizure. He has felt generally tired recently and has a past medical history of colonic carcinoma for which he had an extended right hemicolectomy and hemihepatectomy. An MRI scan of his brain is performed which shows a ring enhancing lesion. What imaging features would favour this lesion being a metastasis rather than an abscess?

a Cerebellar location

b Restricted diffusion on DWI

c Uniformly thick enhancing wall

d Thinning of the medial wall of the lesion

e Vasogenic oedema

70 A 27-year-old female with AIDS presented with a fit and following further investigations, including CT and MRI scans, her symptoms were felt to be attributable to HIV encephalitis. Which region of her brain is most likely to be abnormal on the MRI scan?

a Anteroinferior aspects of the temporal lobes

b White matter of the centrum semiovale

c Corpus striatum (putamen and caudate nuclei)

d Superior cerebellar peduncles

e Hypothalamus

Genito-urinary, adrenal, obstetric, gynaecological and breast radiology

PAPER 1: ANSWERS AND EXPLANATIONS

1 Answer C: Adrenal adenoma

Adrenal adenomas are common, occurring in 1–2% of the population. On unenhanced CT examination if the HU <10 this is 96% specific for adrenal adenoma and in the delayed phase (10–15 minutes after contrast medium) if there is 60% washout or more then diagnosis of adenoma is 97% specific.

2 Answer B: Unenhanced and delayed phase CT examination

Even in a patient with lung carcinoma a small adrenal mass is more likely to be an adenoma than a metastasis (approximately 60–70%) and therefore investigation is to prove if it is an adenoma. If it is not fat containing with washout on CT then PET examination or biopsy may need to be performed.

Boland G, Blake M, Hahn PH, *et al.* Incidental adrenal lesions: principles, techniques and algorithms for imaging characterization. *Radiology*. 2008; **249**(3): 756–75.

3 Answer D: Wolman's disease

Wolman's disease is a very rare autosomal recessive (AR) lipoidosis in which the findings described are typical. It is almost always fatal in the first year of life.

4 Answer A: Myelolipoma

Adrenal myelolipoma are fatty-tissue masses with HU of −30 to −115. Acute retroperitoneal haemorrhage occurs in approximately 12%.

5 Answer A: CT examination with adrenal protocol (unenhanced and delayed phases)

Conn's syndrome is caused by hyperaldosteronism most commonly from a hyperfunctioning adrenocortical adenoma but also can be from bilateral adrenal hyperplasia or adrenocortical carcinoma. These adenomas can be very small and both CT and MRI techniques have been used but CT is currently the most popular technique for detection of adenomas.

Lingam R, Sohaib S, Vlahos I, *et al.* CT of hyperaldosteronism (Conn's syndrome): the value of measuring the adrenal gland. *Am J Roentgenol.* 2003; **181**(3): 843–9.

6 Answer B: Locate an extra-adrenal phaeochromocytoma

MIBG is indicated in the investigation of phaeochromocytoma where there is clear clinical/laboratory evidence of tumour but no adrenal abnormality on CT or MRI. MIBG is also positive for neuroblastoma, carcinoid tumour, paraganglioma, medullary thyroid carcinoma and ganglioneuroma.

7 Answer D: Adrenal haemorrhage

Stress increases secretion of adrenocorticotropic hormone (ACTH), which increases adrenal vascularity and subsequent intraglandular haemorrhage. Surgery, sepsis (Waterhouse-Friderichsen syndrome), burns, hypotension, pregnancy, cardiovascular disease and steroids are all associated with non-traumatic adrenal haemorrhage.

8 Answer E: 1.5 per 100 women over five years

The relative risk is the ratio of the absolute risk of the event occurring in those exposed to the absolute risk in those not exposed. In this example those not exposed have an absolute risk of 1.5 and the relative risk is 2, hence the absolute risk increase is also 1.5.

9 Answer C: Perform ultrasound and ultrasound-guided core needle biopsy if a solid lesion is visible

Although this lesion has the features of a fibroadenoma, ultrasound cannot reliably distinguish between a well-circumscribed carcinoma and a fibroadenoma. Usually, histological confirmation of the benign lesion is made via ultrasound-guided core biopsy. In individual cases, some patients may opt for excisional biopsy without prior biopsy.

10 Answer E: A hyperechoic posterior wall

Strict ultrasound criteria for a simple cyst include well-circumscribed margins, round/oval shape, absence of internal echoes, through transmission and posterior acoustic enhancement with a bright posterior wall.

11 Answer D: Demonstration of eggshell calcification

Both lesions may appear as rounded lucent lesions with a surrounding capsule on mammography. A history of recent lactation and multiple areas of fatty and fibroglandular density would make a galactocoele more likely.

12 Answer C: Upper outer quadrant

Fifty per cent of all breast cancers arise in the upper outer quadrant, which usually contains the most glandular tissue in the breast. The second most common site is the retroareolar region where 18% of cases arise.

13 Answer C: Bone

Most common sites of initial distant metastasis from breast cancer are bone (58%), lung and pleura (26%), and lymph nodes other than ipsilateral axillary nodes (16%). Initial involvement of the liver or brain is less frequent.

14 Answer C: Every six months for the first two years and annually thereafter

Exact follow-up regimes may vary from centre to centre, according to local policy. In patients treated with radiotherapy mammography skin thickening post-irradiation usually decreases within two years following treatment but may persist longer.

15 Answer C: An increase in size in the post-menopausal period, in the absence of HRT

Cyst margins may be completely or partially defined (or even completely obscured) by adjacent fibroglandular breast tissue. Cysts frequently disappear or subside following menopause. Peripheral eggshell calcification is seen in fat necrosis. Tea cup calcification, seen on the floor of the cyst on an erect lateral film, may be seen in cysts containing milk of calcium (rare).

16 Answer A: Ductal carcinoma

Ductal carcinoma accounts for the majority of invasive breast cancers and lobular carcinoma approximately 5–10%. Medullary and mucinous account for around 2% each and <1% of cases are of sarcomatous origin.

17 Answer D: Linear, branching

See discussion for Q.18 below.

18 Answer A: <0.5 mm

Microcalcifications are defined as individual calcific opacities <0.5 mm in diameter. Characteristics suspicious of malignancy include a casting shape, linear, segmental and clustered distribution. Other non-specific characteristics that increase the degree of suspicion include pleomorphism, variation in size, increased density for size, irregular margins, irregular boundaries of the area of calcification, many calcifications per square centimetre (>5/cu cm). Scattered small calcifications bilaterally with radiolucent centres are typical of calcified sebaceous glands of the skin, but may present as a localised cluster of calcification. Irregular coarse 'popcorn' calcification may be seen within a fibroadenoma. Calcification within a fibroadenoma is typically peripheral but may be centrally or eccentrically situated, as may be seen in carcinoma.

19 Answer D: Lymphoma, melanoma, ovarian carcinoma, lung carcinoma

In that order of frequency. Sarcoma can also metastasise to the breast.

20 Answer C

(a) Type 2 curve. (b) Type 1a curve. (d) Type 1b curve. Malignant lesions are associated with a type 3 (approximately 60%) or type 2 curve (approximately 30%). (e) consistent with a benign lesion.

Morris E, Liberman L. *Breast MRI Diagnosis and Intervention.* New York, NY: Springer-Verlag; 2005.

21 Answer E: Phyllodes tumour

Causes of large (>5 cm) well-defined opacities include the following: giant cyst, giant fibroadenoma, lipoma, sebaceous cyst, cystosarcoma phyllodes.

22 Answer C: XXY

This is Klinefelter's syndrome in which there is a 20-fold increased risk of male breast cancer. 45 X0 (Turners) and 47 XXX (triple X) are females. 46 XY is normal and 47 XY 13 is a male with Patau's syndrome (trisomy 13).

23 Answer D: Breast MRI

Breast MRI is indicated when there is an axillary metastasis but no primary is visible on mammography or clinical examination. It is also indicated in a number of other situations: dense breasts plus high risk lesion of LCIS, positive BRCA screen, assessment of response to neoadjuvant chemotherapy and suspected multifocal breast carcinoma. The sensitivity to DCIS is relatively poor.

24 Answer B: Non-visualisation of cardiac activity when crown–rump length (CRL) is 7 mm

At 6.5 weeks the CRL is approximately 5 mm and cardiac movement can be identified. The intradecidual sign is seen in intrauterine pregnancy. The gestational sac can be seen at the fundus from five weeks and is surrounded by an echogenic ring which can be asymmetric. The yolk sac is seen at approximately five to seven weeks when the gestational sac is 6–9 mm.

25 Answer B: CT followed by biopsy

In a patient with a clinical history, ultrasound findings and CA-125 level consistent with ovarian carcinoma, a staging CT examination should be the next investigation. As well as staging the patient this will also need a guided biopsy. Omental biopsy can be undertaken percutaneously via ultrasound or CT guidance but ovarian disease biopsy would usually have to be performed surgically. MRI of the pelvis is used in the investigation of an adnexal mass which is not definitely ovarian in origin as a problem-solving tool.

26 Answer D: Peritoneal metastases

FIGO Staging of Ovarian Carcinoma
Answer (a): FIGO stage IC
Answer (b): FIGO stage IIA

Answer (c): FIGO stage IIC
Answer (e): FIGO stage IV

27 Answer A: Endometrioma

Although ultrasound appearances can be variable approximately 95% of endometriomas demonstrate the above findings. They may be unilocular or multilocular with thick or thin septae. Rarely, they are anechoic, mimicking a functional ovarian cyst.

28 Answer B: Ovarian fibroma

Endometriosis is typically high signal on routine and fat-saturated T1 sequences due to methaemoglobin. Similarly, a haemorrhagic mass would be expected to be bright on T1. Dermoids often contain fat which is high signal on routine T1 sequences and mucinous lesions can also be high signal but not as high as the T1 signal of fat and blood.

Mayo-Smith W, Lee M. MR imaging of the female pelvis. *Clin Radiol*. 1995; **50**(10): 667–76.

29 Answer E: Aching muscles

Occurrence in surgical scars, particularly after gynaecological surgery, is recognised. Catamenial pneumothorax occurring at the onset of menses as well as haemothorax and lung nodules can occur in the chest. In the bladder endometrial deposits can cause haematuria and often biopsy is required for definitive diagnosis. Malignant transformation is rare (<1%) and 75% of the malignancies arise from endometriosis of the ovary.

30 Answer C: Cervix

Normal FDG activity is seen in brain myocardium, liver, spleen, bone marrow, GI tract, testes and skeletal muscle. In the pelvis pitfalls of sites of increased uptake include cyclical uptake in the endometrium and ovaries, renal collecting system (ureters and bladder) and the blood pool.

Subhas N, Patel P, Pannu H, *et al*. Imaging of pelvic malignancies with in-line FDG PET-CT: case examples and common pitfalls of FDG-PET. *RadioGraphics*. 2005; **25**(4): 1031–43.

31 Answer D: Pelvic ultrasound examination after six weeks

Functional cysts are common, and benign features on ultrasound include unilocular thin-walled cysts with no solid component. If the cyst is larger than 3 cm, follow-up ultrasound at a different time in the menstrual cycle is recommended to ensure resolution.

32 Answer A: Endometrial

33 Answer E: Double decidual sac sign

The double decidual sac sign is seen at approximately five weeks of pregnancy and represents the inner rim of chorionic villi surrounded by a thin rim of fluid in the endometrial cavity which is surrounded by the echogenic decidua vera. The double decidua sign is highly reliable for intrauterine gestational sac. Note: intrauterine pregnancy does not exclude heterotopic (ectopic + coexistent intrauterine pregnancy) which occur in 1:6800–30 000 pregnancies.

Levine D. Ectopic pregnancy. *Radiology*. 2007; **245**(2): 385–97.

34 Answer D: Hypertension

Nulliparity is a risk factor as is unopposed oestrogen therapy and obesity.

35 Answer C: Referral to gynaecologist for Pipelle biopsy or hysteroscopy

Measurement of endometrial thickness post menopause: in a patient not on HRT <5 mm homogeneously echogenic, in a patient on HRT <8 mm. In premenopausal patients: menstrual phase (1–4 mm), proliferative phase (5–7 mm), periovulatory phase (up to 11 mm) and secretory phase (up to 16 mm). There are alternative diagnoses that increase endometrial thickness such as endometrial polyps and endometrial hyperplasia and therefore radiological staging is performed once there is a histological diagnosis.

Barwick T, Rockall A, Barton D *et al*. Imaging of endometrial adenocarcinoma. *Clin Radiol*. 2006; **61**(7): 545–55.

36 Answer C

On T2-weighted images three distinct layers can be seen: the endometrium is high signal, junctional zone is low signal and myometrium medium signal. On T1-weighted images the uterus is medium to low signal intensity.

Messiou C, Spencer J, Swift S. MR staging of endometrial carcinoma. *Clin Radiol*. 2006; **61**(10): 822–32.

37 Answer B: II

FIGO staging of endometrial carcinoma is stage II for cervical invasion irrelevant of the depth of myometrial invasion.

38 Answer B: Gestational trophoblastic disease

Gestational trophoblastic disease is a group of disorders that arise from aberrant fertilisation. The spectrum includes benign hydatidiform mole, invasive mole and choriocarcinoma. Maternal age >35 and <20 years, previous molar gestation and previous spontaneous abortion are risk factors.

Allen S, Lim A, Seckl M, *et al*. Radiology of gestation trophoblastic neoplasia. *Clin Radiol*. 2006; **61**(4): 301–13.

39 Answer A: Extracapsular extensions

MRI is used to demonstrate tumour location, extracapsular extension and seminal vesicle invasion. Answer a is T3a, b is T2b, c is T4, d is T2c, and e is T4.

40 Answer D: High signal on T1-weighted images in the peripheral zone

Haemorrhage is high signal on T1-weighted images and therefore can be distinguished from tumour.

41 Answer A: Testicular germ cell tumour

The findings show testicular microlithiasis which is also associated with Klinefelter's syndrome, cryptoorchidism, testicular infarcts, granulomas, infertility, male pseudohermaphroditism, Down's syndrome and alveolar microlithiasis

42 Answer E: Seminoma

Seminoma is the most common pure germ cell tumour and average age is 40.5 years.

43 Answer C: Epidermoid cyst

These are the typical ultrasound appearances of an epidermoid cyst, which is confined to the tunica albuginea.

44 Answer E: Lung

Metastases to the testis are more common than seminoma in a patient over the age of 50 years. The most common sites (in order of frequency) are prostate, lung, kidney, GI tract, bladder, thyroid, melanoma.

45 Answer A: Discharge the patient back to GP with no follow-up

These findings are consistent with an epididymal cyst, which is incidental to management.

46 Answer A: Normal grey-scale appearance of both testes at 12 hours

In acute testicular torsion the typical appearances are of decreased blood flow at one hour and absent blood flow after four hours, but remember that torsion-detorsion and incomplete torsion can give false negative appearances. In cryptoorchidism the testes are arrested along their line of development with a 10× increased risk of torsion. Normal grey-scale appearances of the testes can occur but changes in appearance usually occur after six hours of torsion.

47 Answer C: Staging CT examination

Staging CT examination of the chest, abdomen and pelvis is the most appropriate next step following urological referral.

48 Answer D: Anterior aspect of the base of the bladder

The site of rupture is usually close to the base of the bladder anterolaterally. On contrast examination a flame-shaped contrast extravasation into perivesical fat (best seen on post-void films), which may extend into the thigh or anterior abdominal wall. Eighty per cent of bladder ruptures are extraperitoneal. It is usually caused by penetration of the bladder by a bony spicule from a pelvic fracture or an avulsion tear at the fixation points of the puboprostatic ligaments. Plain film may demonstrate a 'pear-shaped bladder'. Other signs of extraperitoneal bladder rupture are loss of obturator fat planes, paralytic ileus and upward displacement of ileal loops on plain film. Intraperitoneal bladder rupture usually occurs as a result of an invasive procedure (cystoscopy), a stab wound or surgery; or due to blunt trauma.

49 Answer C. Bilateral ureteric obstruction and hydronephrosis from the bladder primary

Collecting system opacification is delayed because of the raised backpressure reducing ultrafiltration of contrast at the glomerulus. Delayed imaging will be required to demonstrate the level of obstruction. Urgent urological opinion should be sought as ureteric stenting or nephrostomies may be required to relieve the obstruction.

50 Answer D. Adrenaline (Epinephrine) 1:1000 0.5 mg intramuscular administration

Management of acute anaphylactoid reaction: Call for help. Secure airway and administer oxygen. Elevate patient's legs if hypotensive. Adrenaline 1:1000 intramuscularly followed by intravenous crystalloid fluid challenge, intravenous H_1 blocker and steroids.

51 Answer A: Unenhanced scan, followed by post-intravenous contrast scans acquired at 60 and 100 seconds

An unenhanced scan detects the presence of calcification, which may otherwise be obscured by contrast. The 60-second acquisition shows the corticomedullary phase, where there is differential enhancement of the cortex and the 100-second acquisition shows the nephrogram phase where the renal parenchyma uniformly enhances.

52 Answer D: Unenhanced CT abdomen and pelvis, performed prone with low mA dose protocol

Virtually all ureteric calculi, even those radiolucent on plain radiography, are detected by CT. A low mA dose protocol is performed without intravenous or oral contrast. The patient lies prone to distinguish between calculi at the vesico-ureteric junction and those that have already passed into the bladder; the latter will lie dependently within the bladder.

53 Answer B: The ureter from the superior pelvis inserts below that from the inferior pelvis, and the upper renal moiety has calyceal dilatation from distal ureteric obstruction

The upper moiety ureter classically inserts ectopically low, below that of the lower moiety, and it is often associated with a stenotic insertion site, which results in dilatation of the intramural ureter, forming an ectopic ureterocoele and subsequent distal ureteric obstruction. The lower moiety ureter has a more horizontal path and is more prone to reflux.

RULE: Upper moiety inserts low and obstructs. Lower moiety refluxes.

54 Answer D: Presence of internal calcification

AML >4 cm are symptomatic in >80%, and bleed spontaneously in 50–60%.

Intratumoural calcifications are virtually never present with AML. Rarely renal cell carcinoma can undergo osseous metaplasia with growth of fatty marrow and associated calcifications.

55 Answer D: Schistosomiasis infection (Bilharziasis)

Schistosoma haematobium is a trematode endemic in parts of Africa. Eggs are deposited in the submucosa of the bladder and ureters leading to granulomas, oedema and strictures. This can result in a fibrotic bladder, with mural calcification, and ureteric dilatation. Squamous cell carcinoma is a recognised complication.

The Candiru fish is found in the Amazon basin and may be able to enter the urethra where it becomes lodged.

56 Answer E: Inferior mesenteric artery

The inferior mesenteric artery limits the ascent of the isthmus, and the pelves lie anteriorly. Renal calculi are more common. Risk of TCC (transitional cell carcinoma) is three to four times the general population. Incidence of horseshoe kidney is 1–4:1000.

57 Answer B: Tuberous sclerosis

The description is of multiple bilateral large angiomyolipomas, which occur in 80% of patients with tuberous sclerosis, usually presenting by the age of 10 years. AML are also associated with neurofibromatosis type 1 and von Hippel-Lindau disease.

58 Answer B: CT abdomen and pelvis with intravenous contrast and instilled intravesical contrast

CT cystography is equivalent or better than standard cystography for detection of bladder injury and should be performed in patients already undergoing CT for pelvic fractures. 400 mL of 4% contrast can be instilled via a drip bladder infusion, and scans performed before and after bladder emptying.

59 Answer A: Renal lymphoma

Renal lymphoma is a common site for extra-nodal non-Hodgkin's lymphoma. It usually shows poorer enhancement than renal cortex in the nephrographic phase.

60 Answer C: Lung

Recurrence of renal cell carcinoma usually occurs within the first six years after surgery. The risk increases with the initial stage. Distant metastases develop in 20–30% of patients, with lungs the commonest site (50–60%), followed by mediastinum, bone and liver.

61 Answer E: Protease inhibitor use in HIV

Indinavir (a protease inhibitor) use results in crystalline stones that are non-opaque on CT. They are demonstrated by contrast-enhanced CT as filling defects in the ureter.

- Hyperparathyroidism – calcium oxalate/phosphate calculi, HU > 1000
- Chronic urinary infection – struvite (magnesium ammonium phosphate) calculi, HU 300–900
- Gout – uric acid calculi, HU 150–500 (radiolucent on plain film)
- Cystinuria – cysteine calculi, HU variable 200–880

62 Answer B: Acute cortical necrosis

Cortical nephrocalcinosis, described as tramline calcification, can be seen in any cause of acute cortical necrosis, including renal vein thrombosis, although obstetric shock is the commonest cause. Renal damage is more severe than in acute tubular necrosis.

63 Answer D: Multiple simple cysts

Multiple simple cysts increase in frequency with age and are the most likely cause in a patient over 50 years with no family history of cysts or cysts in other organs.

64 Answer E: Von Hippel-Lindau disease

Von Hippel-Lindau disease is an autosomal-dominant disorder, manifestations of which include renal and pancreatic cysts, renal cell carcinoma, and cerebellar haemangioblastomas.

65 Answer B: Autosomal-dominant polycystic kidney disease

Autosomal-dominant polycystic kidney disease typically presents clinically with hypertension and renal failure aged 30–50 years, and cysts are present in the liver and pancreas, which along with a family history differentiates this from other causes.

66 Answer A: Acquired renal cystic disease

Acquired renal cystic disease occurs in 90% of patients who have been on dialysis for 5–10 years. Innumerable small cysts form and the kidney enlarges over time. Wall calcification is common and they regress following transplantation. Complications include haemorrhage and renal cell carcinoma.

67 Answer B: Multicystic dysplastic kidney

Multicystic dysplastic kidney is a congenital, non-hereditary renal dysplasia in which there is no functioning renal tissue, instead multiple thin-walled cysts and connective tissue. If bilateral it is fatal at birth.

68 Answer A: Renal tubular acidosis

All are causes of medullary nephrocalcinosis, but distal renal tubular acidosis is the commonest cause in a child. It may be associated with rickets.

69 Answer B: Peripheral renal enhancement

A stretching injury to the renal artery damages the intima and thrombus can then occlude the artery, which causes non-perfusion of the affected kidney. Capsular vessels do not arise from the main renal artery and so result in peripheral renal enhancement (the rim sign). The kidney may appear otherwise intact. Renal revascularisation should be accomplished within two hours of injury, but can be successful later depending on the collateral supply and extent of injury.

70 Answer D: Abdominal and pelvic CT with intravenous contrast

Contrast-enhanced CT is the imaging modality of choice in a stable patient with or without haematuria and with evidence of major flank impact. Both US and IVU have a low sensitivity for detection of renal trauma, which often will not result in free intra-abdominal fluid. No imaging is required for an adult patient with microscopic haematuria, who is haemodynamically stable and with no other indication for CT. Instead observation until haematuria settles is appropriate. However, this does not hold true for the paediatric trauma patient, in whom microscopic haematuria without hypotension can be associated with significant renal imaging and CT imaging is warranted.

Genito-urinary, adrenal, obstetric, gynaecological and breast radiology

PAPER 2: ANSWERS AND EXPLANATIONS

1   Answer A: 20–40 mBq of nanocolloid injected subdermally into the quadrant of the breast where the cancer is located

20–40 mBq is given into the skin in the same quadrant as the tumour depending on whether surgery is that day or the next. Surgeons often use methylene blue at the time of surgery, but it is not radio labelled. The surgeon may use both a detector probe and dye at the time of surgery.

2   Answer A: Previous *tuberculosis* infection

Calcification occurs in 25% of Addison disease caused by TB. Other causes of chronic primary adrenal insufficiency include idiopathic atrophy from an autoimmune disorder (60–70%), fungal infection (histoplasmosis, blastomycosis, coccidioidomycosis), sarcoid and rarely bilateral metastatic disease. Both ganglioneuroma and phaeochromocytoma can have calcifications but would be present with an adrenal mass.

3   Answer B: Isointense/hypointense to liver on T1-weighted images and very hyperintense to spleen in T2-weighted images

Phaeochromocytoma occur in 50% of patients with MEN (multiple endocrine neoplasia) type 2 and these are the typical signal characteristics for a phaeochromocytoma. They are very high signal on T2-weighted images compared to spleen in 60% due to intratumoral cystic areas. They may also contain areas of high signal on T1-weighted images in 20% due to haemorrhage, but in comparison to myelolipoma and adenomas, which contain fat, there is no change in signal intensity between in and out of phase images in phaeochromocytoma. Option (a) is the signal characteristics of a myelolipoma and option (c) of adrenal cortical carcinoma. Options (d) and (e) are adrenal haemorrhage signal characteristics at different stages of evolution.

4   Answer B: Width of the adrenal limb measures 2 cm

The normal width of an adrenal gland is less than 1 cm.

Barwick T, Malhotra A, Webb J, *et al*. Embryology of the adrenal glands and its relevance to diagnostic imaging. *Clin Radiol*. 2005; **60**(9): 953–9.

5   Answer A: Bilateral diffuse enlargement of the adrenals but preservation of their usual morphology

Congenital adrenal hyperplasia is a group of autosomal recessive conditions due to defective enzyme synthesis, which ultimately produces increased ACTH and hyperplasia of the adrenal cortex. As well as adrenal hyperplasia there is also hyperplasia of rest tissue, which is seen in the retroperitoneum and testes.

6   Answer C: Heterogeneous solid mass with low density areas and calcifications displacing the right kidney and encasing the IVC

These findings are typical for neuroblastoma, which contains calcifications on CT in 85%, can extend across the midline and encases rather than invades vascular structures. Option (a) describes a rhabdoid tumour of the kidney, option (b) mesoblastic nephroma (although 90% of these occur before 1 year), option (d) Wilms' tumour and option (e) adrenal haemorrhage.

7   Answer E: Involvement of the IVC

Regional lymph nodes are removed at surgery. Caval involvement is an indicator of unresectability.

8   Answer A: Astrocytoma

The patient is asymptomatic, negative endocrine testing and has a large mass with delayed washout, which are all consistent with a diagnosis of adrenal cortical carcinoma (ACC). Of these, 30% are calcified and the calcifications and large size are suggestive of malignancy. ACC is associated with hemihypertrophy, Beckwith-Wiedemann syndrome and astrocytomas. Phaeochromocytoma is associated with MEN2 and neurofibromatosis. Adrenocortical hyperplasia is associated with the Carney complex; phaeochromocytoma is associated with the Carney syndrome.

9   Answer E: T2-weighted fast spin echo MRI sequences

Intracapsular ruptures are not detectable on mammography because the silicone is contained within the fibrous capsule that forms around the implant. Extracapsular rupture may sometimes be detected on mammography but may also be obscured by the overlying implant or may not be imaged if it occurs in an area of the breast or chest wall not included in the mammogram. Ultrasound has a lower sensitivity (70% vs. 94%) but similar specificity (92–97%) than MRI in detecting implant rupture. The fibrous capsule surrounding the implant is hypointense on T2 and silicone and saline both display high signal intensity on T2. The most effective sequences in evaluating implants are inversion recovery which suppresses fat, with an additional suppression of water for pure depiction of silicone, and with additional suppression of silicone for pure depiction of the saline component.

10 Answer C: 5–10%

Five to ten per cent degenerate into malignant fibrous histiocytoma/fibrosarcoma/liposarcoma/chondrosarcoma/osteosarcoma with local invasion and haematogenous metastases to lung, pleura and bone, with axillary metastases being quite rare. Incomplete excision results in recurrence in 15–20% despite their benign nature.

11 Answer B: Gynaecomastia due to digoxin therapy

The normal male breast appears on mammography as a mound of subcutaneous fat without glandular tissue. Gynaecomastia appears as described. It is NOT a risk factor for breast carcinoma. Thiazide diuretics and spironolactone are also recognised drug-induced causes of gynaecomastia. Invasive lobular carcinoma is distinctly uncommon as tubular structures are usually not found in the male breast. Gynaecomastia occurs in 60–75% of healthy pubertal boys.

12 Answer B: Hamartoma of the breast (fibroadenolipoma)

This description is classical.

13 Answer D: A lesion of mixed density on mammography with a fat-water level on a horizontal beam view

This is a typical appearance in the second phase; a large radiopaque lesion of water density is seen in the first phase. They can also resemble a lipoma (small radiolucent lesion) and may contain a fluid-calcium level. Ultrasound usually demonstrates a complex mass.

Both conditions occur in the retroareolar portion of the breast. A cold abscess is associated with the features described in (b) and (e). Associated raised inflammatory markers, fever and pain are also seen.

14 Answer C: 50–70 years

There are plans to increase the age range to 47–73 years in due course, but staffing considerations and the impact on current resources will have to be taken into account before this can be introduced.

NHS Breast Screening Annual Review 2008. Available at: www.cancerscreen ing.nhs.uk/breastscreen/publications/nhsbsp-annualreview2008.pdf (accessed 15 February 2009).

15 Answer C: Craniocaudal and mediolateral oblique (MLO)

16 Answer C: Post-surgical seroma

Silicone would appear hyperintense on water-suppressed STIR sequences. The appearances are consistent with a localised collection serum after surgery.

17 Answer D: Surgical excision is required for a definite diagnosis

There is no association with trauma or previous trauma. It has a variable appearance in different projections. No skin thickening or retraction is seen. Frozen section, core needle biopsy or fine needle aspiration should be avoided. It is rarely palpable and is usually detected at screening mammography or occasionally in mastectomy specimens.

18 Answer C: The condition is associated with ductal carcinoma *in situ* in 60% of cases

This patient has Paget's disease of the nipple. Associated with invasive ductal carcinoma in 30%, negative mammogram in 50%, and can display linearly distributed subareolar/diffuse malignant calcifications. The diagnosis is often delayed many months as the condition can resemble benign eczema.

19 Answer A: Inflammatory carcinoma

One might expect these changes with recent surgery, but not seven years later, and the findings raises the suspicion of inflammatory carcinoma or lymphatic obstruction in a patient with previous breast malignancy.

20 Answer D: Snowstorm sign posteriorly on ultrasound

The snowstorm sign is a hyperechoic nodule, which is well-defined anteriorly with indistinct echogenic noise posteriorly (= free silicone droplets mixed with breast tissue). The other options are signs of intracapsular rupture.

21 Answer E: Symptomatic treatment only

Mondor disease is a usually self-limited thrombophlebitis of the subcutaneous veins of the breast and anterior chest wall, of unknown cause. It may be associated with carcinoma (in up to 12%) and DVT. There are further possible associations with trauma, exertion, surgery, dehydration and inflammation.

22 Answer D: Plasma cell mastitis

Mammary duct ectasia or plasma cell mastitis is often asymptomatic, but may present with breast pain, nipple discharge and retraction or a subareolar mass. The mean age at which it occurs is 54 years. Duct dilatation is seen up to the nipple, with ducts usually measuring >2 mm on ultrasound. It is often bilateral and symmetric but may be unilateral and focal. It is a rare aseptic inflammation of the subareolar region. Intraductal calcifications associated are fairly uniform, linear, often needle-shaped, of wide calibre and occasionally branching. Periductal calcifications appear as oval/elongated rings around dilated ducts with very dense peripheries (due to surrounding deposits of fibrosis and fat necrosis).

23 Answer C: Choriocarcinoma

Malignant melanoma, renal cell carcinoma and Kaposi sarcoma would be other possible primaries.

24 Answer C: Septate uterus

Uterine anomalies are due to failure of fusion of Mullerian duct. Arcuate uterus is the most common uterine anomaly not associated with reproductive failure. Septate uterus is associated with 90% abortion rate which can be treated with excision of the septum.

Scarsbrook A, Moore N. MRI appearances of Mullerian duct abnormalities. *Clin Radiol.* 2003; **58**(10): 747–54.

25 Answer D: Hypointense rim of cervical stroma

A continuous hypointense rim representing the cervical ring measuring >3 mm is most reliable in excluding parametrial invasion with a quoted specificity of 96–99%. Nodularity and thickening of the parametrial tissue are signs of frank invasion.

26 Answer D: Pedunculated subserosal fibroid

Uterine artery embolisation is recommended only in symptomatic patients (pain, bleeding and pressure symptoms). Subserosal pedunculated fibroids are a relative contraindication as the risk of detachment from the uterus is high, which would require surgical treatment.

Watkinson A, Nicholson A. Uterine artery embolisation to treat symptomatic uterine fibroids. *BMJ.* 2007; **335**(7622): 720–2.

27 Answer C: Distinct hypointense transient bulge in the myometrium on T2-weighted images

Transient areas of low signal in the myometrium are a recognised pitfall in the diagnosis of adenomyosis and reflect myometrial contraction. These areas can also be mistaken for leiomyomas.

Holloway B, Lopez C, Balogun M. A simple and reliable way to recognise the transient myometrial contraction – a common pitfall in MRI of the pelvis. *Clin Radiol.* 2007; **62**(6): 596–9.

28 Answer B: Parametrial invasion

FIGO staging of cervical carcinoma. Stage IA – preclinical invasive carcinoma, stage IB – 1 < 4 cm, stage IB – 2 >4 cm, stage IIA – vaginal extension excluding lower third vagina, stage IIB – parametrial invasion, IIIA – invasion of lower third vagina, stage IIIB – pelvic side wall invasion and hydronephrosis, stage IVA – invasion bladder/rectum, stage IVB – distant organ spread.

29 Answer A: Epithelial ovarian carcinoma

The radiological findings are consistent with a malignant lesion and CA-125 levels are not raised in 20% of malignant ovarian cancers. CA-125 level is raised in 60% for mucinous type, 20% for non-mucinous. In benign processes such as fibroids, pregnancy, endometriosis, liver cirrhosis, pancreatitis and PID raised in 30%. Raised in 1% of normal individuals.

30 Answer A: Right ovarian thrombosis

This is the typical clinical scenario for ovarian vein thrombosis, which is an important differential to consider as it has a mortality of 5%. Eighty per cent occur in right ovarian vein, 14% bilateral and only 6% in left ovarian vein. On CT a tubular structure is seen of low density in the location of the vein.

31 Answer A: Severe growth restriction

Oligohydramnios is when there is less than 500 mL of amniotic fluid at term. It is associated with a 20 times increase in foetal abnormalities and occurs with renal anomalies, intrauterine growth restriction (IUGR) and most commonly with premature rupture of the membranes. The other options are associated with polyhydramnios (amniotic fluid volume >1500–2000 mL at term).

32 Answer A: Maternal diabetes mellitus

Both maternal and foetal disease can cause enlargement of the placenta. Increasing maternal age and multiparity are risk factors for placenta praevia.

33 Answer E: Abdominal radiograph

An abdominal radiograph is indicated if the coil is not definitely identified by ultrasound before referral to gynaecology.

34 Answer C: Polycystic ovary syndrome (PCOS)

PCOS occurs in 2.5% and is associated with elevated LH levels with an increased LH/FSH ratio. The findings on ultrasound of slightly enlarged ovaries (>15 mL) occurs in 70%. The small cysts represent an excessive number of developing follicles and are small in size in comparison to OHSS where the cysts can be >10 cm and the ovaries themselves >5 cm.

35 Answer D: Torsion of the ovary

A pre-existing ovarian lesion is present in torsion in >50% of cases. The appearances on ultrasound are of a complex mass and Doppler ultrasound may demonstrate absence of arterial Doppler waveforms, but this should not be relied upon due to the dual blood supply from both ovarian and uterine arteries. Immediate surgery is indicated in these cases.

36 Answer B: A 'ground-glass' pattern

Haemorrhage into a functional cyst is common and can produce echogenic material within the cyst without Doppler signal.

37 Answer C: Rapid change in size

Malignant transformation is rare (approximately 0.2%) and is very difficult to interpret given the variable appearances and signal characteristics of benign leiomyomas. A rapid increase in size, irregular margin and loss of outer capsule are concerning. High signal on T2-weighted images is seen in cystic degeneration. Low signal on T2-weighted images is seen in hyaline or calcific degeneration.

38 Answer A: Fat density on plain film

Mature teratoma (dermoid) is the most common ovarian neoplasm and is benign. It contains mature tissue from all three germ cell layers with 88% of cases containing sebaceous material. Calcifications (tooth) can be seen but are also seen in other germ cell tumours whereas fat on plain film is specific.

39 Answer D: *Escherichia coli*

M:F = 1:2. CT is the most specific modality. The common causative organism is *E. coli* but a wide range of organisms may be responsible: *Candida albicans*, *E. aerogenes*, *P. mirabilis*, *S. aureus*, *Streptococci*, *Clostridium perfringens* and *Klebsiella*. Gas may extend up the ureter giving an air pyelogram.

40 Answer C: Subserosal bladder rupture

This is a rare form of bladder rupture, which is recognised as an elliptical extravasation adjacent to the bladder on contrast-enhanced CT.

41 Answer C: Reiter's syndrome

Reiter's syndrome classically presents with the triad of conjunctivitis, urethritis and arthritis.

42 Answer D: Markedly increased perfusion through spermatic cord vessels with increased activity of scrotal contents on static images

Option (a) is seen with testicular abscess. Curvilinear increased activity laterally is seen in epididymitis. Option (c) is seen in acute testicular torsion and (e) in testicular tumour.

43 Answer B: Simple ureterocoele

This is the typical 'cobra head' or 'spring onion' appearance on IVP with a radiolucent halo formed by the ureteral wall and adjacent bladder urothelium. A simple ureterocoele is usually an incidental finding in adults; M:F = 2:3. It may be bilateral (33%). An ectopic ureterocoele is usually seen in the upper moiety ureter of a duplex kidney (80%). Twenty per cent of ectopic ureterocoeles are seen in a single non-duplicated system and are usually associated with a small/ poorly functioning, sometimes non-visualised ipsilateral kidney (the further the ureteral orifice is from the normal site of insertion, the more dysplastic the kidney tends to be). (c), (d) and (e) are causes of pseudoureterocoele. No protrusion of the ureter is seen into the bladder lumen.

44 Answer A: An abrupt short segment of narrowing in the bulbous urethra

A saddle injury tends to result in injury to the bulbous urethra, with subsequent development of a urethral stricture being a common complication. Abrupt short-segment strictures tend to be post-traumatic. Long segment strictures may be either traumatic or inflammatory. Traumatic injury to the posterior urethra occurs in about 10% of pelvic fractures, with the junction between the prostatic and membranous urethra being the most common site of injury.

45 Answer C: Torsion of the appendix testis

The appendix testis is the vestigial remnant of the Mullerian duct and is seen as a small projection from the upper testicular pole in up to 80% of ultrasound examinations. It is common in childhood.

Smart JM, Jackson EK, Dewbury KC, *et al*. Ultrasound findings of masses of the paratesticular space. *Clin Radiol*. 2008; **63**(8): 929–38.

46 Answer C: Scrotal haemangioma

Benign paratesticular lesions tend to be well defined, painless and show little or no increase in flow on colour Doppler. Scrotal haemangioma is an exception due to its high vascularity.

47 Answer C: High signal intensity in the prostate bed on axial T2 sequence

The usual post-prostatectomy appearance is low signal fibrosis. Increased signal on T2 sequence in the setting of a rising PSA is indicative of local recurrence.

48 Answer D: Mullerian duct cyst

This is a remnant of the paramesonephric duct which usually regresses by the third foetal month. It is discovered usually in the third to fourth decade. It tends to be midline and does not communicate with the urethra. It is associated with increased incidence of carcinomatous transformation.

49 Answer D. Mesoblastic nephroma

Mesoblastic nephroma is the commonest solid renal mass in a neonate; 90% occur in the first year. It is derived from early nephrogenic mesenchyma and can have a variable appearance on US. Distinguishing features are lack of a well-defined cleavage plane, lack of extension into renal vein (cf. Wilms') or pelvis (cf. multilocular cystic nephroma). Sarcomatous transformation and metastases are rare. Treatment is nephrectomy with an excellent prognosis.

50 Answer E: T3b (perivesical fat invasion) N1 M1

CT is not able to distinguish between layers of the bladder wall. The role of CT is to differentiate between T3a and T3b tumours (although MRI is better at this), invasion of adjacent organs (T4a), extension to the pelvic side wall (T4b), and to stage pelvic nodal and metastatic disease.

51 Answer A: Rise in serum creatinine from 80 μmol/L to 124 μmol/L

The definition of contrast-induced nephropathy is an impairment of renal function (an increase in serum creatinine by more than 25% or 44 μmol/L (0.5 mg/dL)) which occurs within three days following intravascular administration of contrast medium, in the absence of an alternative aetiology.

The ESUR. *ESUR Guidelines on Contrast Media, version 6.0*. The European Society of Urogenital Radiology; 2007. Available at www.esur.org (accessed 15 February 2009).

52 Answer C. Inferior vena caval invasion

The role of MRI in staging renal carcinoma is one of problem solving. Invasion of the renal vein and inferior vena cava is better shown on T1W sequences with and without contrast, particularly in the coronal and sagittal planes.

53 Answer C: Lytic bone metastases

^{18}FDG is not useful in primary renal or urothelial tumour assessment as it is physiologically excreted in the urine. ^{18}FDG PET-CT is useful for the detection of and response to therapy of lytic bone metastases.

54 Answer E: Further assessment during consideration of a cystectomy

MRI is the imaging modality of choice for those patients considered suitable for radical treatment (cystectomy or radical radiotherapy) because of its ability to demonstrate muscle wall invasion or penetration. CT is suitable for patients with clinical suspicion of advanced local disease, or distant metastases, or those not suitable for radical treatment.

55 Answer C: Unilateral acute ureteric obstruction

Vicarious excretion of intravenous iodinated contrast medium is commonly associated with unilateral renal disease such as acute obstruction, although it may be a normal variant. It is also associated with contrast extravasation.

56 Answer D: Hepatic fibrosis

Autosomal-recessive polycystic kidney disease is classified into four subgroups corresponding to the age of onset: perinatal, neonatal, infantile and juvenile. The abnormality lies with the epithelium of the collecting ducts resulting in ductal proliferation and dilatation. The proportion of ducts involved affects the degree of renal impairment and age of onset. Those in the juvenile group have the lowest number of ducts affected, but the degree of hepatic fibrosis is greatest in this group and death occurs from portal hypertension.

57 Answer B: Recent bladder catheterisation

Iatrogenic introduction of air is the commonest cause of incidental gas in the bladder. If the patient has not had recent catheterisation, the causes are more serious and all the choices may result in gas within the urinary tract.

58 Answer D: Cortical depressions between calyces

Foetal lobulation occurs due to incomplete fusion of the foetal lobules, leading to a lobulated contour with depressions/interlobular septa occurring between calyces.

59 Answer C: Normal finding

The normal renal cortex is hypoechoic or isoechoic to the liver parenchyma. Arcuate arteries may be seen as small hyperechoic foci without shadowing at the corticomedullary junction. The medullary pyramids are hypoechoic to the renal cortex.

60 Answer C: Tc-99m-dimercaptosuccinic acid (DMSA)

Tc-99m-DMSA has minimal urinary excretion (<5%) and high cortical binding (50% of dose at four hours post injection), which makes it the ideal agent for assessment of renal cortical activity.

61 Answer C: Umbilical-urachal sinus

The urachus is an embryological remnant of the cloaca and the allantois, and usually closes to become the median umbilical ligament. There are four types of urachal remnant. (1) Patent urachus (continuous connection between the umbilicus and bladder), usually symptomatic and diagnosed in the neonatal period. (2) Umbilical-urachal sinus is a blind dilatation of the urachus at the umbilical end. A small opening into the umbilicus is usually present and trauma from the piercing has opened it up. (3) Vesico-urachal diverticulum is a communication only with the bladder dome. (4) Urachal cyst consists of closure at both ends with isolated dilatation usually in the lower third. Meckel's diverticulum is the remnant of the vitello-intestinal duct.

Yu JS, Kim KW, Lee HJ, *et al*. Urachal remnant diseases: spectrum of CT and US findings. *RadioGraphics*. 2001; **21**(2): 451–61.

62 Answer D: Posterior interpolar calyx

The posterior approach is associated with less bleeding complications. Either an interpolar or lower pole calyx may be used for percutaneous nephrostomy, but the angle made from an interpolar entry site facilitates ureteric stent insertion.

63 Answer D: Focal reflux nephropathy (chronic atrophic pyelonephritis)

Focal reflux nephropathy is the only condition listed that gives a calyceal abnormality with associated cortical loss. It usually results as a consequence of infection associated with reflux in childhood. It may be widespread or focal in which case it is more common in the upper poles and on the right. The kidney is always small and there may be contralateral compensatory hypertrophy.

64 Answer B: Glomerulonephritis

Goodpasture's syndrome is the association of glomerulonephritis and pulmonary haemorrhage secondary to anti-glomerular basement membrane antibodies. The only renal imaging features are symmetrical change in size, initially enlarged, later small, with excessive renal sinus fat.

65 Answer C: *Tuberculosis*

The clinical and radiological features suggest *tuberculosis*. Cloudy high attenuation dilated calyces represents calcification within caseous pyonephrosis.

Calcification is seen in 30% of cases and may result in putty kidney or calcified autonephrectomy. One feature that suggests TB rather than papillary necrosis or focal reflux nephropathy is the relatively poor excretion of contrast in relation to the degree of obstruction.

66 Answer E: A renal pelvic calculus

Xanthogranulomatous pyelonephritis is an uncommon chronic inflammation usually associated with proteus infection and 70% have renal pelvic calculi, in which renal calyces and parenchyma are replaced by lipid-laden macrophages, debris and other inflammatory cells. The nephrogram is totally or focally absent in 80%. The generalised form is commoner but a focal form can mimic a renal tumour.

67 Answer E: Single kidney

The main complication to renal biopsy is haemorrhage and thus the presence of a single kidney is a contraindication in case of catastrophic bleeding, although fortunately this is uncommon. Less than 5% of patients require transfusion or surgery and mortality is 1 in 1000.

68 Answer B: End-to-side anastomosis to the external iliac artery

The transplant kidney is usually placed in the contralateral iliac fossa extra-peritoneal space. Usually, a live donor kidney is anastomosed end-to-side with the external iliac artery, or less commonly end-to-end with the internal iliac artery. An aortic patch is usually removed with a cadaveric transplant; this is not possible with a living donor.

69 Answer E: Percutaneous renal biopsy

Biopsy is inevitably required to make the diagnosis of rejection. Acute tubular necrosis does have a characteristic pattern on dynamic renal scintigraphy, with almost normal first pass perfusion, blood pool uptake only at 80–180 seconds and no excretion. Rejection may be identified by reduced perfusion with or without swelling. Duplex US and MR findings are non-specific indicators of transplant dysfunction.

70 Answer C: (Peak systolic velocity – End diastolic velocity)/Peak systolic velocity

The RI is sensitive to changes in downstream flow resistance and is used to assess changes in diastolic flow in low-resistance vascular beds. The normal limit for a renal transplant is 0.8.

The pulsatility index (PI) is calculated by (Peak systolic velocity – End diastolic velocity)/Temporal mean velocity.

Genito-urinary, adrenal, obstetric, gynaecological and breast radiology

PAPER 3: ANSWERS AND EXPLANATIONS

1   Answer D: Non-traumatic adrenal haemorrhage

Neonatal stress can cause non-traumatic adrenal haemorrhage, which is the most common neonatal lesion of the adrenal gland. Infants who are large for gestational age and those of diabetic mothers are predisposed. It occurs R:L = 7:3 and is bilateral in 10%.

2   Answer C: Attenuation >30 HU

Although phaeochromocytoma may contain intracellular fat (and therefore appear hyperintense on T1-weighted MR images) they are of increased attenuation relative to fat-containing adenomas on CT. Calcification can be present in both as can arterial phase enhancement. Phaeochromocytoma tend to be >3 cm and often appear heterogeneous.

3   Answer A: Presence of large amount of mature fat

Adrenal myelolipomas contain a large amount of mature fat, causing their attenuation to be −30 to −115 HU. Lipid-rich adenomas will also have a HU <10 but contain intracytoplasmic lipid and are of higher attenuation. The mean size of an adrenal adenoma is approximately 2 cm, but the mean diameter of a myelolipoma is approximately 10 cm. Calcification can occur in both.

4   Answer D: India ink effect on chemical shift MRI

The presence of lipid causes the characteristic black lines outlining the interface between organ and adjacent fat and as phaeochromocytoma do not contain fat would be suggestive of an adenoma. Marked hyperintensity on T2 images is typical of a phaeochromocytoma. Similarly, heterogeneous enhancement and slow washout are more suggestive of phaeochromocytoma than adenoma.

5   Answer C: Attenuation of 26 HU on delayed images 15 minutes after contrast injection

Attenuation of <37 HU on delayed images has been suggested to be diagnostic of adenoma.

6 Answer D: CT-guided core biopsy

Biopsy of phaeochromocytoma, which is catecholamine producing, may precipitate life-threatening hypertension or arrhythmia. Non-ionic intravenous contrast medium can safely be used for CT examination without alpha-adrenergic blockade.

7 Answer D: Corticomedullary junction

8 Answer E: Lymphangioma

True adrenal cysts are rare. Endothelial lining 'cysts' such as lymphangioma are more common. Pseudocysts also occur from previous haemorrhage/infarction.

9 Answer C: Invasive ductal carcinoma

This is most likely to appear as a spiculated mass, usually on both mammographic views. It is also the most common histological type of breast cancer. The other types most often appear as rounded lesions with a smooth border and may display a halo sign.

10 Answer D: A normal mammogram three years previously

Neither cysts nor fibroadenomas grow after the menopause and any new mass lesion should be regarded with suspicion, despite an otherwise apparently benign appearance.

11 Answer E: Spiculated lesion with a plateau in the post-initial phase on contrast-enhanced T1-weighted images

Malignant morphology always trumps kinetics. Features of malignancy on breast MR include reduced signal on T2 WI, irregular morphology, lymphangitic bridges, and the following on CE T1 WI: rapid wash-in –90/90 rule (SI increase of >90% in the first 90s), centripetal wash-in, plateau/rapid washout in post-initial phase, markedly higher amplitude than normal parenchymal tissue.

12 Answer D: Six months after open biopsy

Optimal timing of MR of the breast includes 7–20 days after the beginning of the menstrual cycle, six months after open biopsy and 12 months after radiation therapy.

13 Answer B: Upper outer quadrant

Fifty-four per cent occur in the UOQ, 14% in the UIQ, 15% are retroareolar, 7% in the LIQ and 10% in the LOQ.

14 Answer C: Post-surgical haematoma

Deoxyhaemoglobin of subacute haematoma. Seroma and abscess would display high signal intensity on T2 images due to fluid content. Fat necrosis usually occurs up to six months following insult, and would display increased signal intensity on T2 due to reactive oedema in a fresh lesion.

15 Answer D: High signal on T1- and T2-weighted images with avid peripheral enhancement without central uptake on contrast-enhanced T1 images

High T1 SI is due to the high protein content of fluid in a chronic/cold abscess of the breast in a lactating woman. The abscess wall enhances strongly post contrast.

16 Answer C: 6 per 1000 women screened

www.cancerscreening.nhs.uk/breastscreen/publications/nhsbsp-annualreview2008.pdf

17 Answer E: Calcification may be present

The patient has fibrocystic changes of the breast. Tea cup calcification on horizontal beam lateral view, low-density round calcification on CC projection (milk of calcium)/'oyster pearl-like'/psammoma-like/'involutional type' fine punctate calcifications in one or more lobes against fatty background are all described. Symptoms usually occur with ovulation; regress with pregnancy and at menopause. It is the most common diffuse breast disorder, found in 72% of the screening population >55 years of age.

18 Answer A: 0% It is not pre-malignant

Fat necrosis is not pre-malignant but is an important differential for carcinoma, particularly if it causes distortion of the skin or breast tissue or has mammographic features which are indistinguishable from malignancy as in this case.

19 Answer B: Central solitary papilloma

Papillary carcinoma is a rare form of ductal carcinoma. MRI features usually differ slightly in that the lesion is hypointense on T1-weighted images, shows strong initial enhancement with contrast sometimes with ring enhancement and a post-initial plateau or washout. T2-weighted images demonstrate a well-circumscribed intermediate intensity lesion in a signal-intense cyst.

20 Answer B: Haematocolpos

Imperforate hymen at puberty may cause haematocolpos which distends the vagina with blood causing low-level echoes on ultrasound examination.

21 Answer E: Neural tube defect

An elevated alpha-fetoprotein level is associated with foetal anomalies in 61%, of which 51% are neural tube defects. Other causes include a normal pregnancy that is more advanced, twin pregnancy, missed abortion, renal anomalies and anterior abdominal wall defects.

22 Answer C: Multiple further lesions in the pelvis

Multiplicity, multilocularity and adhesions to other organs are features that may distinguish endometriomas. They may also have a hypointense thick wall.

23 Answer E: Vessel visualised within stalk on colour Doppler

Seventy-nine per cent of endometrial polyps have the appearance of a well-defined smooth hyperechoic homogeneous intracavitary mass but the diagnosis can be confusing particularly if there is heterogeneity.

24 Answer A: Adult granulosa cell tumour

Adult granulosa cell tumour is the most common oestrogenic tumour.

25 Answer B: Hypointensity on T2-weighted images

Cervical carcinoma is hyperintense on T2-weighted images but non-degenerated leiomyomas are low signal.

26 Answer D: Central placenta praevia

Central placenta praevia totally covers the internal os. Placenta accreta, increta and percreta are increasing degrees of the placenta growing into the myometrium with contact with the myometrium, myometrial invasion and penetration to the serosa respectively.

27 Answer E: Low signal on T2-weighted images

Fibroids have variable appearances on ultrasound but are commonly hypoechoic and can distort the uterine cavity when large. The typical appearances on MRI examination are well defined areas which are low signal on T2-weighted images and are isointense to myometrium on T1-weighted images. The appearances are variable if there is haemorrhage or cystic degeneration.

28 Answer A: Wilms' tumour

Beckwith-Wiedemann syndrome (omphalocoele, macroglossia, gigantism) is associated with increased risk of benign and malignant tumours of multiple organs: Wilms' tumour >adrenocortical neoplasm >hepatoblastoma.

29 Answer E: Spina bifida

Spina bifida is associated with Arnold-Chiari malformation in 90% and the ultrasound findings of Arnold-Chiari malformation include hydrocephalus, abnormally pointed frontoparietal region (lemon sign) and abnormally shaped cerebellum (banana sign).

30 Answer C: Bartholin's gland cyst

Bartholin's glands are located behind the labia minora and their ducts can become blocked. This can cause retention of secretions and is most common in women of reproductive age.

Lopez C, Baogun M, Ganesan R, *et al*. MRI of vaginal conditions. *Clin Radiol*. 2005; **60**(6): 648–62.

31 Answer A: High signal on T1-weighted images

Melanin has a paramagnetic effect causing shortening of T1 relaxation time and therefore is high signal on T1-weighted images and low signal on T2-weighted images.

32 Answer B: Bilateral disease

Female genital *tuberculosis* causes salpingitis in 94% and is mostly bilateral. It can also cause tuboovarian abscess with extension into extraperitoneal compartment.

33 Answer E: Leads to testicular infarction in approximately 3% of cases

The patient has acute epididymo-orchitis. The commonest causative organisms are *Chlamydia* and *N. gonorrhoea* in <35 year olds, and *E. coli* and *Proteus mirabilis* in >35 year olds. *Staphylococcus aureus* is also a recognised cause. Testicular torsion is most common in <20 year olds, and acute epididymitis is most common after the age of 20. Prostatic tenderness is infrequent and TB accounts for 2% of cases, while *E. coli* and *S. aureus* account for 85%. Testicular infarction is a recognised complication of acute epididymitis from extrinsic compression of testicular blood flow.

34 Answer C: Squamous cell carcinoma (SCC) of the bladder

There are features of schistosomiasis on the control films, but this patient has developed a complication in the form of SCC of the bladder following childhood infection (latency period of 20–30 years). SCC often involves in the posterior wall and rarely involves the trigone. A second complication of schistosomiasis is portal hypertension due to ova migrating into the portal venous system and inciting a fibrosing granulomatous reaction within presinusoidal portal veins. Consequently, the haematemesis is likely to relate to oesophageal varices.

Neurofibroma of the bladder wall tends to cause smooth filling defects and is not associated with bladder calcification. *Tuberculosis* tends to begin in the kidney and spread distally, usually resulting in a scarred, contracted bladder of diminished capacity. Multiple granulomas can give rise to filling defects.

35 Answer B: First year of life

Sixty-five per cent first year, 23% 1–16 years, 8% prenatal, diagnosis by urethrogram.

36 Answer C: Cavernosal aspiration/irrigation

Most cases of priapism are due to veno-occlusive disease with arterial causes being relatively rare and related to trauma. Even with appropriate aspiration and irrigation followed by anticoagulation/shunt surgery there is still 50% impotence.

37 Answer B: Secondary to previous gonococcal infection

Approximately 40% of urethral strictures in males in the USA.

38 Answer D: Fournier gangrene

Necrotising fasciitis of the scrotum. The prognosis is usually very poor.

39 Answer B: Routine urological referral

As the patient is symptomatic the surgeon may discuss surgical options such as marsupialisation. The ultrasound operator needs to be vigilant and thoroughly check the testes for an underlying tumour.

40 Answer A. Time gain compensation

Time gain compensation equalises the image brightness between superficial and deeper structures by progressively increasing the gain from deeper (later) echoes. This is adjusted for average tissue attenuation. If a cyst with lower than average attenuation is imaged, the echoes from deeper tissues are over-amplified. Non-linear waveform propagation is the principle behind harmonic imaging, in that the original pulse is distorted so that it comes to contain higher frequency components or harmonics.

41 Answer A: T1-weighted images

MRI is the staging modality of choice for TCC, with an accuracy of 72–96%. T1-weighted images are optimal for detecting invasion of perivesical fat and metastases to lymph nodes and bone. TCC of the bladder is the most common tumour of the genital tract and is 30–50 times more common than upper urinary tract urothelial cancer. Approximately 30% will have an additional histologically similar bladder tumour. Staging CT should be delayed for up to seven days post-instrumentation as it can result in overstaging and is best used for staging of advanced disease as it is poor at differentiating superficial non-invasive tumours from those invading the bladder wall muscle. Adenocarcinoma of the bladder is rare (<1%) and most cases are associated with bladder extrophy and urachal remnants. Treatment options for early-stage disease include cystoscopic resection and intravesical mitomycin C.

42 Answer E: Central enlargement with calcium and mixed echogenicity

Size greater than 30 cu cm and peripheral changes are more suspicious of carcinoma. PSA generally increases with age: 3 ng/mL is considered the upper limit of normal up to 60 years, 4 ng/mL to 70 years and 5 ng/mL for those over 70.

43 Answer B: Malakoplakia

This is an inflammatory condition that usually presents in the immunosuppressed and most often affects the genito-urinary tract. It is rare and biopsy is necessary for diagnosis but the imaging features described are typical.

44 Answer C: No symptom improvement in approximately 10%

This is usually due to unseen vein duplication or the symptoms not being related to the varicocele.

45 Answer A: T2-weighted static fluid MR urography

MR urography is indicated as there is no risk of ionising radiation exposure to the foetus. Static fluid sequences are appropriate. Gadolinium contrast is contraindicated in pregnancy.

Leyendecker JR, Barnes CE, Zagoria RJ. MR urography: techniques and clinical applications. *RadioGraphics*. 2008; **28**(1): 23–46.

46 Answer C: Alternating bands of hypo- and hyperattenuation of the renal parenchyma

This appearance is analogous to the striated nephrogram seen on excretory urography and reflects the underlying pathology of tubular obstruction, interstitial oedema and vasospasm.

On delayed (3–6 hours) imaging, the hypoattenuating regions show delayed and persistent enhancement due to prolonged accumulation and transit of contrast through the collecting system. In haematogenous seeding of pyelonephritis (from staphylococcal or streptococcal infections), round peripheral hypoattenuating lesions are seen. They can mimic neoplasia if pyelonephritis is not suspected clinically.

Craig WD, Wagner BJ, Travis MD. Pyelonephritis: radiologic-pathologic review. *RadioGraphics*. 2008; **28**(1): 255–77.

47 Answer D: A single central nervous system haemangioblastoma

Criteria for diagnosis of VHL disease include: (1) more than one central nervous system haemangioblastoma, (2) one central nervous system haemangioblastoma and any visceral manifestations of VHL disease, and (3) any manifestation and a family history of VHL disease.

Leung RS, Biswas SV, Duncan M, *et al.* Imaging features of von Hippel-Lindau disease. *RadioGraphics*. 2008; **28**(1): 65–79.

48 Answer D: Ureteral ischaemia

Ninety per cent of post-transplant ureteral obstruction is due to ischaemia, usually at the distal ureter close to the ureterovesical junction. This is the area furthest from the renal artery. The other options are also less common causes of obstruction.

Sandhu C, Patel U. Renal transplantation dysfunction: the role of interventional radiology. *Clin Radiol*. 2002; **57**(9): 772–83.

49 Answer C: Malignant fibrous histiocytoma

Malignant fibrous histiocytoma is the most common soft-tissue sarcoma in adults, and approximately 15% occur in the retroperitoneum. It is one of the few tumours to have a myxoid stroma, the imaging characteristics of which are low T1-weighted signal and very high T2-weighted signal. The admixture of solid components, cystic necrosis, haemorrhage, calcification (in 7–20%), myxoid stroma and fibrous tissue gives the bowl of fruit appearance. The enhancement pattern described is common in malignant tumours and bone metastases are present.

Desmoid tumours are typically low on both T1- and T2-weighted images and display delayed enhancement – this is typical of dense collagen fibres.

Surabhi VR, Menias C, Prasad SR, *et al*. Neoplastic and non-neoplastic proliferative disorders of the perirenal space: cross-sectional imaging findings. *RadioGraphics*. 2008; **28**(4): 1005–17.

50 Answer B: Cystic partially differentiated nephroblastoma

Cystic partially differentiated nephroblastoma (CPDN) and cystic nephroma make up the two forms of multilocular cystic renal tumour (MDCT). They originate from metanephric blastema and have identical imaging features. CPDN is typically seen in boys aged three months to four years (90% <2 years) and blastemal cells are present histologically. Cystic nephroma is seen typically in adult women aged 40–60 years, and no septal blastemal cells are present.

Cystic mesoblastic nephroma is rare after the age of six months (commonest neonatal renal mass), and renal cell carcinoma is uncommon under the age of two years.

Wilms' tumour is the commonest malignant abdominal tumour in children aged one to eight years, and the third most common cause of all renal masses in childhood (after hydronephrosis and multicystic dysplastic kidney).

51 Answer C: Angioplasty without stenting

FMD is commonest in young women and typically involves the mid and distal artery (as opposed to atherosclerotic ostial stenosis), bilaterally in two-thirds. Other aortic vessels are affected in 1–2%. The string of beads sign is caused by alternating areas of stenoses and aneurysms and is seen in the commonest form, medial fibroplasia. Treatment is balloon angioplasty, without stenting.

52 Answer C: Bull's-eye appearance of central treated tumour surrounded by a
     thin soft tissue rim, with thin halo of fat separating the two

The typical appearance of RF-ablated renal tumours is of a central non-enhancing mass, clearly demarcated from normal enhancing renal parenchyma. Peripheral or exophytic tumours additionally have a thin double halo of outer soft-tissue density and inner normally appearing fat. This finding is likened to a bull's-eye appearance, and is seen on CT and MR. The central ablation zone is typically hypointense on T2-weighted images. Any nodular enhancing tissue is likely to represent residual or recurrent disease.

Cryoablated renal tumours often show a thin rim of enhancement, however, and are often not detectable at two years, unlike RF-ablated lesions when a mass is invariably still present

Wile GE, Leyendecker JR, Krehbiel KA, *et al*. CT and MR imaging after imaging-guided thermal ablation of renal neoplasms. *RadioGraphics*. 2007; **27**(2): 325–39; discussion 339–40.

53 Answer D: Type 4: Extraperitoneal bladder rupture

Extraperitoneal bladder rupture is the commonest type (80–90%) of bladder rupture and usually occurs from penetrating trauma (from pelvic fractures) or blunt trauma (disruptions of ligamentous attachments to the pelvic floor), in which case rupture occurs at the anterolateral aspect near the neck. Intraperitoneal bladder rupture frequently occurs at the dome with blunt trauma to a distended bladder. Accurate diagnosis is important as types 1, 3 and 4 are treated conservatively but types 2 and 5 require immediate surgery.

Wah TM, Spencer JA. CT of adult urinary tract trauma. *Imaging*. 2005; **17**: 53–68.

54 Answer C: Gadodiamide is contraindicated in patients with a glomerular filtration rate (GFR) of <30 mL/min

There is a causal link between gadolinium-based media and NSF, but no direct proof. There are >200 cases reported, all in patients with renal failure. No cases have been reported in patients with normal renal function. The incidence in at risk patients given Gadodiamide is 3–7%. Gd-based agents are not recommended as replacements for iodinated contrast.

The UK regulatory position as of February 2009 is summarised:

1 Gadodiamide and Gadopentetic acid (Magnevist®) are currently contra-indicated in patients with GFR <30 mL/min, including those on dialysis. Gadodiamide is also contraindicated in all patients with renal impairment awaiting liver transplantation. Both agents should be used with caution in patients with GFR 30–59 mL/min, and in children <1 year old.

2 Careful consideration should be given before using other Gd-based media in patients with GFR <30 mL/min

3 All patients should be screened by history/laboratory tests before administration of Gd-based media

4 Haemodialysis after administration of Gd-based media may remove contrast but there is no evidence that this affects the development or treatment of NSF.

55 Answer B: HIV-related nephropathy

The US findings suggest HIV-related nephropathy, a form of glomerulosclerosis, which is the commonest cause of renal impairment in the HIV-positive population. It particularly affects young black males and is the third leading cause of end stage renal disease in African-Americans aged 20–64 years. Malignancy, HAART therapy and *P. jirovecii* associated nephrocalcinosis are all recognised renal manifestations of HIV infection.

Symeonidou C, Standish R, Sahdev A, *et al*. Imaging and histopathologic features of HIV-related renal disease. *RadioGraphics*. 2008; **28**(5): 1339–54.

56 Answer E: A wedge-shaped non-enhancing parenchymal area

The renal arteries are clamped during the surgery. Damage to the intima may cause local thrombosis and wedge-shaped non-enhancing renal parenchymal infarcts. To promote haemostasis, fat or haemostatic material may be placed in the surgical bed. Fat may later be confused with an angiomyolipoma, and gas bubbles can be present with the latter which may be confused with a gas containing abscess in the early post-operative period. Residual haematoma may have an attenuation of 50–60 HU.

57 Answer D: It has a much better prognosis than conventional RCC

Papillary RCC is the second commonest form (10–15%) of RCC after clear cell RCC (70%). Both arise from the proximal convoluted tubule. It is more homogeneous and relatively hypovascular; this is a key imaging finding, and is more frequently multifocal and bilateral. It has the best prognosis of all forms of RCC.

Prasad SR, Humphrey PA, Catena JR, *et al*. Common and uncommon histologic subtypes of renal cell carcinoma: imaging spectrum with pathologic correlation. *RadioGraphics*. 2006; **26**(6): 1795–806.

58 Answer D: Ureterocoele

The classic appearance of a ureterocoele is likened to that of a cobra's head due to a dilated distal ureter surrounded by a thin radiolucent line of ureteric wall and prolapsed bladder mucosa.

59 Answer C: Membranous urethra

Retrograde urethrography shows the anterior urethra, VCUG shows the posterior urethra: 300–350 mL is required for reliable voiding. US may be useful in assessment of length and thickness of bulbar strictures.

60 Answer A: Early filling images

Early filling during VCUG is essential as bladder tumours or a ureterocoele may be missed when the bladder is full. A single AP image will suffice. During voiding steep oblique views are necessary to visualise the VUJ. AP voiding images increase gonadal radiation dose.

61 Answer B: Prophylactic antibiotics

The majority of children with Grade II vesico-ureteric junction (VUJ) reflux where there is no pelvicalyceal or ureteric dilatation will outgrow reflux within five years.

62 Answer C: Split renal function

Split renal function is assessed with Tc-99m-DMSA or Tc-99m-MAG3 scintigraphy. Dual-phase MDCT with 3-D post-processing is a quick and accurate method for living donor laparoscopic nephrectomy assessment. Of critical importance in the planning and performance of the operation is the renal arterial and venous anatomy.

63 Answer A: Retroperitoneal fibrosis

The findings on IVP are typical. The sensitivity and specificity of CT tissue characteristics are poor for the differentiation of benign from malignant disease. US can be helpful in demonstrating additional features such as bile duct dilatation, portal hypertension and sclerosing pancreatitis. The high T2-weighted signal, and radionuclide uptake within the retroperitoneal soft tissue, reduce with successful treatment and these can be used as markers of response.

64 Answer D: Periprocedural intravenous hydration

Randomised controlled studies and/or meta-analyses have demonstrated reduction in incidence of CIN with periprocedural hydration, low- versus high osmolar and iso- versus low osmolar contrast media. The role of N-acetylcysteine is currently inconclusive.

65 Answer E: Ureteral erosion

Ureteral erosion is a rare but serious complication of stent insertion. Fistulation may occur between the ureter and an adjacent vessel, particular an artery, due to ischaemia in the ureter and pulsations from the vessel. Presentation is with intermittent, or occasionally life threatening, haematuria. Demonstration with imaging may be difficult and angiography may be both diagnostic and allow therapeutic embolisation.

Yu NC, Raman SS, Patel M, *et al.* Fistulas of the genito-urinary tract: a radiologic review. *RadioGraphics.* 2004; **24**: 1331–52.

66 Answer C: Autosomal dominant

The patient has adult polycystic kidney disease which is autosomally dominantly inherited. Patients are also at risk of mitral valve prolapse and have an increased frequency of renal calculi, urinary tract infections and renal cell carcinoma. Bleeds into cysts are common and painful.

67 Answer B: Sarcoma

Overall 75% of urachal tumours are adenocarcinomas but in young patients 75% are sarcomas.

68 Answer A: Conservative management

This is a typical description for a subcapsular haematoma which can usually be managed conservatively.

69 Answer E: Enlarged kidney with loss of cortico-medullary differentiation

The patient has a renal vein thrombosis and the kidney is enlarged due to oedema. There are often hyperechoic areas representing haemorrhage.

70 Answer: C: Posterior urethral valves

Posterior urethral valves are the most common cause of bilateral hydronephrosis in a male infant. There are three types described of which type I is the most common and represents vestiges of the Wolffian duct extending anteroinferiorly.

Paediatric radiology

PAPER 1: ANSWERS AND EXPLANATIONS

1 Answer C: Hirschsprung disease

Hirschsprung disease is the absence of parasympathetic ganglia in the muscle and submucosal layers of the colon. It usually presents in the first six weeks of life of a full-term infant. It is very rare in preterm infants. Eighty per cent involve the rectosigmoid.

2 Answer B: Temporal lobe high signal on T2-weighted images, low signal on T1-weighted images

Herpes simplex encephalitis most commonly affects the temporal lobe with a propensity for the limbic system. A CT may be negative for three days but the MRI should be positive within two days. The signal increases on diffusion weighting, as it is cytotoxic oedema. Small focal haemorrhages are common.

3 Answer D: Slipped upper femoral epiphysis

These are the characteristic radiographic findings in slipped upper femoral epiphysis. Approximately 50% of patients have bilateral involvement.

4 Answer C: Hyperinflation with course linear densities and focal areas of emphysema

The infant described has bronchopulmonary dysplasia, which is caused by oxygen toxicity and barotrauma in infants on assisted ventilation at >21% oxygen for >28 days. Appearances change with time:

Stage	Time	CXR appearances
I	0–3 days	Similar to respiratory distress syndrome, bilateral patchy ground-glass opacities with air bronchograms
II	4–10 days	Complete opacification with air bronchograms
III	10–20 days	Small round cystic lucencies and areas of irregular opacity
IV	>1 month	Hyperinflation, coarse linear densities and focal areas of emphysema

5 Answer A: Liver ultrasound

The description is that of autosomal-recessive polycystic kidney disease. This is associated with congenital hepatic fibrosis. The less severe the renal involvement, the more severe the hepatic involvement.

6 Answer E: Atlantoaxial subluxation

Hypoplastic posterior arch of C1 and abnormal odontoid peg can also be found in Down's syndrome but with the clinical history this child is most likely to have atlantoaxial subluxation.

7 Answer C: Developmental dysplasia of the hip (DDH)

Infants at risk of developmental dysplasia of the hip include those born in a frank breech position, infants with a family history of DDH and those with generalised joint laxity. DDH is more common in girls than boys.

8 Answer C: Widespread patchy consolidation and air trapping

Meconium aspiration is the most common cause of neonatal respiratory distress in full-term or post-term infants. Severe hypoxaemia induces a gasping reflex with resulting inhalation of meconium, which causes medium and small airway obstruction and chemical pneumonitis.

9 Answer D: Right paraumbilical abdominal wall defect

	Gastroschisis	Omphalocoele
Position of defect	Right paramedian	Midline
Cord insertion	Normal	At apex of defect
Peritoneal covering	No	Yes
Ascites	No	Common
Liver herniated	Infrequently	Common
Bowel complications	Common	No
Associated abnormalities	Intestinal atresia	Chromosomal, IUGR, Beckwith-Wiedemann syndrome, cardiac, neural tube, GU

10 Answer C: A soft-tissue erosion into the cochlear, which is isodense on T1-weighted images and hyper-dense on T2-weighted images relative to brain

Cholesteatoma is an epithelial-lined sac of desquamated epithelium that can lead to erosion of the surrounding bones. The MRI imaging characteristics are of a mass emanating from the middle ear invading the temporal bone that is isodense on T1-weighted images and hyper-dense on T2-weighted images as opposed to cholesterol granuloma, which is hyper-intense on T1-weighted images.

11 Answer C: Eosinophilic granuloma

Eosinophilic granuloma is the most benign variety of Langerhans cell histiocytosis that is localised to bone. Fifty per cent of cases are found in the skull.

12 Answer C: DMSA in four to six months

NICE guidelines on management of UTI recommend ultrasound within six weeks and a DMSA scan at four to six months for investigation of recurrent UTI in children over three years and makes very similar recommendations for children six months to three years with recurrent UTIs.

13 Answer A: I123 MIBG study with planar and SPECT images

Although neuroblastoma can be detected on octreotide studies MIBG is the first line of investigation. Whole body images with I123 are used in the treatment and assessment of thyroid malignancy and have no place in this scenario.

14 Answer A: Abdominal ultrasound every three months

Ten to twenty per cent of patients with Beckwith-Wiedemann syndrome develop Wilms' tumour. There is also an increased risk of developing Wilms' tumour in patients with sporadic aniridia, hemihypertrophy and genito-urinary disorders such as Drash syndrome (male pseudohermaphroditism and glomerulonephritis).

15 Answer B: Aneurysmal bone cyst

Aneurysmal bone cysts are benign expansile lytic lesions containing thin-walled cystic cavities filled with chronic blood products. They present with pain, increasing in severity over 6–12 weeks. The peak age of presentation is 16 years.

16 Answer C: Swyer-James syndrome

Swyer-James syndrome is a chronic complication of viral bronchiolitis with recurrent infections preventing normal development of the lung. HRCT appearances include areas of normal lung attenuation within hypoattenuating lung, air trapping and bronchiectasis

17 Answer D: Interhemispheric subdural haematoma

This child has had many non-accidental injuries. Head trauma is the most common cause of death and disability following non-accidental injury. The CT brain findings include: subdural haematoma (most common finding and is most common in the interhemispheric region), subarachnoid haemorrhage, epidural haemorrhage, cerebral oedema and acute cerebral contusions.

Rao P, Carty H. Non-accidental injury: review of radiology. *Clin Radiol*. 1999; **54**(1): 11–24.

18 Answer C: Oesophageal duplication cyst

Oesophageal duplication cysts account for 10–20% of all duplication cysts in the gastrointestinal tract. They are associated with vertebral anomalies, oesophageal atresia and small bowel duplication. They are most commonly found in the distal oesophagus where they are frequently asymptomatic.

19 Answer C: Pyknodysostosis

Pyknodysostosis is an autosomal-recessive condition. Other features include widened hands and feet and characteristic facies with a beaked nose and receding jaw.

20 Answer A: Hypoplastic left heart syndrome

Hypoplastic left heart syndrome or aortic atresia is the underdevelopment of the left side of the heart and is characterised by hypoplastic aortic and mitral valves, left ventricle and ascending aorta. It is twice as common in males as females and the most common cause of congestive heart failure in the neonate.

21 Answer B: Distal intestinal obstruction syndrome

Otherwise known as meconium ileus equivalent, distal intestinal obstruction syndrome occurs in children and adolescents with cystic fibrosis. It occurs due to impaction of inspissated stool in the distal ileum and proximal colon.

22 Answer C: III

The Salter-Harris classification is used for growth plate injuries.
I   A slip of the epiphysis due to a shearing force separating the epiphysis from the physis.
II   A fracture through the physis and extending through the margin of the metaphysis separating a triangular metaphyseal fragment, 'corner sign'.
III A fracture through the growth plate and epiphysis.
IV   A fracture through the metaphysis, physis and epiphysis.
V   A compression fracture through the growth plate.

23 Answer D: Interruption of aortic arch

This child has interruption of aortic arch which is a rare congenital anomaly characterised by interrupted aortic arch, VSD and patent ductus arteriosus. The aortic knuckle and oesophageal impression are absent on CXR.

24 Answer C: Posterior urethral valve

These are congenital thick folds of mucosa within the posterior urethra. They are the most common cause of urinary tract obstruction and end-stage renal disease in boys.

25 Answer E: Subdural empyema

The patient has bacterial meningitis that is complicated with a subdural empyema. There are many potential complications of bacterial meningitis including subdural effusions (which may become secondarily infected becoming subdural empyemas), cerebritis and ventriculitis, atrophy, infarction, hydrocephalus and cranial nerve dysfunction.

26 Answer C: Mucopolysaccharidosis

Mucopolysaccharidoses are a group of inborn errors of metabolism resulting in accumulation of mucopolysaccharides. The mucopolysaccharidoses exhibit common skeletal manifestations. These are collectively called dysostosis multiplex. In addition to the findings described above, features include: short wide metacarpals with narrowed proximal ends, dysplastic changes at the femoral head, macrocephaly and oar shaped ribs.

27 Answer D: Tricuspid atresia

Tricuspid atresia is the second most common cause of neonatal cyanosis after transposition of the great arteries. It is characterised by an absent tricuspid valve, ASD, and a small VSD. Most occur in the absence of transposition (80%), but it may also occur in the setting of transposition. The heart may be normal in size or moderately enlarged with enlargement and hypertrophy of the left ventricle and enlargement of the right atrium.

28 Answer A: Complete ureteric duplication with infrasphincteric insertion of the upper moiety ureter

In complete ureteric duplication, there is an increased risk of obstruction of the upper moiety ureter and of vesicoureteric reflux of the lower moiety ureter. The upper moiety ureter has a suprasphincteric insertion in boys, resulting in no enuresis but epididymitis and urge incontinence. In girls, the upper moiety ureter has an infrasphincteric insertion and causes both wetting in the upright position and intermittent or constant dribbling of urine.

29 Answer C: Acute disseminated encephalomyelitis

Acute disseminated encephalomyelitis is a post-infectious encephalitis, usually following an exanthematous viral illness or vaccination. It is a diffuse inflammatory process leading to areas of demyelination caused by an autoimmune response to the patient's white matter. Acute inflammatory demyelinating polyradiculoneuropathy is often called Guillain-Barré and does not cause changes in the brain.

30 Answer C: Cupping and fraying of the metaphyses with coarse trabeculation

The findings are those of rickets, the causes of which include: vitamin D deficiency, abnormalities in vitamin D metabolism and phosphate metabolism, and calcium deficiency. Radiographic findings include:

- periosteal **R**eaction
- **I**ndistinct cortex
- **C**oarse trabeculation
- affects mainly **K**nees, wrists and ankles
- **E**piphyseal plates are widened and irregular
- **T**remendous metaphysis (cupping, fraying, splaying)
- **S**pur (metaphyseal).

31 Answer C: Echocardiogram

The infant has Kawasaki disease, a multisystem vasculitis with a predilection for the coronary arteries. Fifteen to twenty-five per cent of patients have associated coronary artery aneurysms, most commonly of the left coronary artery. An echocardiogram is advised at the time of diagnosis, at two weeks and six to eight weeks after diagnosis. Contrast-enhanced CT of the chest and MR can also demonstrate the aneurysms.

Newburger JW, Takahashi M, Gerber MA, *et al*. Diagnosis, treatment, and long-term management of Kawasaki disease. *Circulation*. 2004; **110**(17): 2747–71.

32 Answer A: Good hepatic activity within five minutes and no visualisation of bowel at six hours or 24 hours

The DISIDA nuclear scintiscan is 90–97% sensitive and 60–94% specific for biliary atresia. In addition it shows delayed clearance from the cardiac pool and increased renal excretion and bladder activity.

33 Answer B: HIV parotitis

In HIV parotitis the swellings are chronic, firm and non-tender and are associated with an improved prognosis. In mumps the parotid swellings are tender. Warthin's tumours are mixed solid/cystic lesions that usually present in adults.

34 Answer A: Decreased grey and white matter density, decreased grey/white matter differentiation and increased density of the basal ganglia, thalami and cerebellum

The 'reversal' sign occurs in hypoxic ischaemic cerebral injury. It carries a poor prognosis. There is a high association with non-accidental injury, but it can also result from events such as significant accidental trauma, near drowning, cardiac arrest, status asthmaticus and status epilepticus.

35 Answer B: Asthma

The CXR is often normal in the early stages of asthma with abnormalities developing with increasing severity (e.g. hyperinflation, bronchiectasis, scars from recurrent infections).

36 Answer C: Blood flow within the intussusceptum on colour Doppler

The 'target' sign is due to the hyperechoic mesentery of the intussusceptum surrounded by hypoechoic and hyperechoic rings of the intussuscipiens and is classic for intussusception. It is not a predictor of reducibility. Fluid inside the intussusception is associated with irreducibility and ischaemia. The absence of blood flow within the intussusceptum is suggestive of bowel necrosis.

37 Answer A: Squared patella with widening of the intercondylar notch

Patients develop haemophilic arthropathy following repeated bleeding into a joint. Additional features seen at the knee include medial slanting of the tibiotalar joint and flattening of the condylar surface.

38 Answer C: Cystic fibrosis

Cystic fibrosis is an autosomal-recessive disease characterised by mucous plugging of exocrine glands secondary due to exocrine gland dysfunction producing thick obstructing mucus and reduced mucociliary clearance.

39 Answer C: Oesophageal atresia without tracheoesophageal fistula

The inability to pass a feeding NG tube is suggestive of oesophageal atresia; it is seen coiled in the oropharynx on chest radiograph. Neonates with tracheoesophageal fistulae tend to aspirate during feeding with coughing and choking.

40 Answer C: III

The St Jude classification is used to stage NHL. There are four stages:
I   Single extranodal tumour/single anatomic area
II   (a) Single extranodal tumour + regional nodes
      (b) Two or more nodal areas on same side of diaphragm
      (c) Two extranodal tumours +/– nodes on same side of diaphragm
      (d) Primary gastrointestinal tumour +/– nodes
III   (a) Two extranodal tumours on opposite sides of diaphragm
      (b) Two or more nodal areas on both sides of diaphragm
      (c) Primary intrathoracic tumours
      (d) Extensive primary intra-abdominal disease
      (e) Paraspinal/epidural tumour
IV   Any of above + CNS/bone marrow involvement

41 Answer C: Homocystinuria

Homocystinuria is an autosomal-recessive disorder causing a defect in collagen and elastin structure. Other bony abnormalities particularly seen in children include metaphyseal cupping and delayed ossification.

42 Answer C: Duodenal atresia

This is the most common cause of congenital duodenal obstruction. It is associated with Down's syndrome.

43 Answer C: Reactive airways disease

Reactive airways disease (RAD) may be precipitated by respiratory syncytial virus (commonest cause of pneumonia in infants) and *Aspergillus*. Asthma is diagnosed on the basis of recurrent RAD and is not diagnosed within the first year. Apparent severity of RAD on CXR does not correlate with clinical severity.

44 Answer D: Frontal lobe abscess

Causes of brain abscesses include:

- extension from paranasal sinus infection
- septicaemia originating in the lung (e.g. bronchiectasis)

- septicaemia originating in the heart (e.g. congenital heart disease with right to left shunt, bacterial endocarditis)
- septicaemia originating with osteomyelitis
- penetrating trauma or surgery
- cryptogenic.

45   Answer D: Enchondromatosis

Enchondromatosis, or Ollier disease, is a non-hereditary failure of cartilage ossification. It can involve the long bones, causing leg or arm shortening, or the tubular bones of the hands and feet, resulting in deformity.

46   Answer B: Pneumothoraxw

The rupture of subpleural metastatic nodules into the pleural space can cause spontaneous pneumothorax. Cavitating metastases classically occur in squamous cell carcinoma. Osteosarcoma lung metastases can calcify.

47   Answer C: Stage III

Neuroblastoma staging:
Stage I: Limited to organ of origin
Stage II: Regional spread, not crossing the midline
Stage III: Extending across the midline
Stage IV: Metastatic spread to liver, bone, brain, lung, distant lymph nodes
Stage IVs: Stages I and II, with disease confined to the skin, bone marrow and liver with no radiographic evidence of skeletal metastases

48   Answer A: Several 'ground-glass' medullary lesions within the proximal femur with endosteal scalloping

The girl has McCune-Albright syndrome, which consists of at least two out of the triad of: polyostotic fibrous dysplasia, café au lait spots and endocrinopathy including precocious puberty. The café au lait spots in McCune-Albright syndrome tend to be fewer in number and more prominent than the smooth-edged lesions seen in neurofibromatosis. The other radiographic findings listed above are all seen in neurofibromatosis.

49   Answer A: Hyperlucency

Foreign bodies are usually non-radioopaque. Many present with hyperlucency, caused by air trapping and hyperinflation distal to the foreign body. Chronic foreign body aspiration can present as atelectasis, recurrent pneumonia, or bronchiectasis. CT is the most sensitive method to detect obstruction.

50   Answer A: 2 months

Myelination occurs through the infant's brain and peripheral nervous system from caudal to cranial and from posterior to anterior.
   Myelination milestones:

- term birth – brainstem, cerebellum, posterior limb of the internal capsule
- 2 months – anterior limb of the internal capsule
- 3 month – splenium of corpus callosum
- 6 months – genu of corpus callosum.

51 Answer E: Turner's syndrome

Madelung's deformity is a shortening of the ulna or absence of the ulnar styloid process. Other features of Turner's syndrome on a hand radiograph include a positive carpal sign, which is narrowing of the scaphoid-lunate-triquetrum angle to <117 degrees and shortening of the second and fifth middle phalanges (also seen in Down's syndrome).

52 Answer A: Radial dysplasia

VACTERL is an association of congenital defects. V – Vertebral anomalies; A – Anal atresia; C – Cardiac defect; for example, ventricular septal defect or Tetralogy of Fallot; T – tracheoesophageal fistula; E – oesophageal atresia; R – renal anomalies; for example renal agenesis, ectopic kidney; L – limb defects; for example, radial aplasia/dysplasia, triphalangeal thumb, syndactyly, radioulnar synostosis.

53 Answer C: Ewing's sarcoma

The four paediatric tumours that tend to metastasise to the lungs are:

- rhabdomyosarcoma primarily affects children ages 1–5 and 15–19
- osteogenic sarcoma primarily affects children under age 15
- Wilms' tumour primarily affects females under five years of age with a high incidence in African Americans.

54 Answer C: Thalassaemia major

This is an inherited disorder of haemoglobin synthesis and is the more severe, homozygous, form. Manifestations include hypochromic microcytic anaemia, susceptibility to infection and retarded growth.

55 Answer D: Double aortic arch

In double aortic arch, the right arch is usually higher than the left. The right arch passes posterior to the trachea and the left arch passes anterior to the trachea. The right arch supplies the right common carotid artery and right subclavian artery. The left arch supplies the left common carotid artery and left subclavian artery. Double aortic arch is rarely associated with congenital heart disease. A left arch with aberrant right subclavian is the most common arch anomaly and causes a posterior impression on the mid-oesophagus. A right arch with aberrant left subclavian also causes a posterior impression on the mid-oesophagus. Innominate artery compression syndrome causes anterior tracheal compression 2 cm above the carina. An aberrant right pulmonary artery causes an anterior oesophageal impression.

56 Answer E: Ewing's sarcoma

Ewing's sarcoma is the most common bone tumour in children. The lesions are characteristically ill-defined mottled 'moth eaten' areas of bone destruction with a periosteal reaction that has an 'onion skin' appearance. There is usually an associated soft-tissue mass. Osteomyelitis can have similar appearances but usually a shorter history. In eosinophilic granuloma there is a solid periosteal reaction. Osteosarcoma does not cause a lamellar periosteal reaction and frequently has ossification in the soft tissues.

57 Answer D: Haemangioendothelioma

This is the most common benign hepatic tumour seen in infants under six months old. It commonly presents with congestive heart failure due to high-output circulation. They can be solitary or multiple. Haemangioendotheliomas have a natural history of regression within 12–18 months and the initial management is medical.

58 Answer C: Ultrasound of the hip

In children septic arthritis most commonly involves the hip, followed by the knee and then the ankle joint. Less frequently the site is the upper limb. Septic arthritis is usually associated with a joint effusion. Ultrasound is sensitive and specific for diagnosing hip effusions in children.

59 Answer C: Situs inversus

In situs inversus, the heart, stomach, and visceral organs are all on the opposite side to normal. It is associated with sinusitis and bronchiectasis (Kartagener's syndrome) with a slight increase in incidence of congenital heart disease. Situs solitus is where all structures are concordant; that is, in the normal position. Situs solitus with dextrocardia is where the cardiac apex is on the right with the stomach bubble on the left and most cases are associated with congenital heart disease. Levoversion with abdominal situs inversus is always associated with congenital heart disease.

60 Answer A: A line between the anterior margins of C1 and C3 spinous processes passing within 2 mm of the anterior margin of the C2 spinous process

Pseudosubluxation is normal mobility of the upper cervical spine, particularly at C2/3 and C3/4, which occurs in approximately 40% of children younger than eight years old. It results from immature lax ligaments and horizontally aligned facets. Swischuck's line, drawn between the anterior margins of the spinous processes of C1 and C3, should pass through or lie within 2 mm of the anterior margin of the spinous process of C2. More than 2 mm is suggestive of pathological subluxation. In pseudo-subluxation the anterior displacement occurs in flexion and should reduce with neck extension.

61 Answer B: Torsion of the appendix testis

Torsion of the appendix testis and torsion of the appendix epididymis are the most common causes of acute scrotal pain in 6–12 year olds. It is not a real surgical emergency as symptoms usually resolve with supportive care.

62 Answer D: Turner's syndrome

This girl has Turner's syndrome. The findings include aortic coarctation, aortic stenosis, and horseshoe kidneys.

63 Answer E: Collapsed vena cava, increased enhancement of the adrenal gland and decreased splenic enhancement

Hypoperfusion complex is seen in children with hypovolaemic shock who maintain blood pressure with increased sympathetic response causing vasospasm and adequate perfusion to vital organs. It carries a very poor prognosis. On CT there is a small-calibre aorta due to vasospasm, flattening of the inferior vena cava due to decreased venous return, dilated bowel loops with increased wall enhancement due to vasoconstriction of mesenteric vessels, increased enhancement of the adrenal glands, decreased splenic enhancement and dense nephrograms due to lack of contrast excretion by the kidneys.

64 Answer B: 3-cm round hyperechoic left suprarenal mass

The ultrasound appearances are those of an adrenal adenoma. These are usually functional and result in the overproduction of adrenocorticotrophic hormone or aldosterone, resulting in Cushing syndrome or Conn syndrome.

65 Answer A: Dextroposition

Cardiac abnormalities of Trisomy 13 include VSD, ASD, PDA, and dextroposition.

66 Answer B: Multiple cysts of varying sizes, an absent renal pelvis and dysplastic renal parenchyma

Calcifications may be seen in the cyst walls or in the septations between the cysts. The contralateral kidney often shows compensatory hypertrophy.

67 Answer D: Repeat CXR in six weeks

The infant has a round pneumonia, most commonly caused by *Haemophilus influenzae* and *Streptococcus*. Although uncomplicated pneumonia in children does not require follow-up imaging, those patients with round pneumonia, pneumatocele or pulmonary abscess should have a repeat frontal CXR in six weeks to confirm resolution.

68 Answer D: Laparotomy

These findings are consistent with necrotising enterocolitis (NEC). Congenital heart disease is a risk factor for NEC. Gas in the portal venous system can be transient and does not necessarily imply a hopeless outcome.

69 Answer C: Supine

An abnormal position of the duodenojejunal flexure on a barium meal confirms the diagnosis of malrotation, most commonly to the right of the spine.

70 Answer A: Bochdalek hernia

Bochdalek hernia is a posterolateral defect in the diaphragm. It presents in the neonatal period and is more commonly (80%) on the left. Morgagni hernia rarely presents clinically at birth and is an anteromedial congenital diaphragmatic hernia.

Paediatric radiology

PAPER 2: ANSWERS AND EXPLANATIONS

1   Answer D: Pyloric transverse diameter of 20 mm

Pyloric stenosis manifests itself between two and eight weeks of life and is more common in boys. Positive findings on ultrasound include:

- pyloric muscle wall thickness >3 mm
- pyloric canal length >17 mm
- pyloric transverse diameter >13 mm
- exaggerated peristaltic waves
- delayed gastric emptying.

2   Answer A: Retinoblastoma

Retinoblastoma is a rare congenital malignant tumour of the retina. There is a non-inherited (66% of cases) and an inherited form. They usually present between one year and 18 months old with leukocoria or squint. The cysts are due to tumour necrosis. Retinal detachment is present in all cases; acoustic shadowing is only present in 75%. Vitreous haemorrhage is frequent. Persistent hyperplastic primary vitreous is a band from the retina to the posterior surface of the lens or central anechoic line. Retinal astrocytoma is commonly confused with retinoblastoma but is much less common. Rhabdomyosarcoma is the commonest tumour of the orbit in childhood but originates from the orbit, not the retina, and usually presents with exophthalmos at a much later age.

3   Answer C: Frog leg lateral of pelvis

The radiographic findings are those of slipped upper femoral epiphysis. This usually occurs in overweight and tall children between 12 and 15 years old in boys and 10 to 13 years old in girls. Both anteroposterior and frog-leg or true lateral radiographs are essential for diagnosis.

4   Answer B: Scimitar syndrome

Scimitar syndrome is a rare congenital abnormality characterised by a hypogenetic lung with anomalous venous drainage of all or the lower part of the lung. There are variations in the drainage of the anomalous vein; it most commonly drains into the IVC below the right diaphragm, the right atrium or the suprahepatic IVC. Scimitar syndrome is almost exclusively found on the right. Scimitar syndrome is often an incidental finding in older children and adults.

5   Answer C: III

The diagnosis is a second branchial cleft cyst. The internal structure is from haemorrhage or infection. The Bailey classification is:

I   Along anterior surface of the sternocleidomastoid, just deep to the platysma
II   Along anterior surface of sternocleidomastoid, lateral to carotid space, posterior to submandibular gland and adherent to vessels
III   Extends medially between the internal and external carotid arteries to the lateral pharyngeal wall
IV   Within pharyngeal mucosal space.

Type II is the most common.

6   Answer D: Noonan's syndrome

Noonan's syndrome has a phenotype similar to Turner's syndrome but with a normal karyotype. It occurs in both sexes.

7   Answer A: Perthes disease

Perthes disease is an idiopathic avascular necrosis of the femoral capital epiphysis. Bilateral disease occurs in approximately 10% of cases.

8   Answer B: Round pneumonia

Round pneumonia is seen in children. The most common causative organisms are *Haemophilus influenzae*, *Streptococcus* and *pneumococcus*.

9   Answer A: 9/10

The positive predictive value (PPV) is the fraction of positive results that are correct. In this case there are 18 true positives, 2 false positives and the PPV is 18/(18 + 2) = 90%. The negative predictive value (NPV) is similar and is the fraction of patients with a negative result who do not have the disease.

10   Answer B: Renal tract ultrasound

Prune belly syndrome is a congenital non-hereditary disorder that almost exclusively affects males. It is a triad of abdominal wall muscle insufficiency, non-obstructed distended ureters (+/– hydronephrosis and a degree of renal dysplasia) and bilateral undistended testes.

11   Answer C: Hip ultrasound at one month

Positive Barlow and Ortolani tests are suggestive of developmental dysplasia of the hips. Hip ultrasound is too sensitive during the first two weeks of life due to the effect of maternal hormones and is not practical after six months of age. AP pelvic radiographs are not reliable in the first three months of life.

12   Answer B: Normal thymus

The normal thymus can be very large and have extreme asymmetry. The edge is often wavy due to anterior rib end impressions. The thymus appears largest at about two years old, although it continues to grow into adolescence.

13   Answer B: *Streptococcus* group A

The child has epiglottitis. If imaging is required, the imaging of choice is a lateral radiograph with the child erect. Apart from the imaging characteristics described in the question there can be ballooning of the hypopharynx and pyriform sinuses. The classical pathogen is *Haemophilus influenzae* B, but this is now rare due to vaccinations. Of the answers listed *Streptococcus* group A is the most common cause.

14   Answer B: Meconium ileus

Meconium ileus presents with small bowel obstruction secondary to meconium impacted in the distal ileum. Almost all patients with meconium ileus have cystic fibrosis. It is the earliest clinical presentation of meconium ileus (10–15% of cystic fibrosis patients present with meconium ileus).

15   Answer E: Talipes equinovarus

This is otherwise known as congenital clubfoot and is a common severe deformity of the foot.

16   Answer E: Neuromuscular disease

The normal newborn chest is broader than the adult with near parallel lateral margins.

17   Answer A: Tc-99m pertechnetate

Meckel's diverticulum is a persistence of the omphalomesenteric duct and is the most common congenital abnormality of the gastrointestinal tract. Tc-99m pertechnetate is >85% sensitive and >95% specific for Meckel's diverticulum.

18   Answer C: Rickets

Rickets is due to deficient calcification of the osteoid. The metaphyses of the long bones subjected to stress (ankles, wrists and knees) and the costochondral junctions of the ribs show the greatest changes.

19   Answer B. Neurofibromatosis type 1

The imaging findings are those of an optic nerve glioma. The change in iris pigmentation described is likely to be due to Lisch nodules (pigmented iris hamartomas).

20   Answer C: Extralobar pulmonary sequestration

This is an accessory lobe with its own pleural sheath, which prevents collateral air drift, resulting in an airless round mass. Both intralobar and extralobar pulmonary sequestrations have systemic arterial supplies.

Bronchopulmonary sequestrations:

	Intralobar	Extralobar
Pleura	Visceral pleura	Own pleura
Venous drainage	Pulmonary veins	Systemic veins
Symptomatic	Adulthood	First six months

21 Answer A: Turner's syndrome

The diagnosis is Turner's syndrome. This is a condition caused by either a complete absence or abnormal second sex chromosome. The clinical findings and ultrasound appearance are classical for cystic hygroma, the majority of which are associated with chromosomal abnormalities, the commonest of which is Turner's syndrome.

22 Answer B: Multicystic dysplastic kidney

Multicystic dysplastic kidney is the second most common cause of an abdominal mass in a neonate after hydronephrosis. The unilateral form is more common on the left and is associated with anomalies of the contralateral kidney. The bilateral form is fatal.

23 Answer A: Simple bone cyst

Simple bone cysts or unicameral bone cysts are most frequently found in the metaphyses of long tubular bones, particularly the proximal humerus, femur and tibia. Fracture is a common complication with the fractured piece of cortex falling to the dependent part of the cyst, the 'fallen fragment sign', described above.

24 Answer B: Group B Streptococcal pneumonia

Group B *Streptococcus* is the most common cause of neonatal pneumonia. Pleural effusions are seen in two-thirds of cases. Risk factors include prolonged rupture of membranes, maternal fever during labour and preterm labour.

25 Answer C. Congenital toxoplasmosis infection

The presentation of congenital toxoplasmosis infection is very non-specific, as with most of the congenital infections. The ultrasound characteristics are different from congenital *Cytomegalovirus* in that the calcifications are in the basal ganglia and thalamus as well as the periventricular region. The calcifications can be lobulated or curvilinear and can be present in the choroid plexus. The location also differentiates the findings from tuberous sclerosis. Periventricular leukomalacia findings are a broad zone of periventricular echogenicity.

26 Answer A: Abdomen distended by bowel gas

Oesophageal atresia, no fistula	10%
Oesophageal atresia with proximal fistula	1%
Oesophageal atresia with distal fistula	80%
Oesophageal atresia with proximal and distal fistula	1%
H-type fistula with no oesophageal atresia	10%

27 Answer A: Osgood-Schlatter disease

Osgood-Schlatter disease is a traumatically induced disruption of the attachment of the patellar ligament to the tibial tuberosity. It is most common in boys between 10 and 15 years and associated with sports that involve kicking and jumping. Jumper's knee may have similar appearances but affects the proximal end of the patella tendon, not the insertion into the tibial tubercle.

28 Answer C: Bilateral patchy ground-glass opacities with air bronchograms

Respiratory distress syndrome, or hyaline membrane disease, is caused by surfactant deficiency due to immature type II alveolar cells. Premature infants, multiple gestations, perinatal asphyxia and infants of diabetic mothers are at risk. The onset of symptoms is up to five hours after birth.

29 Answer D. Vein of Galen malformation

The vein of Galen malformation is a central arteriovenous malformation that drains directly into a secondarily enlarged vein of Galen. It is a cause of high-output cardiac failure and should be considered if no cardiac or great vessel abnormalities are seen.

30 Answer B: Intestinal atresia

The description is that of gastroschisis. Gastroschisis has associated anomalies in 5%, most of which are intestinal atresia or stenosis. Omphalocoele has a high incidence of associated anomalies including chromosomal, genito-urinary, cardiac (particularly VSD), neural tube defects, IUGR and Beckwith-Wiedemann syndrome.

31 Answer C: Osteogenesis imperfecta

Osteogenesis imperfecta is a group of connective tissue disorders with deficient collagen formation. There is a spectrum of clinical findings and severity. The clinical and radiological findings described above are those of Osteogenesis imperfecta Type I. This is the most common form of mild to moderate disease. It is autosomal dominant and usually presents between two and six years old.

32 Answer D: The left ventricle lies on the right and the stomach bubble lies on the right

The findings are those of Kartagener's syndrome. This is a familial disorder characterised by situs inversus, nasal polyposis with chronic sinusitis and bronchiectasis.

33 Answer D: Wilms' tumour

Wilms' tumour is the most common malignant abdominal neoplasm in one to four year olds. Ninety per cent of cases present with a painless abdominal mass. The Rule of 10s applies to Wilms' tumours:

- 10% unfavourable histology
- 10% bilateral
- 10% vascular invasion
- 10% calcification
- 10% pulmonary metastases at presentation.

34 Answer B: Posteriorly concave vertebral margin

Achondroplasia is an autosomal-dominant disorder with a high rate (80%) of sporadic mutations. Patients have normal intelligence and motor function and multiple skeletal abnormalities.

35 Answer A: Fontan procedure

This is performed between three and five years old for tricuspid atresia. It causes raised central venous pressure and frequently chronic pleural effusions.

36 Answer D: Intussusception

Intussusception is the invagination of a segment of bowel (intussusceptum) into the lumen of the adjacent bowel (intussuscipiens). Ninety-five per cent of cases are idiopathic in children.

37 Answer A: Hand-Schüller-Christian disease

Hand-Schüller-Christian disease is the chronic disseminated form of Langerhans cell histiocytosis. The classic triad is: exophthalmos, diabetes insipidus and destructive bony lesions. Langerhans cell histiocytosis is a group of disorders characterised by Langerhans cell proliferation.

38 Answer D: Left aortic arch with aberrant right subclavian artery

A left arch with aberrant right subclavian affects 0.5% of the population and is usually asymptomatic.

39 Answer C: Duodenojejunal junction low and in the midline

All of the above are found in malrotation. The most common findings associated with the diagnosis of malrotation are: duodenum and jejunum to the right of the spine, corkscrew duodenum and jejunum and the duodenojejunal junction low and in the midline.

40 Answer B: Klippel-Feil syndrome

Klippel-Feil syndrome is caused by failure of normal segmentation of the cervical vertebrae. Features include a short neck, low hairline and reduced mobility of the upper spine. Any of the cervical vertebrae can be involved but fusion of the C2/C3 vertebrae is the most common.

41 Answer A: Ebstein's anomaly

Ebstein's anomaly is caused by apical displacement of the posterior and septal tricuspid valve leaflets, leading to part of the right ventricle becoming part of the right atrium. It is the only cyanotic heart disease to have a hypoplastic aorta and pulmonary trunk.

42 Answer B: DMSA four to six months after the acute infection

NICE guidelines refer to age group, recurrent, typical or atypical infections and the investigations vary accordingly. A retrograde study should never be performed during an infection.

43 Answer C: Fibrolamellar hepatocellular carcinoma

This is a subtype of hepatocellular carcinoma found in older children and adolescents, which is less aggressive. The central scar can calcify.

44 Answer C: Avulsion of the rectus femoris muscle

Apophyseal avulsion injuries are more common in children than adults. Young athletes, in particular hurdlers and sprinters, are at particular risk.

45 Answer A: Large VSD, overriding aorta, right ventricular outflow tract obstruction and right ventricular hypertrophy

This boy has Tetralogy of Fallot. The four cardinal features are right ventricular outflow obstruction (usually the pulmonary infundibulum), large VSD, right ventricular hypertrophy (secondary to raised right ventricular systolic pressure), and an overriding aorta straddling the VSD (receiving blood from both ventricles).

46 Answer C: Pneumoperitoneum

These are all radiological findings seen in necrotising enterocolitis. This is an ischaemic bowel disease secondary to hypoxia, perinatal stress and infection. It is the most common gastrointestinal emergency in premature infants. Portal venous gas is often a transient feature.

47 Answer D: 3 mm

Signs of an effusion are bulging of the anterior joint capsule, >3 mm distance between the bony femoral neck and joint capsule and >2 mm difference from the contralateral side. Ultrasound is almost 100% sensitive at detecting effusions.

48 Answer C: Forked ribs

This neonate has truncus arteriosus, which is the failure of septation of the conotruncus, leaving only a single outlet from the heart. A left to right shunt occurs after birth with the decrease in pulmonary vascular resistance, which leads to congestive heart failure. The truncus arteriosus appears as a widened mediastinal shadow on CXR. Forked ribs can be seen in truncus arteriosus and Tetralogy of Fallot.

49 Answer D: Unilateral undescended testis post-orchidopexy in a nine month old

Testes are normally within the scrotum by 28–32 weeks gestational age. Crypto-orchidism is the arrested descent of testes along their normal course and is associated with an increased risk of testicular cancer (most commonly seminoma). Orchidopexy does not decrease the cancer risk and the risk extends to the contralateral testis.

50 Answer C: 7 years

It is important to be aware of the normal order of ossification of the elbow so as not to mistake an epicondylar fracture for a normal ossification centre. The order and ages of ossification are:

- capitellum one year
- radial head five years
- medial epicondyle seven years
- trochlea 10 years
- olecranon 10 years
- lateral epicondyle 11 years.

51 Answer C: Choroid plexus papilloma

Choroid plexus papillomas account for 2–5% of intracranial tumours in childhood. There is a male sex predominance and up to 80% present before the age of one year old. They are a large collection of choroid plexus fronds, which produce excess CSF leading to hydrocephalus. Five per cent transform into malignant choroid plexus carcinomas, which show signs of invasion. This is an uncommon site for astrocytomas.

52 Answer A: Dilated cystic spaces with air-fluid levels

This child has bronchiectasis, which is an irreversible dilatation of bronchi often with bronchial wall thickening. In severe cases a honeycombing pattern may be seen.

53 Answer D: Grade IV vesicoureteric reflux

Grade	Findings on micturating cystourethrogram
I	Reflux into ureter
II	Reflux into pelvicalyceal system (no evidence of calyceal dilatation or blunting)
III	Reflux into pelvicalyceal system with mild dilatation of ureter and pelvicalyceal system
	Distinct forniceal angles and papillary impressions
IV	Reflux into tortuous ureter with moderately dilated pelvicalyceal system
	Blunted forniceal angles and distinct papillary impressions
V	Reflux into markedly dilated and tortuous ureter with markedly dilated pelvicalyceal system
	Obliteration of forniceal angles and papillary impressions

54 Answer D: Rhabdomyosarcoma

Lung metastases in children most commonly come from rhabdomyosarcoma, osteosarcoma, Wilms' tumour and Ewing's sarcoma.

55 Answer B: Loss of anterior vertebral height and Schmorl's nodes

Scheuermann's disease or adolescent kyphosis is the second most common paediatric spinal deformity, which has its onset at puberty. In the forward flexed position there is abrupt angulation in the mid to lower thoracic region. Additional radiographic features include disc space narrowing, end plate irregularities and kyphosis >40 degrees.

56 Answer A: 'Triangular cord' sign in porta hepatis

This is due to fibrous tissue and is pathognomonic for biliary atresia. The other options can all be seen in both neonatal hepatitis and biliary atresia.

57 Answer D: Non-accidental injury

Subdural haematomas are suspicious for non-accidental injury if they are bilateral, present without a skull fracture, of different ages, present with retinal haemorrhage or are within the interhemispheric fissure or falx.

58 Answer A: Hypothalamic glioma

These are the most common hypothalamic masses accounting for 10–15% of supratentorial tumours in children and present between the ages of two and four years old. This child is showing visual deficits and diencephalic syndrome, which is present in up to 20% of cases. The inhomogeneous enhancement is caused by tumour necrosis. Craniopharyngioma and astrocytomas are uncommon in these sites. Hypothalamic hamartomas are rare and usually present before the age of two years old. They are round isodense lesions that do not enhance on CT.

59 Answer B: Transient tachypnoea of the newborn

Cardiomegaly in neonates has multiple causes including hypoglycaemia, congenital heart disease, asphyxia and infants of diabetic mothers.

60 Answer D: Chondroblastoma

Chondroblastoma is a benign cartilaginous tumour that normally occurs before closure of the growth plates and is characteristically found in the epiphyses of long bones, particularly the femur and tibia. Patients tend to present with a long history of pain. They may become locally aggressive and rarely metastasise.

61 Answer A: Hereditary spherocytosis

Gallstones are rare in neonates without predisposing factors. These include: total parenteral nutrition, furosemide, short gut syndrome, obstructive congenital biliary anomaly, dehydration and haemolytic anaemia.

62 Answer B: Osteosarcoma

Osteosarcoma usually presents with a one- to two-month history of painful swelling and often with associated fever. Ewing's sarcoma rarely contains any calcification.

63 Answer E: *Mycoplasma pneumoniae*

Mycoplasma pneumoniae is the commonest cause of pneumonia in children of school age. There is a spectrum of CXR findings from interstitial infiltrates through to dense consolidation. It is often multifocal. Small effusions are seen in 20% and hilar adenopathy may be seen. *Bordetella pertussis* causes whooping cough in incompletely immunised or very young infants. CXR findings include a 'shaggy heart' caused by central patchy infiltrates and bronchial wall thickening. *Chlamydia trachomatis* causes a barking cough and is associated with conjunctivitis in infants (6–12 weeks of age) due to transvaginal inoculation at birth. Adenovirus is the most frequent viral pneumonia; CXR findings include adenopathy, peribronchial thickening, hyperinflation, and scattered bilateral subsegmental infiltrates. RSV (respiratory syncytial virus) is the most common cause of lower respiratory infection in children under two years of age.

64 Answer D. Hypointense on T1-weighted images, variable on T2-weighted images, homogeneous enhancement with a hypointense rim post gadolinium

Medulloblastoma is the most malignant infratentorial neoplasm. The duration of symptoms is usually less than one month prior to presentation. The most common site of tumour in this age group is the vermis cerebelli and the roof of the fourth ventricle.

65 Answer C: Still's disease

This is a typical presentation of Still's disease, systemic onset juvenile chronic arthritis. The arthritis may not be immediately apparent, but develops with time and persists once the systemic symptoms have resolved.

66 Answer C: Haemolytic uraemic syndrome

This is commonly caused by *E. coli* infection and is the most common cause of acute renal failure in children requiring dialysis. The classic triad is microangio-pathic haemolytic anaemia, thrombocytopaenia and acute oliguric renal failure leading to uraemia.

67 Answer A: ASD

In an ASD there is acyanosis with increased blood flow secondary to a left to right shunt. This results in right-sided cardiac enlargement, which rotates the heart. The CXR appearances therefore show a straightening of the left heart border and the SVC overlies the spine or in many cases is not seen at all on frontal images. There is no left chamber enlargement. Sixty per cent of ASDs are located at the foramen ovale (septum secundum) and 35% are located below the foramen ovale (septum primum).

68 Answer D: Fracture due to non-accidental injury

The plain radiograph findings are a subtle sign of rib fractures. This finding is pathognomonic for non-accidental injury. Accidental rib fractures are rare.

69 Answer A: Rectal duplication cyst

These account for 4% of all gastrointestinal tract duplications; 20% of patients develop perianal fistulae.

70 Answer E: Aortic coarctation

Children with aortic coarctation can present at any age with a murmur, headaches from hypertension or claudication from hypoperfusion. On CXR the 'three' sign may be seen; that is, dilated subclavian artery, which is the upper convexity; narrow point at the coarctation; and post-stenotic dilatation, which is the lower convexity. Rib notching is usually seen by six to eight years of age. Aortic coarctation can also present with congestive heart failure secondary to critical stenosis.

Paediatric radiology

PAPER 3: ANSWERS AND EXPLANATIONS

1   Answer B: Heterogeneous suprarenal mass containing calcification displacing the left kidney

The findings are those of a primary adrenal neuroblastoma with multiple metastatic skin lesions, so called Blueberry Muffin syndrome. Thirty-six per cent of neuroblastomas arise in the adrenals and are almost always unilateral. Common sites of metastases in decreasing order of occurrence are: bone, regional lymph nodes, orbits, liver, brain and lung.

2   Answer E: Lumbar myelomeningocele

The child has Arnold Chiari malformation (Chiari II malformation), which has the above characteristic features. It is associated with lumbar myelomeningocele in >95% of cases and syringohydromyelia. In addition it is associated with the following supratentorial anomalies:

- dysgenesis of corpus callosum (80–85%)
- obstructive hydrocephalus secondary to closure of myelomeningocele (50–98%)
- absence of septum pellucidum (40%)
- excessive cortical gyration.

It is notably not associated with basilar impression, C1 assimilation and Klippel-Feil deformity.

3   Answer C: Trisomy 18

Trisomy 18 or Edward's syndrome is associated with multiple abnormalities including holoprosencephaly and congenital heart defects. The prognosis is poor with death by one year of age.

4   Answer B: Renal vein thrombosis

Risk factors for renal vein thrombosis in neonates include advanced maternal age, diarrhoea, sepsis, birth trauma, adrenal haemorrhage and dehydration from vomiting. It is more common on the left due to the longer left renal vein.

5 Answer A: Transient tachypnoea of the newborn

Transient tachypnoea of the newborn is caused by inadequate clearance of the lung fluid before the first breath. It occurs typically in infants born by Caesarean section or precipitous delivery.

6 Answer A: Intraventricular haemorrhage with ventricular dilatation, 20% mortality

The grading system is:
1 Subependymal haemorrhage, no long-term abnormality
2 Intraventricular haemorrhage without ventricular dilatation, 10% mortality
3 Intraventricular haemorrhage with ventricular dilatation, 20% mortality
4 Intraparenchymal haemorrhage, 50% mortality.

7 Answer D: Posterior scalloping of vertebral bodies

Homocystinuria and Marfan's syndrome have similar phenotypes and are both disorders of connective tissue structure. Scoliosis is found in both disorders. Biconcave vertebrae are a feature of homocystinuria. The important differences are:

	Homocystinuria	Marfan's syndrome
Inheritance	Autosomal recessive	Autosomal dominant
Biochemical defect	Cystathionine synthase	Not known
Lens dislocation	Downward	Upward
Osteoporosis	Yes	No

8 Answer C: Oesophageal atresia without tracheo-oesophageal fistula

The diagnosis is made incidentally in this instance, as the patient has not required feeding yet. Nasogastric tubes are passed routinely when the neonate is intubated. The nasogastric tube does not pass into the stomach and coils in the neck. The lack of air within the abdomen differentiates it from patients with a tracheo-oesophageal fistula.

9 Answer D: Appendicitis

The appendix is frequently not visualised in appendicitis due to retrocaecal position, the inability to compress the abdomen adequately or prior perforation.

10 Answer E: 41 degrees

The alpha angle is the angle between the straight lateral edge of the ilium and the bony acetabular margin.

Hip type	Alpha angle	Description
1	>60 degrees	Mature hip
2A	50–59 degrees	Physiological <3 months

(continued)

Hip type	Alpha angle	Description
2B	43–49 degrees	Concentric but unstable
3	<43 degrees	Dislocated

11 Answer A: Giant cell astrocytoma

The diagnosis is tuberous sclerosis. It usually presents with a classic triad of facial angiofibroma, epileptic seizures (these are usually the first sign but decrease in frequency with age) and mental retardation. There are a number of associated CNS abnormalities: subependymal hamartomas, giant cell astrocytomas, cortical/subcortical tubers and heterotopic grey matter islands in the white matter.

12 Answer E: Bronchogenic cyst

Bronchogenic cysts are relatively rare but are the commonest cystic lesion of the mediastinum causing partial obstruction of the trachea or bronchus, which may lead to emphysema. Eighty-five per cent of bronchogenic cysts occur in the mediastinum; 15% are intrapulmonary.

13 Answer E: Fusiform cyst beneath the portal hepatis, separate from the gallbladder

The clinical and ultrasound findings are those of a choledochal cyst. This is the most common congenital lesion of the gallbladder and is a segmental dilatation of the common bile duct. It does not involve the gallbladder or cystic duct.

14 Answer A: Superior and lateral

In a frontal view of the hip, the line of Klein (described above) should normally intersect the femoral head. This does not happen in slipped capital femoral epiphysis, where the physis is displaced posteromedially in relation to the femoral neck. In addition the physis is wider with indistinct margins.

15 Answer C: Truncus arteriosus

In truncus arteriosus there is a single artery arising from the heart giving rise to the coronary, pulmonary and systemic arteries and straddling a large VSD. The widened mediastinum is caused by the truncus arteriosus. Affected infants usually present with severe congestive heart failure in the first days or months of life due to a large right to left shunt.

16 Answer D: Adrenocortical carcinoma

These are rare in children, with an incidence of 3:1 000 000. They present with a palpable abdominal mass and/or virilisation in females and precocious puberty in males. Approximately 20% contain calcification.

17 Answer D: Supracondylar fracture

Elevation of the anterior and posterior fat pads indicates an elbow joint effusion in association with a supracondylar, lateral condylar or proximal ulnar fracture.

The humerus is involved in 80% of paediatric elbow fractures; of these supra-condylar fractures are the most common.

18 Answer E: Transposition of great arteries

This baby has transposition of great arteries, which is the most common cause of cyanosis in the neonate. Patients with transposition of great arteries become symptomatic at one to two weeks of age.

19 Answer E: Agenesis of the corpus callosum

Dandy-Walker malformation is characterised by an enlarged posterior fossa with a high tentorium, agenesis or hypoplastic cerebellar vermis and cystic dilatation of the fourth ventricle. It is associated with other CNS abnormalities: 20–25% have dysgenesis or agenesis of the corpus callosum, 25% have holoprosencephaly and 25% have malformation of the cerebral gyri.

20 Answer A: Ultrasound during the acute infection, DMSA four to six months after the acute infection and MCUG

Recommended imaging schedule for infants younger than six months:

Test	Responds well to treatment within 48 hours	Atypical UTI	Recurrent UTI
Ultrasound during the acute infection	No	Yes	Yes
Ultrasound within 6 weeks	Yes	No	No
DMSA 4–6 months following the acute infection	No	Yes	Yes
MCUG	No	Yes	Yes

An atypical infection includes septicaemia and failure to respond to appropriate antibiotics within 48 hours. National Institute for Health and Clinical Excellence. *Urinary Tract Infection in Children: NICE guideline 54.* London: NIHCE; 2007. www.nice.org.uk/guidance/CG54

21 Answer B: Osteochondritis dissecans

Osteochondritis dissecans is an osteochondral fracture caused by chronic injury. It most commonly affects the lateral aspect of the medial femoral condyle. Early in the disease, radiographs demonstrate either no abnormality or a joint effusion. In more advanced disease there is a completely detached, loose osteochondral fragment.

22 Answer B: Teeth

This child has a pericardial teratoma, which is a benign germ cell tumour. It can cause respiratory distress and cyanosis due to pericardial tamponade and compression of the SVC, right atrium, aortic root, and pulmonary artery. Calcified pericardial cysts are extremely rare in children and usually asymptomatic.

23 Answer A: Enlarged hyperechoic left testis with increased peritesticular flow and absent parenchymal flow

The diagnosis is subacute or missed testicular torsion when symptoms are present for >24 hours and <10 days. The salvage rate is dependent on the time interval between onset of pain and surgery and is 80–100% at <6 hours and near 0% at >24 hours.

24 Answer A: Femoral metaphysis

Osteomyelitis is often the result of haematogenous spread in the paediatric population. In neonates there is commonly multicentric involvement. In children from 18 months to 18 years the metaphyseal vessels loop sharply without penetrating the growth plate, therefore the metaphysis is most commonly affected.

25 Answer C: Kawasaki syndrome

Kawasaki syndrome is an idiopathic acute febrile multisystem vasculitis involving large, medium and small arteries with a predilection for the coronary arteries. It typically occurs in children under five years old and is associated with a fever for greater than five days. Further features include cervical lymphadenopathy and erythema of palms and soles with desquamation.

26 Answer B. Ataxia telangiectasia

Ataxia telangiectasia is a rare autosomal-recessive disorder characterised by telangiectasias, cerebellar ataxia, sinus and pulmonary infections, immunodeficiencies and increased risk of developing malignancies. Cerebral infarcts are caused by emboli shunted through the vascular malformations in the lung. Ruptured telangiectatic vessels can cause cerebral haemorrhage. Wolman disease is a very rare autosomal-recessive lipid storage disease, which is almost always fatal in the first year of life. Friedreich's ataxia shows atrophy of the cervical spinal cord but the cerebellum is usually spared. Multiple sclerosis shows plaques within the brain and cerebral atrophy, not cerebellar atrophy. Niemann-Pick disease is lipid storage disorder; there are multiple sub-types, most of which would have been fatal by the age of presentation of this child and there is also no imaging CNS abnormalities involved.

27 Answer B: Intussusception

Other findings on abdominal radiograph include an abdominal soft-tissue mass in the right upper quadrant, normal appearances and small bowel obstruction.

28 Answer B: CT head without intravenous contrast

In suspected non-accidental injury a skeletal survey and an AP and lateral skull radiograph should be performed. Once the patient is stable a CT brain, initially unenhanced, should be performed. If the fontanelle is patent, cranial ultrasound should be performed. MRI should be used if there are neurological signs but the CT brain is equivocal or normal.

29 Answer A: Differential function can be measured

Differential function can be measured and assessment of split function in duplex systems can be made. A horseshoe kidney may be demonstrated but it is not a primary indication for a DMSA. GFR is an entirely different study using Tc-99m-labelled DTPA and serial blood tests. No dynamic images are obtained on DMSA and obstruction or reflux of urinary flow is not a feature. However, the sequelae of infection, such as cortical scarring and reduced differential function, can be accurately demonstrated.

30 Answer B: Henoch-Schönlein purpura

This is a hypersensitivity-related acute small-vessel vasculitis, which often begins as an upper respiratory tract infection. It causes a proliferative glomerulonephritis with IgA deposits and can lead to renal insufficiency and rarely to end-stage renal disease.

31 Answer B: Late-phase Perthes disease

Perthes disease is avascular necrosis of the femoral head. Early in the disease there is widening of the joint space, a small femoral epiphysis and sclerosis of the femoral head. On radionucleotide imaging there is reduced uptake in the femoral head. Later in the disease a radiolucent crescent line is seen, which represents a subchondral fracture, there is femoral head fragmentation and femoral neck cysts. On radionucleotide imaging there is increased uptake in the femoral head.

32 Answer A: Dandy-Walker malformation

Dandy-Walker malformation is characterised by an enlarged posterior fossa with a high tentorium, agenesis or abnormal cerebellar vermis and cystic dilatation of the fourth ventricle.

An arachnoid cyst is an ultrasound differential for Dandy-Walker but the anatomy and source of the cystic structure should be evident on CT. This child is too young and displaying incorrect symptoms for a diagnosis of epidermoid cyst. The cyst fluid in an astrocytoma is denser than CSF and shows some degree of solid tumour thus allowing differentiation.

33 Answer E: Air trapping and hyperinflation

This child has aspirated a foreign body, which often causes air trapping and hyperinflation, and less often gives rise to pulmonary infiltrates.

34 Answer C: Malrotation of the ileum

The other options can all give false positive results. False negative results can be caused by a recent barium enema, irritable bowel in the right lower quadrant causing rapid transit or presence of only a small amount of ectopic gastric mucosa.

35 Answer B: Chondromyxoid fibroma

Chondromyxoid fibroma is a rare benign cartilaginous tumour that presents with pain. It is usually found in the metaphysis of the long bones, most commonly in the proximal tibia. There is no associated periosteal reaction unless it is fractured.

36 Answer B: Morgagni hernia

This boy has a Morgagni hernia, which is an anteromedial parasternal defect caused by the maldevelopment of the septum pellucidum and tends to present in older children. Bochdalek hernias are posterolateral defects and tend to present in babies. The chronic cough may have been misdiagnosed as asthma but may well be related to the hernia.

37 Answer C: Stage 2B

The staging system for Hodgkin's lymphoma is:
Stage 1: One group of lymph nodes involved.
Stage 2: Two or more groups of lymph nodes involved on one side of the diaphragm.
Stage 3: Lymph nodes involved on both sides of the diaphragm. The spleen may be involved.
Stage 4: Spread beyond lymph nodes to, for example, liver, lungs or bone marrow.
A: No systemic symptoms
B: Night sweats, weight loss >10% or fever.

38 Answer C: Ewing's sarcoma

Forty per cent of Ewing's sarcoma are found in the flat bones and usually have a disproportionately large soft-tissue mass. They have a large intrathoracic component and a minimal extrathoracic component.

39 Answer B: Pilocytic astrocytoma

Pilocytic astrocytoma is one of the most common childhood cancers of the posterior fossa. It is also the most benign astrocytoma and is associated with neurofibromatosis type I. The symptoms are dependent on the position of the tumour. T2-weighted images are the differentiating sequences, as PNETs and ependymomas are isointense. Medulloblastomas are isointense on T1-weighted images and usually have a ring of vessels between the tumour and the brain.

40 Answer A: Respiratory distress syndrome

This baby has respiratory distress syndrome, which is an acute pulmonary disorder characterised by generalised atelectasis, intrapulmonary shunting, ventilation-perfusion abnormalities and reduced lung compliance due to surfactant deficiency. Term infants of diabetic mothers are predisposed to the condition.

41 Answer B: Turner's syndrome

Turner's syndrome is a monosomy 45, XO. It is associated with renal ectopia and horseshoe kidney. Neonates with Turner's may be born with lymphoedema of the hands and feet.

42 Answer A: Osteoblastoma

Approximately half of osteoblastomas are found in the spine, most of which arise in the posterior elements. They typically present with painful scoliosis, worse at night.

43 Answer B: Scintigraphy

Scintigraphy should be considered if non-accidental injury is suspected in children with single fractures who have a negative skeletal survey, if there is a high index of suspicion of non-accidental injury but skeletal survey is negative, when radiographic findings are ambiguous and to demonstrate occult fractures before changes are seen on plain radiographs. Scintigraphy is sensitive in detecting soft-tissue injury and rib, scapular, spinal, diaphyseal and pelvic fractures. In older children scintigraphy can be used as an initial screening test for non-accidental injury.

44 Answer A: Respiratory syncytial virus bronchiolitis

Respiratory syncytial virus (RSV) causes 75% of cases of bronchiolitis, most commonly affecting infants between three and six months old.

45 Answer E: Blount disease

Early onset Blount disease is a form of osteochondrosis of the medial proximal tibial metaphysis. There is increase in the normal physiological bowing of the lower limbs at onset of weight bearing. It is progressive, present bilaterally in 80% and is more common in obese black children. Physiological bowing of the legs involves both the tibia and distal femur and is normal in children less than two years old.

46 Answer C: Wilson's disease

Wilson's disease is an autosomal-recessive disease that causes excessive copper retention. The dark ring around the iris is a Kayser-Fleischer ring and is diagnostic of Wilson's disease. Wilson's disease causes cirrhosis, neurological, renal and ophthalmological dysfunction. Children usually present with hepatic dysfunction.

47 Answer C: Congenital lobar emphysema

This newborn has congenital lobar emphysema of the middle lobe. Congenital lobar emphysema mainly presents in the neonatal period and most commonly affects the left upper lobe, then the middle lobe, followed by the right upper lobe. Initially, there is opacity due to slow clearance of foetal lung fluid, which clears over the first days of life, then hyperinflates.

48 Answer D: Tangential to the superior end plate of the superior end vertebra and tangential to the inferior end plate of the inferior end vertebra

The Cobb angle is the most commonly used method of measuring the scoliotic curve on an AP view. It divides severity of curvature into seven categories and is used to aid selection of patients for surgical treatment and monitoring results of treatment. The vertebrae used in measurement must be noted and the same vertebrae used in subsequent measurements to allow comparison. The Risser-Ferguson method, which is used less commonly, is measured as described in answer A. The result is not comparable with the Cobb angle.

49 Answer A: Acute splenic sequestration crisis

This occurs in patients with sickle cell disease when the intrasplenic veins become obstructed leading to a sudden trapping of a large amount of blood in the spleen.

50 Answer C: Soft-tissue swelling, juxta-articular osteopenia and periosteal reaction

Juvenile rheumatoid arthritis commonly involves the large joints initially. Radiographic appearances later in the disease include erosions, epiphyseal over-growth and ankylosis.

51 Answer E. Repetitive subarachnoid microhaemorrhage

The most common cause of communicating hydrocephalus is repetitive sub-arachnoid microhaemorrhage mainly due to repetitive trauma. The other causes are less frequent but can cause hydrocephalus.

52 Answer A: Right upper lobe apical segmental bronchus originates from the trachea rather than the right upper lobe bronchus

This is also known as a 'pig bronchus' since in a pig the right upper lobe bronchus normally arises from the trachea. There is also an association with tracheal stenosis. Rarely, there may be a duplicated bronchus with a normally located right upper lobe apical segmental bronchus present as well.

53 Answer A: Anterolateral bowing of the tibia

Anterolateral bowing of the tibia is seen in patients with neurofibromatosis type I; this is secondary to deossification. The tibial shaft is often narrowed.

54 Answer B: Osteogenesis imperfecta

Osteogenesis imperfecta is a group of connective tissue disorders with deficient collagen formation. There is a spectrum of clinical findings and severity. The clinical and radiological findings described above are those of osteogenesis imperfecta type II. This is the more severe form and the disease is manifest at birth (and in utero on antenatal ultrasound). Osteogenesis imperfecta can be difficult to differentiate from non-accidental injury, which is far more common. Fractures in osteogenesis imperfecta tend to involve the shafts of long bones and result in deformity. In addition, children with osteogenesis imperfecta usually have blue sclerae, wormian bones and impaired hearing.

55 Answer C: She is unlikely to have aspirated

Hydrocarbon aspiration can occur from emesis post ingestion of gasoline, kerosene, household cleaners and polishes. CXR findings are usually significant at two to eight hours after ingestion, which includes pulmonary infiltrates due to pneumonitis. Pneumatoceles may develop as sequelae.

56 Answer C: Budd-Chiari syndrome

This is the syndrome of clinical and pathological abnormalities seen with acute hepatic vein occlusion. Most cases are idiopathic but it can be related to radiation, chemotherapy, toxins and other causes. Hepatic veno-occlusive disease refers to occlusion of the post-sinusoidal venules with the inferior vena cava and major hepatic veins remaining patent.

57 Answer A: A well-demarcated low-attenuation lesion a few millimetres in size, surrounded by an area of high attenuation

Osteoid osteoma is a common benign bone tumour. Its commonest location is within the cortex of long bones. It characteristically presents with pain that is worse at night and is relieved by non-steroidal anti-inflammatory drugs. On plain radiographs it is a small (<1.5 cm) lytic lesion, which is surrounded by reactive sclerosis. The nidus may not be visible on plain radiographs due to the density of the surrounding sclerosis. CT shows the nidus in these cases. Osteoblastoma is a rare benign tumour that can undergo malignant transformation. It is similar histologically to osteoid osteoma. It has a nidus of >1.5 cm that ranges from lytic to densely sclerotic in appearance.

58 Answer B: Great vessel aneurysm

Mediastinal lesions by location:

- anywhere in the mediastinum – lymphoma/leukaemia, adenopathy, mediastinitis, haematoma
- anterior mediastinum – teratoma, thyroid, thymoma
- middle mediastinum – bronchopulmonary foregut malformations, hiatal hernia/other gastric or oesophageal abnormality, cardiac/pericardiac tumours and cysts, great vessels aneurysms/anomalies
- posterior mediastinum – neurogenic tumours, neurenteric cysts, lateral meningoceles, spinal tumours/osteomyelitis/discitis, descending aortic or azygous anomaly/aneurysm, extramedullary haematopoiesis.

59 Answer E: Leydig cell tumour

Leydig cell tumours usually present between three and six years of age. They produce oestrogens or testosterones, resulting in gynaecomastia or virilisation.

60 Answer B: Cystic fibrosis

In cystic fibrosis the lungs are initially normal but abnormal chloride secretions result in viscoid airway mucus, which predisposes to infection, inflammatory response and airway obstruction of small and large airways. There is progressive bronchiectasis and chronic obstruction, resulting in hyperinflation. Adenopathy may develop causing hilar enlargement and later pulmonary hypertension with dilated central pulmonary arteries may be seen. Increasing cardiac size indicates cor pulmonale and poor survival without transplantation. Pneumomediastinum and pneumothorax can also occur.

61 Answer B: Pyloric stenosis

This occurs most frequently in boys aged three to six months and presents with non-bilious vomiting.

62 Answer D: RSV

The commonest organisms causing pneumonia at different ages:

- Premature infants – (1) Group B *Streptococcus*, (2) *E. coli*, (3) *Listeria*, (4) CMV
- Infants – (1) RSV, (2) *Chlamydia*, (3) *Streptococcus pneumoniae*, (4) *Haemophilus influenzae* type B
- School age – (1) *Mycoplasma*, (2) *Influenza* A, (3) *Streptococcus pneumoniae*.

63 Answer C: Midgut malrotation

Midgut malrotation usually presents within the first month of life with bilious vomiting. The pathognomonic finding of midgut malrotation is an abnormally positioned ligament of Treitz with the duodenojejunal junction lying to the right or below the expected normal position, shown on a barium meal. Duodenal atresia obstructs near the ampulla of Vater and results in bilious vomiting in the first 24 hours of life. Plain radiograph findings of duodenal atresia are of a 'double bubble' sign of a dilated stomach and duodenal bulb with no gas seen distally.

64 Answer E: Craniopharyngioma

Craniopharyngioma can also present with diabetes insipidus from compression of the pituitary gland. Epidermoids of the CNS usually present at a later age (10–60 years old) with different symptoms but can have bony destruction and calcification. Rathke's cleft cysts and pituitary adenomas do not cause bony destruction and are unlikely to contain calcification.

65 Answer C: PDA

Surfactant decreases atelectasis and pulmonary vascular resistance, and allows a PDA to shunt left to right. An enlarged aorta, left atrium and left ventricle are seen in PDA.

66 Answer C: Necrotising enterocolitis

Necrotising enterocolitis is the most common surgical emergency in neonates. Inflammation and mucosal ulceration of the bowel leads to widespread transmural necrosis.

67 Answer B: Poland syndrome

Poland syndrome is a congenital defect with unilateral underdevelopment or absence of pectoralis muscles. There is usually ipsilateral syndactyly. The right side is more commonly affected. In pectus excavatum there is a depressed sternum with left-sided displacement of the heart and loss of definition of the right heart border (resembling right middle lobe pneumonia) on CXR. In pectus carinatum there is a 'pigeon breast' with prominence of the sternum. Askin tumour is an aggressive neuroectodermal chest wall tumour, which is destructive and invasive.

68 Answer B: Ectopic thyroid tissue seen in the suprahyoid position

The condition described is congenital hypothyroidism. Ectopic thyroid is the most common cause of congenital hypothyroidism.

69 Answer D: Down's syndrome

Eleven pairs of ribs are seen in cleidocranial dysplasia, campomelic dysplasia and in 5% of normal individuals. Ninety per cent of babies with Down's syndrome have a hypersegmented manubrium and 25% have 11 pairs of ribs.

70 Answer D: Rhabdomyosarcoma of the biliary tract

This a rare tumour, most commonly arising from the common bile duct. It is more common in males.

Neuroradiology, head and neck and ENT radiology

PAPER 1: ANSWERS AND EXPLANATIONS

1 Answer D: PTH level

This patient has hyperparathyroidism and the lytic mass is a brown tumour. Generalised loss of the lamina dura is seen in osteoporosis, osteomalacia, Paget's disease, scleroderma and hyperparathyroidism. The description is typical for a brown tumour and these are most commonly seen in primary hyperparathyroidism. The jaw is the most common site for these tumours.

2 Answer A: Coloboma

A Coloboma is a congenital defect in the orbit, which is caused by incomplete closure of the choroidal fissure. They are typically cone or notched shaped and commonly affect the inferomedial portion of the globe. They are bilateral in 50% and can occur in association with other congenital abnormalities such as encephalocele, agenesis of the corpus callosum or as part of a syndrome (CHARGE syndrome).

3 Answer C: Pineoblastoma

Leukokoria is a white papillary light reflex. This can be caused by tumours (retinoblastomas, retinal hamartomas), developmental (PHPV, Coat's disease), infections and trauma. These bilateral orbital masses are retinoblastomas and this is a very typical description. The peak age is 18 months and males and females are affected equally. Two-thirds are sporadic and of these only 30% are bilateral while in the hereditary form 70% are bilateral. When bilateral retinoblastomas are associated with pineoblastomas they are called trilateral retinoblastomas.

4 Answer B: Drusen

Drusen are the accumulation of calcified hyaline material typically in the region of the optic nerve. It is bilateral 75% of the time and is often familial. Typically, on CT they are flat discs of calcification overlying the optic nerves. Patients present with headaches and visual field defects.

5 Answer B: Microphthalmia

Persistent hyperplastic primary vitreous (PHPV) is a rare condition caused by persistence of the primary vitreous, which presents in newborns with leukocoria. The orbit is small and deformed with a flattened lens and the optic nerve is small. PHPV is hypervascular and prone to bleeding hence the vitreous is dense due to repeated haemorrhage. No calcification is demonstrated. Retinoblastomas cause expansion of the globe, are calcified and cause bony destruction. Both tumours can be high signal on T1-weighted imaging.

6 Answer E: Kinking and bucking of the optic nerve

Features	Meningioma	Optic glioma
Age	Middle-aged females	Children under 5 years
Uni/bilateral	Typically unilateral	May be bilateral, if so consider NF1 (25%)
Symptoms	Slow progressive painless loss of vision	Slow progression painless loss of vision. Central scotoma
Bone reaction	Hyperostosis	No hyperostosis
Optic canal widening	10%	90%
Optic nerve	Straight optic nerve with eccentric thickening	Kinking and buckling of optic nerve. Smooth outline
Calcification	Calcification common	Calcification uncommon
MRI signals	Similar signal characteristic to the optic nerve	Isointense on T1 and bright on T2
Enhancement	Diffuse uniform enhancement, train track sign	Variable enhancement

7 Answer A: High signal on both T1- and T2-weighted imaging

Orbital melanomas are high signal on both T1- and T2-weighted imaging. They are the commonest intraocular primary in adults, arise from the choroids plexus and are associated with retinal detachment, vitreous haemorrhage and glaucoma.

8 Answer B: Precocious puberty

The imaging features are typical of fibrous dysplasia. Fibrous dysplasia, multiple café au lait spots and endocrine disorder such as precocious puberty and hyperthyroidism are seen in McCune-Albright syndrome.

9 Answer D: Antrochoanal polyp

An antrochoanal polyp is a benign expansile lesion of the maxillary sinus, which usually arises from the maxillary antrum and causes bone remodelling due to mass effect. On CT the mass is of homogeneous low density reflecting the oedematous nature of the polyp. They fill the antrum, expanding through the secondary ostium into the ipsilateral nasal cavity and may even extend through the posterior choana into the nasopharynx. The oedematous mass displays low signal intensity on T1 weighting and high signal on T2. There may also be peripheral enhancement post gadolinium. By definition an antrochoanal polyp extends into the nasal cavity and the diagnosis is aided by the evidence of bony remodelling rather than erosion, the latter being suggestive of a malignant process. A mucocele can be expansile but would not extend beyond the cavity of the sinus. An inverted papilloma displays moderate enhancement on CT and intermediate signal intensity on T1W images with definite enhancement post contrast.

10 Answer E: Congenital cholesteatoma

Cholesteatomas can be classed as either congenital or acquired. They appear as relatively well-circumscribed masses, which sometimes contain cystic areas and do not enhance post contrast. A congenital cholesteatoma typically occurs in childhood as a result of inclusion of squamous epithelium within the temporal bone during development. An intact TM is visible on both examination and on radiological images and the patient is often asymptomatic. An acquired cholesteatoma arises from a retraction pocket of the tympanic membrane, usually causing a chronically discharging ear and grossly abnormal tympanic membrane. In 70–80% of cases of acquired cholesteatoma the mass is seen lateral to the ossicular chain. Conversely, in the congenital form it is medial and fills the oval window niche. Cholesterol granulomas are granulomatous lesions, which are thought to arise as a result of an inflammatory process, and contain both cholesterol and haemosiderin deposits. The appearances on CT are very similar to those of cholesteatomas and may even be indistinguishable. On MRI, however, cholesterol granulomas can be differentiated from congenital cholesteatomas. Cholesterol granulomas display high signal intensity on both T1- and T2-weighted images as a result of the presence of haemoglobin breakdown products. Cholesteatomas are of low signal intensity on T1 and high intensity on T2W images. Glomus tympanicum are a type of paraganglioma arising from the paraganglion cells around Jacobson's nerve in the middle ear. They are the most common primary neoplasms of the middle ear and on examination can be seen as a pulsating cherry red mass behind the tympanic membrane. On CT the mass can be seen arising from the wall of the middle ear and as a result of its hypervascular nature displays intense enhancement post contrast on both MRI and CT.

11 Answer A: Persistent stapedial artery

A persistent stapedial artery (PSA) is a vascular anomaly that arises from the petrous part of the internal carotid artery. It can present with hearing loss, pulsatile tinnitus or a mass seen over the promontory in the middle ear on otoscopic examination but is often an incidental finding. The prevalence is approximately 0.05%. The stapedial artery develops from the hyoid artery during early foetal life and divides into upper and lower branches. The upper branch becomes the middle meningeal artery and the lower leaves the cranial cavity via the foramen spinosum and becomes the inferior alveolar and infraorbital arteries. If the stapedial artery persists then the middle meningeal artery arises from it and the foramen spinosum is aplastic, hence absence of the foramen spinosum is an indirect sign of PSA. A small vessel arising from the petrous part of the internal carotid artery and coursing through the middle ear cavity may be visible on CT and if not recognised, injury can cause haemorrhage during middle ear surgery. PSA can also be associated with an aberrant internal carotid artery.

Jain R, *et al*. Persistent stapedial artery. *Radiology*. 2004; **230**(2): 413–16.

12 Answer B. Enhancement following gadolinium

Acoustic neuromas are also known as vestibular schwannomas and are the most common tumours of the cerebellopontine angle. They arise from the perineural Schwann cells of the vestibular division of the VIII cranial nerve and are usually unilateral. In Type II neurofibromatosis they are, by definition, bilateral. A vestibular schwannoma displays the characteristic imaging appearances that are common to all schwannomas; on CT imaging they are isointense with brain parenchyma, exhibiting enhancement post contrast and containing cystic components. On MRI the lesion is isointense with brain parenchyma on T1W images, hyperintense on T2 and displays enhancement post gadolinium.

13 Answer B: High signal intensity on T2-weighted images

A Tornwaldt's cyst is a benign submucosal lesion found in the midline of the posterior nasopharynx. It is a diverticular remnant lined by squamous epithelium and occurs due to a persistent communication between the notochord and the nasopharyngeal epithelium during development. As a result it can become filled with proteinaceous secretions then intermittently discharge its contents into the nasopharynx. A midline mass is seen on CT along the posterior wall of the nasopharynx that exhibits high attenuation due to its increased protein content. This high protein content is also reflected in the MRI findings of a thin-walled, cystic structure seen within the pharyngeal bursa between the longus coli muscles that displays a high signal intensity on T1W and T2W. Characteristically, the cyst does not enhance with contrast.

14 Answer B. Frontal sinus mucocele

A sinus mucocele is an expansile lesion, which develops as a result of obstruction of the sinus ostium, containing mucoid secretions and lined by respiratory epithelium. Mucoceles can arise from any of the sinuses but most commonly affect the frontal sinus (65% of cases) with the sphenoid being the least affected. On CT scan there is complete opacification of the sinus as it is filled with mucoid secretions causing the sinus cavity to enlarge and the walls to undergo remodelling and thinning due to pressure necrosis. The diagnosis is confirmed if there is complete absence of any remaining air within the sinus. These appearances are in contrast to mucous retention cysts, which occur because of blockage and swelling of a mucous gland within the sinus mucosa and therefore air remains within the sinus cavity itself. Characteristic appearances on CT are that of an expanded frontal sinus cavity filled with homogeneous low-attenuation matter. The peripheral rim enhancement enables it to be differentiated from other pathologies such as inverted papilloma. Due to the high water content (>95%) of the secretions the signal intensity on MR is of low intensity on T1 and high on T2W images. A malignant pathological process would be expected to cause bone destruction as opposed to remodelling. A frontal mucocele can extend into the upper orbit causing the patient to experience a range of symptoms such as proptosis, nasal obstruction and bossing of the forehead.

15 Answer A: On MRI the granulation tissue would be expected to be low intensity on both T1- and T2-weighted images

Malignant otitis externa is a potentially fatal infection of the external ear, which presents with severe, deep otalgia and tends to affect immunocompromised individuals, particularly those with diabetes. It is almost always associated with *pseudomonas aeruginosa*. A high index of suspicion is required and if left undiagnosed the infection can result in osteomyelitis of the skull base causing erosion of the mastoid and temporal bones. This can result in lower cranial nerve palsies, sigmoid sinus thrombosis as well as meningeal and intracranial involvement. On CT an abnormal soft-tissue mass is visualised in the external auditory canal with associated bony destruction and opacification of the mastoid air cells. On MRI the granulation tissue is classically low intensity on both T1- and T2-weighted images. MRI is generally superior to CT with regard to detection of skull base involvement due to its ability to identify bone marrow oedema. The radiological appearances usually lag behind the clinical and pathological findings.

16 Answer B. Level II

See table below of the anatomical boundaries of the six cervical lymph node levels.

Cervical lymph node level	Anatomical boundaries
Level IA (submental)	Anterior belly of digastric muscles and hyoid bone
Level IB (submandibular)	Anterior belly of digastric muscle, hyoid bone, the stylohyoid muscle and the body of the mandible
Levels II (upper jugular)	Anterior triangle from skull base superiorly to the inferior aspect of the hyoid bone inferiorly
Level III (midjugular)	Anterior triangle from hyoid bone superiorly to the cricoid cartilage inferiorly
Level IV (lower jugular)	Anterior triangle cricoid cartilage superiorly to the clavicle
Level V	Posterior triangle
Level VI (anterior triangle)	Lymph nodes of the anterior central compartment group

Harrison L, Sessions RB, Waun Ki Hong. *Head and Neck Cancer: a multidisciplinary approach*. Baltimore, MD: Lippincott, Williams and Wilkins; 2008. p. 183.

17 Answer E. Perineural extension

The most common malignant tumour of the parotid gland is mucoepidermoid carcinoma and in children it is the most frequently occurring salivary gland malignancy. This tumour type is composed of both mucoid and squamous (epidermoid) cells, the latter forming the majority of the cell population in the more high-grade tumours. On both CT and MRI the imaging appearances can vary depending on the grade of the tumour, with low-grade lesions appearing well circumscribed while higher grade lesions are poorly defined and infiltrative. Signal intensities on both T1- and T2-weighted images are low to intermediate, and enhancement is clearly evident post contrast. A hypointense signal intensity on T2W images enables differentiation between a parotid malignancy and a pleomorphic adenoma. Both adenocystic and mucoepidermoid tumours can exhibit perineural extension.

18 Answer A: Le Fort I

All Le Fort fractures involve the pterygoid process. Le Fort I is a transverse fracture through the maxilla, Le Fort II is more extensive and the separated fragment is pyramidal while in Le Fort III there is complete craniofacial disjunction. In practice fractures do not fit these descriptions exactly and maybe asymmetrical or coexist. The classification is still in general use and aids in subsequent surgical management. In Le Fort I and II the fractured maxillary fragment is usually wired to the zygomatic arches, but if these are fractured as in Le Fort III, a more complex pin and rod fixation to the skull vault is undertaken.

19 Answer B: *Staphylococcus aureus*

The most common pathogens that result in a retropharyngeal abscess are *Staphylococcus aureus* or Group A beta haemolytic *Streptococcus*. The retropharyngeal space is an important potential space posterior to the pharyngeal mucosa extending from the skull base to the T4 and is important as it is the route through which infection can spread to the mediastinum. Retropharyngeal abscesses typically follow an upper respiratory tract infection and present in children with general malaise, anorexia and stridor. On lateral neck plain X-rays there is thickening of the retropharyngeal space and blebs of air maybe seen in the abscess. A false positive result may occur if the child's neck is flexed or if the film is taken in expiration. On CT there is typically thickening of the retropharyngeal space, fat streaking, abscess and enlarged cervical lymphadenopathy.

20 Answer A: Facial nerve schwannoma

The intratemporal segment of the facial nerve is affected in this case. A facial nerve schwannoma is the only lesion that can be limited to this region. Acoustic neuromas can involve CN VIII while brain stem gliomas are likely to involve other cranial nerves, such as VI. Parotid malignancy and malignant otitis media could compromise the extracranial parotid segment of the facial nerve but would not be expected to be associated with the loss of lacrimation and taste.

21 Answer A: En plaque spread along the skull base

It is assumed she has a meningioma. Erosion of the jugular foramen is suggestive of a glomus jugulare tumour while smooth expansion would be expected in a vagal schwannoma. Enhancement occurs in both neuromas and meningiomas, and therefore is not a distinguishing feature. Thickening of the dura is seen in meningitis or dural metastasis and is an unlikely finding in a jugular foramen meningioma.

22 Answer A: Giant cell granuloma

GCG is thought to be a reactive inflammatory process resulting in overgrowth of tissue in response to trauma or infection. They are more common in the mandibular region than the maxillary region and are less than 2 cm in size. Patients with GCG typically present early in adult life with a male to female ratio of 1:1. GCG is associated with Paget's disease and fibrous dysplasia. Gingivitis is a risk factor.

Nackos JS, *et al.* CT and MR imaging of giant cell granuloma of the craniofacial bones. *Am J Neuroradiol.* 2006; **27**(8): 1651–3.

23 Answer C: Round shape

Size alone is a relatively poor criterion in defining a neck lymph node to be possibly malignant. Oval nodes with a fatty hilum tend to be benign. The orientation of the node is irrelevant. Further features such as calcification, necrosis, extracapsular spread and increased Doppler flow could represent malignant spread.

24 Answer A: Ranula

These are the classical findings of a ranula. The most important differential diagnosis to exclude is a pleomorphic adenoma, which would enhance on fat saturated T1-weighted images. B would appear in the posterior triangle, while a thyroglossal duct cyst is likely to be in the midline. D is not normally sublingual and normally multiloculate.

25 Answer B: Vein of Galen (VoG) malformation

VoG malformation is used to describe enlarged deep venous structures of the galenic system fed by abnormal midline AV communications. Presentation is usually early in life with high output cardiac failure and obstructive hydrocephalus. Seizures, focal neurologic deficit and haemorrhage can occur. Spontaneous thrombosis is known.

26 Answer B: Neurofibromatosis type 1

Involvement of the optic tracts is typically seen in NF-1. Histologically, most lesions are low-grade astrocytomas although 20% of chiasmal gliomas may behave aggressively. Imaging is best on MRI where lesions are usually hypo to isointense on T1 and hyperintense on T2 with variable contrast enhancement.

27 Answer D: Spinal cord

The underlying condition is von Hippel-Lindau syndrome (VHL). Differentials for intra-axial cystic lesions in the posterior fossa in adults include metastases, haemangioblastoma, lymphoma and lipoma. Most haemangioblastomas occur sporadically while 10–20% occur in VHL. In VHL 75% of haemangioblastomas occur in the cerebellum and 25% in the spinal cord. Appearances in the spinal cord are those of a syrinx-like cyst with an isointense nodule that enhances strongly after contrast.

28   Answer B: Morquio syndrome

The condition described is os odontoideum which is either orthotopic with a normal position of the odontoid tip or dystopic with the tip near the basioccipital bone in the area of the foramen magnum. It may be fixed to the anterior ring of the atlas and the two move as a unit. Subluxation and instability are common. It is often discovered incidentally and associated syndromes include Morquio syndrome and multiple epiphyseal dysplasia. Differentiation from non-union may be difficult.

29   Answer C: Chiari II malformation

Chiari II is the most common and serious complex of anomalies resulting from a small posterior fossa. Chiari I is not associated with a myelomeningocele and is an isolated hindbrain anomaly without supratentorial abnormalities. Chiari III is rare and thought to be unrelated to Chiari I and II. It is associated with occipital/cervical meningomyelocele. Dandy-Walker is characterised by a large posterior fossa, vermian anomalies and cystic dilatation of the fourth ventricle.

30   Answer C: Dandy-Walker malformation

Dandy-Walker malformations are characterised by a large posterior fossa, vermian anomalies and cystic dilatation of the fourth ventricle filling the entire posterior fossa. Midline CNS anomalies are seen in >60%. Differentials include a posterior fossa extra-axial cyst, arachnoid cyst and a mega cisterna magna.

31   Answer C: Neurofibroma

The condition described is NF-1. Abnormalities within the spine occur in about 60% of patients. Most of these are secondary to a neurofibroma which maybe dumbbell shaped along an exiting nerve root. Lateral thoracic meningoceles are also known to occur. Meningiomas and ependymomas are more common in NF-2.

32   Answer E: Sturge-Weber syndrome

Sturge-Weber syndrome is a sporadically occurring phakomatosis in which facial port wine naevi, leptomeningeal venous angiomatosis and orbital manifestations are described. Presentation is usually with seizures contralateral to the site of facial naevus. The underlying aetiology is probably an abnormality in the development of cortical venous drainage. Cortical atrophy, tram track gyral calcification, enhancing pial angioma and prominent draining veins may be seen.

33   Answer A: Mineralising angiopathy

Mineralising angiopathy is widespread perivascular calcification which typically occurs in children receiving both irradiation and chemotherapy for acute leuk-aemia. The commonest sites include basal ganglia and junction of the cortex and subcortical white matter.

34 Answer E: Axial T2*-weighted MRI images

The history is typical of a subarachnoid haemorrhage (SAH). A month after the event the blood would have be degraded to haemosiderin, which is low signal on T2, T1, FLAIR and T2*. Blooming artefact occurs with T2*, which can help detect small amounts of blood and would be the most useful test to perform. Lumbar puncture would not be helpful as it is too long since the bleed. Once a diagnosis of a subarachnoid bleed has been made then the cause for the bleed can be diagnosed using CT cranial angiogram.

35 Answer E: Left superior cerebellar artery

Left-sided cerebellar symptoms are caused by ipsilateral lesions in the cerebel-lum, while left-sided cerebral symptoms are due to contralateral lesions. The most superior aspect of the cerebellar hemisphere, vermis and tectum is supplied by the superior cerebellar artery. The posterior inferior cerebellar artery supplies the inferoposterior surface of the cerebellar hemisphere. The anterior inferior cerebellar artery supplies the middle cerebellar peduncle, floccular region and the anterior petrosal surface of the cerebellum.

36 Answer D: Dehydration

This child has a transverse sinus thrombosis described on the CT as high density within the dural sinus. A contrast CT reveals a filling defect in the dural sinus, descried as the delta sign. On MR in the acute phase there is low signal on T2 and isointense signal on T1. Dural sinus thrombosis can result in venous infarcts which on CT appear as parenchymal haemorrhage involving both grey and white matter typically in an unusual position such as bilaterally affecting the parasagit-tal parenchyma. Thirty per cent of all dural sinus thrombosis are spontaneous. The rest are either due to infection from mastoiditis, sinusitis, encephalitis and meningitis and from non-infective causes such as trauma, tumour compressing the dural sinus or from low flow states such as dehydration and congestive heart disease. On the CT, there is no opacification of the mastoid air cells or sinuses; therefore, the most likely cause is dehydration.

37 Answer C: 1.3%

The risk of stroke due to an angiogram is approximately 1.3%.

Willinsky PW, *et al*. Neurologic complications of cerebral angiography: prospective analysis of 2,899 procedures and review of the literature. *Radiology*. 2003; **227**(2): 522–8.

38 Answer E: Insular ribbon sign

Thrombosis of the deep cerebral veins may cause relatively symmetric infarction of the basal ganglia, thalami and midbrain. Involvement of the grey-white matter may occur in a non-arterial distribution. MRI demonstrates loss of flow void in the venous sinuses and depending on the age of the clot a high signal on T2 and FLAIR images in the venous sinuses. Pitfalls include slow flow states and arachnoid granulations. The insular ribbon sign is seen in early arterial infarcts and indicates loss of grey-white differentiation.

39 Answer D: Right common femoral artery

Patients who are undergoing a coiling have a general anaesthetic as they need to keep completely still for the procedure. For simple cerebral angiograms patients do not have to have general anaesthetics if they are cooperative. The right femoral approach is used because it is easier to manoeuvre the wires into position from this approach. The right brachial approach is not used as the neuroradiologist tries to minimise the amount the aorta is crossed. A 5–6 French catheter is used and hand injection rather than pump injection. Typically, only small volumes of contrast are needed (7–8 mL over two seconds).

40 Answer D: Diffuse low uptake

This hypothyroid patient has Hashimoto's disease. The ultrasound features of a heterogeneous diffusely enlarged low-reflectivity thyroid with increased vascularity are very typical of Hashimoto's disease. On Tc-99m imaging there is generalised low uptake of tracer within the thyroid. The pyramidal lobe can be prominent and there may be a single or multiple cold nodules within the thyroid.

41 Answer A: Middle meningeal artery

Extradural haematomas (EDH) are biconvex/lentiform in shape and result from a lacerated middle meningeal artery/dural sinus in 70–85%. Associated fractures are seen in 85–95%. EDH occur between the skull and the dura and cross dural attachments, but not sutures. Subdural haematomas are crescentic and are generally caused by stretching/tearing of bridging cortical veins. They occur between the dura and arachnoid and cross sutures but not dural attachments.

42 Answer D: Grey-white matter junction

Diffuse axonal injury (DAI) occurs in severe trauma as a result of shearing stress along the course of the white matter tracts especially at the grey-white matter junction. The injury is usually microscopic and initial CTs are usually normal despite profound clinical impairment. Acute DAI may also be seen as small petechial haemorrhages at the grey-white matter junction (67%), internal/external capsule, corona radiata, corpus callosum (21%) and brainstem. MR features depend on the age of the haemorrhage. Prognosis is poor.

43 Answer C: Caroticocavernous fistula (CCF)

A CCF is a dural AV fistula characterised by abnormal arteriovenous shunting within the cavernous sinus. It can result from blunt/penetrating trauma, although the majority are thought to be spontaneous. Classical presentation is with pulsatile proptosis; chemosis, diplopia and cranial nerve palsies can also occur. CT and MRI show a markedly enlarged superior ophthalmic vein and prominent cavernous sinus. Congestion of the extraocular muscles may be seen. Angiography is required for confirmation and treatment. Balloon occlusion of the fistula is the treatment of choice.

44 Answer A: *Cryptococcus neoformans* is the most common fungal infection in AIDS

Cryptococcus neoformans is the most common fungal CNS infection in AIDS and is the third most common CNS pathogen after toxoplasmosis and HIV. It is inhaled from bird excrement and spread haematogenously to the brain. It typically results in meningitis, which is poorly appreciated on imaging as the pathogen does not exhibit a strong inflammatory response. A gelatinous mucoid material is produced, which results in widening of the subarachnoid spaces. Cryptococcomas are another feature of *Cryptococcus* infections. They present as small non-enhancing low-density lesions within the basal ganglia with variable enhancement. These lesions represent dilated perivascular spaces filled with gelatinous cryptococcomas. MRI has a greater sensitivity for the detection of cryptococcomas.

Offiah CE, Turnbull IW. The imaging appearances of intracranial CNS infections in adult HIV and AIDS patients. *Clin Radiol*. 2006; **61**(5): 393–401.

45 Answer D: The typical imaging feature of a tuberculoma is a target lesion

CNS *tuberculosis* has increased in the developed world secondary to the increasing incidence of AIDS. It is typically spread haematogenously from a pulmonary source and most commonly presents as meningitis. On cross-sectional imaging there is thick enhancement of the meninges and ependyma. Communicating hydrocephalus is common due to reduced resorption of CSF. Tuberculomas typically arise in the corticomedullary region and are supratentorial. They commonly appear as target lesions on both CT and MRI.

Offiah CE, Turnbull IW. The imaging appearances of intracranial CNS infections in adult HIV and AIDS patients. *Clin Radiol*. 2006; **61**(5): 393–401.

46 Answer B: Subependymal giant cell astrocytoma

Fifteen per cent of patients with tuberous sclerosis develop subependymal astrocytomas. They typically occur at the foramen of Monro and are usually a well-defined rounded mass with some calcification. They usually enhance uniformly with contrast and can degrade to a high-grade astrocytoma. Ninety-five per cent of tuberous sclerosis patients have subependymal hamartomas. These occur in the periventricular region, are isointense to white matter on T1 and calcified on CT. Fifty-five per cent of patients have cortical tubers, which are high signal on T2-weighted imaging.

47 Answer A: Pilocytic astrocytoma

Pilocytic astrocytoma is the most likely diagnosis as it is low density on CT with calcification and nodular enhancement. They are commonly located in the vermis (50%) and are complicated by hydrocephalus. They commonly occur before the age of nine and are characteristically a cyst with an enhancing nodule. Haemangioblastoma is a serious consideration, but more commonly occurs in the paravermian position; the nodule is hyperdense on non-contrast CT and they virtually never calcify. Both lesions can be cystic with a solid enhancing nodule. Haemangioblastomas occur more commonly in adults and as part of Von Hippel-Lindau syndrome.

48 Answer B: Renal cell carcinoma

Malignant melanoma, choriocarcinoma, oat cell, thyroid and renal cell carcinoma all cause hyperdense cerebral metastases. They all enhance brightly with contrast.

49 Answer D: Arising from the vermis

	Medulloblastoma	Ependymoma
Site	Vermis Roof of the fourth ventricle	Floor of the fourth ventricle
Unenhanced CT	Hyperdense	Isodense
Enhancement	Moderate	Minimal
Calcification	10%	50%
Cyst	Rare	Common
Spread	40% CSF seeding	Through the foramen of Luschka and Magendie

50 Answer A: Dural tail

This woman has a parasagittal meningioma. Evidence of a dural tail is very typical of meningiomas but it can also occur in dura metastasis.

51 Answer B: Gliomatosis cerebri

Gliomatosis cerebri is a grade 3 WHO classification cerebral tumour, which affects at least two or more lobes and is principally centred in the cortex and has little mass affect or architectural distortion. It typically affects patient aged 40–50 years of age. On CT imaging it can be easily missed but features are loss of the grey-white matter differentiation with minor enlargement of the cortex. On MRI imaging bright signal is seen within the affected area and contrast is minimal. Prognosis is poor with 50% one-year survival.

52 Answer B: Pleomorphic xanthoastrocytoma

Pleomorphic xanthoastrocytoma is a superficial grade 2 tumour and accounts for 1% of all intracranial tumours. It occurs in a younger group of patients with a mean age of 26 years. It preferentially affects the superficial temporal lobe and is cystic with an enhancing nodule and with peritumoral vasogenic oedema.

53 Answer A: Low signal

This patient has an arachnoid cyst, which typically has similar signal characteristics to CSF (bright on T2W, low on T1W and FLAIR). On DWI the signal characteristic is similar to CSF and hence is low.

54 Answer C: High signal within the periaqueductal region

Chronic alcohol results in atrophy of the cerebellum, particularly the vermis. This patient has Wernicke's encephalopathy, which is characterised by confabulation, delusions, ataxia, ophthalmoplegia and confusion and is caused by thiamine deficiency. High signal is seen in the periaqueductal region, paraventricular thalamic regions and mammillothalamic tract on MR imaging on FLAIR and T2W.

55 Answer E: Pick's disease

Striking disproportional atrophy of the frontal and anterior temporal lobes in a young patient is typical of Pick's disease, which is also known as frontotemporal atrophy. In Alzheimer's disease there is medial temporal lobe atrophy with compensatory enlargement of the temporal horns. Parkinson's disease results in a generalised cerebral atrophy. Progressive supranuclear palsy results in atrophy of the midbrain, globus pallidus and frontal lobes.

56 Answer B: High signal in the caudate and putamen on T2-weighted MR images

This patient has Huntington's chorea which has autosomal-dominant inheritance and is characterised by involuntary choreoathetoid movements and severe memory impairment. The age at which symptoms occur is dependent on the length of the trinucleotide CAG-repeat mutation on chromosome 4, but is typically around 40 years. On imaging there is bilateral atrophy of the caudate lobe with compensatory enlargement of the frontal horns of the lateral ventricles. High signal is seen within the caudate and putamen in the juvenile form.

57 Answer D: Tuberous sclerosis

Phenytoin, alcohol, ataxic telangiectasia and paraneoplastic syndrome from a bronchial tumour all result in cerebellar atrophy. Other causes are marijuana, steroids, radiation, multisystem atrophy and gluten insensitivity.

58 Answer C: Right temporal lobe resection

This patient has temporal lobe epilepsy caused by mesial temporal sclerosis. On MRI there is atrophy of the hippocampus, amygdala, mammillary bodies and fornix. High signal within the hippocampus is seen on T2-weighted imaging which may be bilateral in 20% of cases. Nuclear medicine imaging can be used to diagnose the site of the epilepsy focus. On interictal FDG-PET imaging there is decreased uptake of radiotracer at the site of fit focus. On ictal SPECT scanning there is increased uptake of tracer at the focus of the fit. If epilepsy is refractory to antiepileptics, a temporal lobectomy can be performed. Approximately 50% of all temporal lobe resections are for epilepsy.

59 Answer B: Antihypertensives

This patient has infarcts in the regions of the watershed areas between the anterior and middle cerebral arteries and the middle and posterior cerebral arteries. This patient must have taken something to reduce the cerebral perfusion. Antihypertensive medication is the best answer.

60 Answer D: Oedema extending across the corpus callosum

Vasogenic oedema is oedema associated with either a primary or secondary tumour. It is caused by increased vascular permeability. On imaging there is oedema within the white matter not affecting the cortex. It can extend across vascular territories and the corpus callosum. Cytotoxic oedema is caused by ischaemia and results in arrested metabolism of cells. It appears as oedema conforming to a vascular territory with well-demarcated edges and involves the cortex. It does not cross the corpus callosum. There is restricted diffusion on DWI.

61 Answer D: Lymphoma

The term ivory vertebra describes single or multiple very dense vertebrae and all the options listed are causes. Paget's disease and haemangiomas show coarse reticulation and some expansion. Low-grade infections are associated with end-plate destruction, disc narrowing and paraspinal masses. Sclerotic metastases generally do not show expansion but a history of underlying malignancy is often available and there may be evidence of metastatic disease elsewhere.

62 Answer B: Morquio syndrome

Anterior vertebral body beaks are seen at the thoracolumbar junction and usually associated with kyphosis. All the options listed are associated with anterior beaks, but most occur in the lower third of the vertebral body, except Morquio syndrome where this is seen more centrally. Other manifestations include hypoplastic dens, dorsal scoliosis, irregular ossification of the femoral capital epiphyses and short wide tubular bones with irregular metaphyses.

63 Answer E: Right L4/L5 lateral disc bulge

Intervertebral disc herniation and degeneration is the most common source of compressive radiculopathy. The lumbar roots emerge from below their respective vertebrae. Different nerves are compressed depending on the location of the disc protrusion.

To avoid confusion, nerve roots are designated as 'exiting' and 'descending/traversing' nerve roots. The exiting nerve is the nerve leaving the spinal canal through the neural foramen below the pedicle of the vertebral body sitting on top of the disc. At each intervertebral disc level, there is usually only one spinal nerve root outside the dural sac in the spinal canal descending behind the intervertebral disc to exit below the pedicle of the vertebral body forming the lower surface of that disc.

At the L4-L5 disc, for example, the exiting nerve would be the L4 nerve, which usually leaves the dural sac at about the level of the lower part of the body of L3, descends behind the L3-L4 disc, and exits the spinal canal below the pedicle of L4 through the top of L4-L5 neural foramen. The descending nerve would be the L5 nerve root.

64 Answer C: Basilar invagination

McGregor's line extends from the posterior limits of the hard palate to the base of the occipital region. The odontoid peg should lie 5 mm below this level. If it is at the level of the McGregor's line, this is basilar invagination. Causes of basilar invagination are rickets, osteomalacia, fibrous dysplasia and developmental such as Klippel-Feil. Platybasia is flattening of the skull base and it commonly occurs with basilar invagination. The basal angle is greater than 140 degrees in platybasia.

65 Answer C: Normal pedicles

Features that are suggestive of a bony metastasis are: a bowed posterior border of the vertebral body, abnormal signal in the pedicles, an epidural or paraspinal mass and multiple lesions. Features suggestive of osteoporotic wedge fractures are: low signal on both T1- and T2-weighted imaging, spared normal marrow signal and multiple compression fractures.

Jung HS, *et al*. Discrimination of metastasis from acute osteoporotic compression spinal fractures with MR imaging. *RadioGraphics*. 2003; **23**(1): 179–87.

66 Answer C: Ependymoma

Ependymomas are the most common primary spinal cord tumour. They most commonly occur in the cervical region followed by the thoracic region and extend over a large area (average of four vertebral bodies). They are well-defined and central lesions. They often have a low signal rim around the outside due to haemosiderin from repeated bleeds. As they are slow-growing tumours they are associated with bone remodelling. They metastasise to the lung, retroperitoneum and lymph nodes. There is an 80% five-year survival.

67 Answer B: Metastatic breast cancer

Drop metastases are most commonly seen in the paediatric population and are most commonly due to PNETs, medulloblastomas, ependymomas, germinomas and pinealoblastomas. In adults metastatic breast and melanoma are common causes. The above description is very typical. Irregularity along the surface can also be seen.

68 Answer E: Chordoma

This is a typical description of a sacral chordoma. Chordomas originate from embryonic remnants of the notochord. They arise in patients aged between 30 and 70 years of age and are more common in males. The most commonly occur in the sacrum then the clivus. They metastasise to the liver, lung and lymph nodes and tend to recur despite radical surgery.

69 Answer C: Spinal cord cavernous angioma

Spinal cavernomas are uncommon, unlike cerebral cavernomas. They typically present in women (M:F = 1:4) between 30 and 50 years of age and are most common in the cervical and thoracic regions. They are intramedullary lesions, which are well defined and are bright on both T1 and T2 as they contain methaemaglobin. Blooming artefact is present because of the presence of haemosiderin from previous bleeds. Little mass effect is seen. A common presentation of spinal cavernomas is with Brown-Séquard syndrome (hemiparaplegia, ipsilateral loss of proprioceptive sensation, hyperesthesia and contralateral loss of pain and temperature). Progression of symptoms is common.

70 Answer D: Wormian bones

This patient has cleidocranial dysostosis, an autosomal-dominant condition which results in delayed ossification of midline structures. Patients typically have absent or hypoplastic lateral clavicles, supernumerary ribs, hemivertebrae, widened symphysis pubis, absent or short radius and elongated second metatarsals. In the skull patients typically have wormian bones, widened anterior fontanelles, large mandible and small paranasal sinuses.

Neuroradiology, head and neck and ENT radiology

PAPER 2: ANSWERS AND EXPLANATIONS

1   Answer C: Gorlin's disease

The description is very typical of a dentigerous cyst. They are cyst associated with the crown of an unerupted cyst and affect the molars and canine teeth. Gorlin's syndrome is associated with multiple dentigerous cysts, multiple basal cell naevi, rib abnormalities and heavy calcification of the falx cerebri. It is an autosomal-dominant condition.

2   Answer B: Cherubism

Cherubism is also known as familial fibrous dysplasia and is seen in children but is more severe in boys. Fibrous dysplasia is characterised by generalised bone expansion and ground-glass changes. Multicystic lesions are common in fibrous dysplasia. Children with cherubism have problems with their dentition but it usually regresses in adolescence.

3   Answer C: Generalised tram track enhancement

This patient has an optic nerve sheath meningioma. These typically demonstrate uniform bright enhancement with a non-enhancing optic nerve. Patchy enhancement of the optic nerve is seen in optic nerve gliomas.

4   Answer C: III, IV, V1 and VI

The oculomotor (III), trochlear (IV), ophthalmic branch of the trigeminal nerve (V1) and abducens (VI) and sympathetic filaments of the internal carotid plexus all pass through the superior orbital fissure. The superior and inferior ophthalmic veins, the meningeal branch of the lacrimal artery and the orbital branch of the middle meningeal artery also pass through the superior orbital fissure.

5   Answer E: Left optic radiation

Monocular visual loss is due to a defect in the optic nerve.

Bitemporal hemianopia is due to a defect at the optic chiasm level.

Right-sided homonymous hemianopia is caused by a defect in the contralateral optic tract or through any part of the contralateral optic radiation.

Right upper outer quadrantanopia is due to a defect in part of the optic radiation.

Central bilateral homonymous hemianopia is due to a defect in the contralateral primary visual cortex.

6 Answer A: Neuroblastoma

The most common orbital metastases in children are from neuroblastomas followed by Ewing's tumours and leukaemia. In adults breast and lung are the most common primaries causing intraorbital lesions. The deposits are typically intraocular.

7 Answer D: Right carotid artery

A painful partial right-sided Horner's syndrome is due to a disruption of the sympathetic nerves within the wall of the ipsilateral carotid artery caused by dissection.

8 Answer A: Ivory osteoma

Ivory osteomas are benign hamartomas of the bone, which are relatively common. They may be associated with other conditions such as Gardener's syndrome. They most commonly occur in the frontal and ethmoid sinuses and may cause obstruction of the sinus ostium. Ivory osteomas are dense areas of compact bone and are well-defined sclerotic bone on CT and low signal on T1-weighted imaging.

9 Answer E: Bilateral choanal atresia

Choanal atresia is failure of perforation of the oronasal membrane. Bilateral choanal atresia is a paediatric emergency because babies are obligate nasal breathers until two to six months. The septation is either bony (85%) or membranous (15%). The bilateral form is slightly more common. It is associated with other congenital anomalies such as malrotation, DiGeorge syndrome and foetal alcohol syndrome. With bilateral disease babies are intubated and endoscopic perforation is performed.

10 Answer A: Glomus tympanicum

Glomus tumours are rare tumours arising from the paraganglionic tissue and can occur anywhere between the skull base and pelvis. Glomus tympanicum tumours present with pulsatile tinnitus and hearing loss and are seen on otoscopy as a reddish blue mass behind the tympanic membrane. They are typically sited along the lateral aspect of the cochlear, particularly the cochlear promontory. The globus tympanicum does not erode the ossicles but engulfs them.

11 Answer C: Retromandibular vein

The parotid gland is divided into superficial and deep lobes by the facial nerve. As the portion of the nerve which traverses the gland is not readily seen on routine imaging the retromandibular vein, which lies just medial to the nerve, can be used as an anatomical landmark. The external carotid artery is also present within the parotid gland and gives off its terminal branches, maxillary and superficial temporal arteries within the gland parenchyma.

12 Answer B: Dermoid cyst

Dermoid cysts usually occur along the midline and are commonly found at this location. They are thought to occur within the region where the neural tube closes. A nasal dermoid cyst can be associated with a deep sinus with potential communication with the intracranial cavity. Dermoid cysts contain skin and sebaceous material, giving them a density similar to fat on CT. On MRI they display high signal intensity on T1W images and are hyperintense on T2. An encephalocele also usually arises in the midline but more than 90% occur posteriorly in the region of the occiput and they are associated with a defect in the skull table allowing herniation of meninges, brain parenchyma and CSF. Potts puffy tumour can occur as a complication of frontal sinusitis and consists of osteomyelitis of the frontal bone, which can progress to an extradural abscess.

13 Answer B: Inverted papilloma

Inverted papillomas arise from the lateral nasal wall and appear macroscopically similar to nasal polyps but with frond-like projections. The underlying respiratory epithelium exhibits an endophytic growth pattern. Even though these are benign lesions there is a possibility of focal malignant transformation and therefore regular surveillance is usually undertaken. The avid enhancement post contrast differentiates an inverted papilloma from a mucocele. Nasal polyps, mucoceles or mucous retention cysts would not be expected to exhibit bony destruction.

14 Answer E: Isointense to grey matter on T1-weighted images

A trigeminal nerve schwannoma displays the characteristic imaging appearances that are common to all schwannomas. On CT imaging they are isointense with brain parenchyma, exhibiting enhancement post contrast and containing cystic components. On MRI imaging the lesion is likely to be isointense with brain parenchyma on T1, hyperintense on T2-weighted images and shows enhancement post gadolinium.

15 Answer A: Gradenigo's syndrome

This patient has developed an abscess in the aerated petrous apex, which typically spreads from the middle ear. The infected phlegm irritates the fifth and sixth nerves as they pass the petrous apex causing the triad of symptoms called Gradenigo's syndrome (otitis media, retro-orbital pain and a sixth nerve palsy). Typically, infective agents are pseudomonas and enterococcus. The petrous apex is aerated in approximately 30% of the population. Korsakoff's syndrome is typically seen in alcoholics with thiamine deficiencies that have an inability to produce new memories, and confabulate. Riley-Day syndrome is an inherited condition resulting in dysautonomia. Gerstmann's syndrome is characterised by four primary symptoms of dysgraphia, dyscalculia, finger agnosia and left to right disorientation. Chilaiditi's syndrome describes interposition of the colon between the liver and the diaphragm.

16 Answer C: Embolisation

Given the presentation and radiological features the mass is most likely to be a juvenile angiofibroma. These tumours typically arise from the region of the sphenopalatine foramen and extend into the pterygopalatine and infratemporal fossa. On CT there is characteristic erosion of the medial pterygoid plate, which is a useful distinguishing feature between juvenile angiofibromas and other nasopharyngeal mass lesions. Angiography is not necessary for diagnostic purposes, but may be carried out prior to pre-operative embolisation. Therapeutic embolisation is an adjunct to surgery as the whole supply to the tumour cannot generally be embolised.

17 Answer A: <1%

Thyroglossal cysts occur along the path of migration of the foetal thyroid from its position at the base of the tongue to its adult position in the mid-neck. The majority of these occur in the midline and in an infrahyoid location. Less than 1% undergoes malignant change. Thyroglossal duct carcinoma has a slight female predilection and histologic findings of thyroglossal duct carcinoma are most commonly papillary carcinoma (75–80%).

Branstetter BF, *et al.* The CT appearance of thyroglossal duct carcinoma. *Am J Neuroradiol.* 2000; **21**(8): 1547–50.

18 Answer B: Le Fort II fracture

All Le Fort fractures involve the pterygoid process. Le Fort I is a transverse fracture through the maxilla, Le Fort II is more extensive and the separated fragment is pyramidal while in Le Fort III there is complete craniofacial disjunction. In practice fractures do not fit these descriptions exactly and may be asymmetrical or coexist. The classification is still in general use and aids in subsequent surgical management. In Le Fort I and II the fractured maxillary fragment is usually wired to the zygomatic arches, but if these are fractured as in Le Fort III, a more complex pin and rod fixation to the skull vault is undertaken.

19 Answer A: Keratosis obturans

Keratosis obturans is a bilateral process of inflammatory ear masses in association with chronic sinusitis and bronchiectasis. Van der Hoeve syndrome is characterised by osteogenesis imperfecta and osteosclerosis. Malignant otitis externa, surfer's ear and cholesteatoma could all account for inflammatory external ear masses but have no other clinical associations.

20 Answer A: Sinus hypoplasia

All the conditions can cause opacification of the maxillary sinus. Sinus hypoplasia is the most likely answer given the CT features. Maxillary dentigerous cyst contains a tooth or crown whereas primordial dentigerous cyst does not. In acute sinusitis one would expect an air/fluid level in radiological investigations representing the disease process. Classical CT findings of ameloblastoma are of multilocular lesion with scalloped borders on a background of diffuse ground-glass changes within the bone.

21 Answer A: Croup

These are the classical XR findings in croup. In supraglottitis one would expect to see the 'thumb sign' of a short, broad epiglottis. Plain films in congenital tracheal stenosis would reveal a narrowed tracheal lumen. In subglottic haemangioma, indicative findings are a soft-tissue mass in the subglottic region extending inferiorly, narrowing the airway. Laryngomalacia is a clinical and endoscopic diagnosis, but findings consistent with laryngomalacia are anterior bowing and inferior displacement of the aryepiglottic folds. Films taken during expiration would show abnormal persistent dilatation of the oropharyngeal airway, which is indicative of laryngomalacia.

22 Answer C: 50%

Sensitivity is a measure of how well the test picks up the disease if it is present; that is, true positives/(true positives and false negatives). Specificity is a measure of how often the test is negative when the disease is not present; that is, true negatives/(true negatives + false positives).

23 Answer A: Within foramen lacerum

Answer A is incorrect as all the other answers are on the normal course of thyroid descent from the back of the tongue (foramen caecum) inferiorly to its normal position in the neck. Foramen lacerum transmits the internal carotid artery.

24 Answer D: 32 mL

The appropriate dose is 2 mL/kg up to an adult dose of 50 mL. Usually, a hand injection is sufficient and the patient is imaged within the next few minutes. It is possible to estimate a child's weight between 1 year and 10 years by the formula Weight = (Age + 4) × 2.

25 Answer C: Corpus callosum agenesis

Agenesis of the corpus callosum can be partial or complete. The rostrum and splenium are absent or hypoplastic in the partial variety. Widely separated lateral ventricles, with longitudinal white matter mater tracts (Probst bundles) indenting the medial margins of the lateral ventricles and dilated occipital horns (col-pocephaly) are seen. Associated abnormalities include Chiari II, Dandy-Walker malformation, migration disorders and lipomas.

26 Answer A: Schizencephaly

Schizencephaly describes a full thickness CSF cleft lined by grey matter extending from the subarachnoid space to the subependyma of the lateral ventricle. This can be either open lipped (the walls of the cleft are separated) or closed lipped (the walls are opposed). The clefts may be unilateral or bilateral and asymmetric. The important differential is porencephalic cyst, which results from insult to a normally developed brain.

27 Answer C: Bilateral nodular subependymal grey matter

Heterotopic grey matter occurs secondary to developmental arrest of migrating neuroblasts from the ventricular walls to the surface of the brain. Nodular and laminar forms are described. Signal is isointense to grey matter on all sequences.

28 Answer A: Diastematomyelia

Diastematomyelia is characterised by a developmental sagittal cleft, which splits the spinal cord or filum terminale. The septum is either bony, osteocartilagenous or fibrous. This usually occurs between T9 and S1 and has a distinct female preponderance. It is associated with other anomalies including Chiari II, tethered cord, neurenteric cyst and dermoids.

29 Answer E: Scaphocephaly

Craniostenosis is the premature closure of sutures. At birth all sutures are normally open. Typically, only one suture is fused but in a quarter of cases more than one fuses. Early fusion results in an abnormally shaped head. Boys are more commonly affected and it may be part of a syndrome. Scaphocephaly is the premature fusion of the sagittal suture, is the most common and leads to a long thin head. Brachycephaly is premature fusion of the lambdoid or coronal suture producing a short wide head. Plagiocephaly is unilateral fusion of the coronal and lambdoid suture producing a lopsided skull. Trigonocephaly is the fusion of the metopic suture producing a forward-pointing skull. A cloverleaf skull typically occurs in thanatophoric dysplasia and is due to premature closure of the sagittal, coronal and lambdoid suture.

30 Answer C: Transsphenoidal encephalocele

This patient has a transsphenoidal or basal encephalocele. Basal encephaloceles account for 10% of all encephaloceles. They typically present with a soft-tissue mass within the nasal cavity, which can increase in size during the Valsalva manoeuvre. Affected patients may be obligate mouth breathers due to nasal obstruction. It is associated with agenesis of the corpus callosum, pituitary and hypothalamic dysfunction and hypoplasia of the optic nerves.

31 Answer D: Atrophy of the amygdala

This boy has mesial temporal sclerosis, which is characterised by atrophy of the hippocampus, and high signal on T2-weighted MRI. There is also loss of the normal interdigitation of the hippocampal head. It is associated with atrophy of the ipsilateral mammillary bodies and fornix.

32 Answer D: Mass effect with a midline shift

CT findings in stroke evolve with time. Although 60% of scans obtained within

12 hours are normal, early signs like a hyperattenuating MCA and obscured lentiform nuclei may be seen. Loss of grey-white matter interface along the lateral insula is termed the insular ribbon sign. Mass effect increases between 24 and 72 hours and is not an early sign.

Osborn AG. *Diagnostic Neuroradiology*. St Louis, MO: Mosby; 1994. pp. 344–7.

33 Answer C: Right PCA territory

Features described are those of descending transtentorial herniation where the uncus and parahippocampal gyrus protrude over the free tentorial margin. With progressive herniation, the ipsilateral PCA may become compressed against the tentorial incisura resulting in occipital ischaemia or infarction. Other manifestations of descending transtentorial herniation include periaqueductal necrosis, Duret haemorrhage and compressive cranial neuropathies.

Osborn AG. *Diagnostic Neuroradiology*. St Louis, MO: Mosby; 1994. pp. 222–7.

34 Answer D: Venous bleed

If there have been two negative angiograms, the likely cause of the cerebral bleed is venous in nature. When there has been a single negative angiogram a repeat angiogram is usually performed after a period of time as vasospasm in an artery adjacent to an aneurysm may have occurred, leading to a false negative during the first angiogram.

35 Answer B: Sagittal sinus thrombosis

Sagittal sinus thrombosis can result in venous infarcts. These typically present as bilateral parasagittal haemorrhage affecting both the grey and white matter. The patient also has hydrocephalus as a result of the venous infarct. Hypertensive angiopathy typically produces haemorrhage within the basal ganglia. Amyloid angiopathy results in lobar haemorrhage within the frontal and parietal lobes the deep grey matter is typically spared. Metastasis occurs within the corticomedullary region; haemorrhage can occur within them. It would be unlikely that there were two metastases that resulted in haemorrhage.

36 Answer D: Moyamoya disease

The Moyamoya pattern of collateral blood flow is non-specific and can be seen in slowly progressive intracranial occlusive vascular disorders such as atherosclerosis, radiation-induced angiopathy and sickle cell disease. It is classically described in the Japanese; there is occlusion of the supraclinoid ICA with progressive collateralisation to supply the ischaemic areas. Angiography demonstrates a 'puff of smoke' appearance and multiple flow voids are seen on MRI.

37 Answer C: Anterior inferior cerebellar artery

The SCAs supply the entire superior surface of the cerebellar hemispheres, vermis, much of the cerebellar white matter and the dentate nuclei. The AICAs supply the anterolateral surface of the cerebellum, the middle cerebellar peduncles, flocculus and inferolateral pons. The PICAs supply the postero-inferior surface of the cerebellum, inferior vermis, tonsils and the posterolateral medulla.

38 Answer C: Multinodular goitre with prominent nodule

Multinodular goitre can give rise to heterogeneous uptake in both types of scan as a functioning thyroid nodule will take up both tracers. The presence of smooth uniform uptake on the thyroid scan would have been more consistent with a functioning parathyroid adenoma. Salivary gland uptake is seen with Tc-99m pertechnetate but not I131. Thyroid malignancy presents as a cold (nonfunctioning) nodule in 90% of scans.

39 Answer D: Hyperflexion

Hyperflexion injury of the spine accounts for 46–79% of all cervical spine injuries. The anteroinferior teardrop fracture is the most severe and unstable injury of the spine. The widening of the posterior elements indicates disruption of the posterior ligament complex. It is an unstable injury, which results in ligamentous damage and spinal cord compression. Typically, these occur at C6 to C8. Hyperflexion injuries are the most common injury accounting for between 50 and 75% of injuries. The anterior height of the vertebral body is reduced with anterior reduction in disc space and there is diffuse prevertebral soft-tissue swelling. Extension teardrop fractures occur at the anteroinferior corner of C2 and this may occur in isolation or with a hangman's fracture. Here there is widening of the anterior disc space.

40 Answer C: 3–7 days (intracellular methaemoglobin)

The appearance of blood clot on MRI is dependent on several factors including the relaxivity and susceptibility effects of the iron-containing haemoglobin. Accurate dating of haematoma is contentious, particularly in the setting of suspected NAI, and should only be attempted by experts, although the temporal evolution of haemoglobin degradation products does occur in a predictable fashion.

	Age	Haemoglobin	T1	T2
Hyperacute	>24 hours	Oxyhaemoglobin	Iso	Hyper
Acute	1–3 days	Deoxyhaemoglobin	Hypo	Hypo
Subacute early	3–7 days	Intracellular methaemoglobin	Hyper	Hypo
Subacute late	7–14 days	Extracellular methaemaglobin	Hyper	Hyper
Haemosiderin	>14 days	Haemosiderin	Hypo	Hypo

41 Answer B: Ossicular dislocation

The fracture described is a longitudinal fracture of the petrous temporal bone, which runs parallel to the axis of the bone. Ossicular dislocation, most commonly incudostapedial, is usually present. Facial paralysis occurs in 10–20% secondary to oedema but resolves spontaneously. Otorrhoea may be seen. In transverse fractures, which run perpendicular to the axis of the pyramid, there is irreversible sensorineural hearing loss and facial paralysis in 50%.

42 Answer B: Diffuse avid uptake in a uniform pattern

Graves' disease usually shows avid uniform uptake. Patchy uptake may indicate Hashimoto's thyroiditis or multiple hot nodules. Radioactive thyroid therapy is contraindicated in poorly controlled thyrotoxicosis as it may precipitate a thyroid storm and can worsen eye symptoms but a diagnostic scan is appropriate.

43 Answer B: Herpes encephalitis

Herpes simplex encephalitis results in fulminant necrotising encephalitis and is due to the herpes simplex virus (HSV). A third of patients have a primary infection while the rest are due to reactivation. Patients present with acute confusion and disorientation which can progress to fits, loss of consciousness and death. HSV has a predilection for the temporal lobes, insula, frontal lobes and cingulated gyrus. The putamen is typically spared. On early imaging on FLAIR and T2W there is high signal in these areas. There may be restricted diffusion in the affected areas due to infarction and lack of restrictive diffusion suggests reversibility. At 10 days the extent of the tissue involved is known, and parenchymal haemorrhage can be seen at this stage. The prognosis is poor with only 2.5% of treated HSV patients returning to a normal life. If untreated there is a 70% mortality.

44 Answer B: Cerebral abscess

Cerebral abscesses typically result in a thin uniformly enhancing rim of contrast while metastasis and GBM have thick walls and incomplete enhancement. The DWI characteristics are of restrictive diffusion, which occur in infarcts and cerebral abscesses, although not all abscesses demonstrate these signal characteristics. Sometimes the abscess may have a thin rim of high signal on T1 and low signal on T2-weighted imaging, which is caused by haemorrhage or free radicals.

45 Answer B: Primary CNS lymphoma

Primary lymphoma is the most likely answer because of the position, the hyperdensity on CT and the necrotic centre. Cerebral lymphoma is often hyperdense due to the dense cellularity, although this may not be the case in patients who are immunocompromised. Toxoplasmosis is also a consideration but these are more often multiple. Herpes encephalitis is an unlikely diagnosis as the patient is relatively well and the typical imaging features are asymmetric high signal in the frontal and temporal lobes on T2W imaging.

46 Answer A: Arachnoid cyst

Arachnoid cysts are common incidental findings, which are CSF-filled cystic lesions within the arachnoid space. They are found within the middle fossa, perisellar cisterns, retrocerebellar cisterns and cerebellopontine angle. They are thin-walled cystic lesions which are CSF density (0–20 HU) and do not enhance with contrast. There is often bone remodelling and compression of the underlying parenchyma. On MR imaging it has the same signal characteristics as CSF on T1, T2, FLAIR and DWI. They can be complicated by haemorrhage. Epidermoids appear very similar to arachnoid cysts on CT but on FLAIR and DWI they are bright and will be brighter than CSF on T1-weighted images.

47 Answer A: Lipoma

Intracranial lipoma is an uncommon mass accounting for 1% of all intracranial tumours. They commonly present in the callosal cistern but can occur in any cistern. On CT they are well defined, of similar density to fat (–100 HU) with peripheral calcification and no enhancement. On MRI the signal characteristics are similar to fat but inhomogeneous on PD. Craniopharyngiomas are usually sellar or suprasellar. Arachnoid cysts have the same signal characteristics as CSF. Epidermoids are usually lobulated and off midline. Dermoids are usually more heterogeneous.

48 Answer B: Craniopharyngioma

Craniopharyngiomas are intrasellar or suprasellar lesions and most commonly occur in the first two decades of life. They are high signal on T2 and can be either high or low signal on T1-weighted imaging, the low signal areas being due to calcification. Bony destruction occurs in 75% of cases and also in 75% of cases the mass is principally cystic.

49 Answer D: Hypothalamic hamartoma

Hypothalamic hamartoma is a tumour of the tuber cinereum. Patients are typically less than two years of age and present with precocious puberty and gelastic seizures (spasmodic laughter). They are most commonly seen in the tuber cinereum or mammillary bodies. On CT they present as a round well-defined homogeneous mass with no enhancement. On MRI they tend to be isointense on both T1- and T2-weighted imaging.

50 Answer C: Suprasellar cistern

This patient has a germinoma and the second most common site is in the suprasellar region (20%). Germinomas account for 2% of all paediatric brain tumours and are commonly seen in males aged between 10 and 25 years of age. Patients commonly have Parinaud's syndrome (paralysis of upward gaze). On CT there is a well-defined hyperdense mass within the pineal gland and on MRI it is isointense on T1 and low signal on T2-weighted imaging. On both CT and MRI there is bright enhancement with contrast.

51 Answer C: Intracranial hypotension

Intracranial hypotension can occur spontaneously, post-operatively or following a lumbar puncture and presents with postural headaches. On MRI there is dural thickening with uniform enhancement, subdural fluid collections, engorgement of the veins, sagging of the brain and increased enhancement of the pituitary gland. The likely cause for this patient's postural haemorrhage was an unintended dural puncture during insertion of her epidural. These are often treated by a 'blood patch' (injecting the patient's own blood at the level of the puncture to seal the defect). Meningitis and sarcoid can cause diffuse dural thickening with enhancement but as the patient is well this is unlikely. En plaque meningioma and dura metastasis are unlikely as she is a bit young and the whole of the dura is affected.

Wouter I, Schievink MD. Spontaneous spinal cerebrospinal fluid leaks and intracranial hypotension. *JAMA*. 2006; **295**(19): 2286–96.

52 Answer A: Rathke's cleft cysts

Rathke's cleft cysts are embryological remnants of the Rathke's pouch. The cysts are lined by columnar and cuboidal cells and occur in the intrasellar region. They are high signal on T2 and can be high or low signal on T1-weighted imaging. Rathke's cleft cysts can compress the pituitary gland. They are usually asymptomatic but may cause hypopituitarism. Treatment is either with cyst aspiration or cystectomy.

53 Answer C: Autosomal dominant

This patient has Huntington's disease, which is an autosomal dominantly inherited disease. The age at which symptoms occur is dependent on the length of the trinucleotide CAG repeat sequence.

54 Answer C: Telangiectasia

Ataxic telangiectasia is an autosomal recessive disease, which is characterised by multiple telangiectasia, cerebellar ataxia, pulmonary infections and immunodeficiency. Brain imaging demonstrates vermian atrophy, cerebral infarcts and cerebral haemorrhage secondary ruptured telangiectatic vessels. Patients are susceptible to upper respiratory infections and malignancy such lymphoma and leukaemia in children. Adults have a very high incidence of breast and bowel cancers.

55 Answer A: Wilson's disease

Wilson's disease is an autosomal recessively inherited condition, which results in abnormal caeruloplasmin metabolism. Copper is deposited within the liver, cornea and brain. Dysarthria, dystonia and tremors are commonly early clinical findings. On imaging there is atrophy of the caudate lobe and high signal within the outer margin of the putamen, caudate and lateral aspect of the thalami. High signal is often seen within the pons. Treatment is with a collating agent.

King AD, Walshe JM, Kendell BE, *et al.* Cranial imaging in Wilson's disease. *Am J Roentenol*. 1996; **167**(6): 1579–84.

56 Answer A: Ruptured dermoid cyst

Dermoid cysts are usually midline and are well-defined masses with fat, skin, sebaceous glands and sweat glands. They are fat density on CT and high signal on both T1- and T2-weighted imaging. These are prone to rupture and as the fat molecules are less dense than CSF they tend to lie in the most superior areas of the ventricles (temporal and frontal horn of the lateral ventricles).

57 Answer A: Axial T2

FLAIR and T2 sequences are good at identifying MS plaques. T2 sequences are better at identifying lesions within the spinal cord and posterior fossa.

Pretorius PM, Quaghebeur G. The role of MRI in the diagnosis of multiple sclerosis. *Clin Radiol.* 2003; **58**(6): 434–48.

58 Answer D: Eosinophilic granuloma

Eosinophilic granuloma is also known as histiocytosis X and Langerhans cell histiocytosis. It results from proliferation of the reticulohistiocytic elements. It is most commonly a monostotic disease (50–75%) affecting young children (5–10 years). The most commonly affected bone is the skull, but lesions can occur in both flat and long bones. In long bones it most commonly occurs in the diaphyseal region. Skull lesions are punched out, well-defined lytic masses most commonly occurring in the parietal and temporal bones. Once treatment has been instigated a thin sclerotic margin is seen in 50% of cases. On CT there is often an enhancing soft-tissue within the lytic area.

59 Answer C: Meningeal biopsy

This patient has sarcoid, which is most common is females and West Africans and the most common presentation is with bihilar lymphadenopathy. The CNS is affected in 1–8% of patients with sarcoid. The leptomeninges, dura, subarachnoid space, peripheral nerves and ventricular system are affected and the most common findings are cranial neuropathies with the facial and acoustic nerves being the most commonly affected. Patients can present with aseptic meningitis, fits and MS-like plaques. On imaging there is diffuse enhancement of the meninges, which is sometimes nodular and is most common in the basal cisterns, but can affect any region. Hydrocephalus may be present and small vessel change can occur. Definitive diagnosis is made by meningeal biopsy and ACE levels may not be raised.

60 Answer D: Ependymoma

The lesion described is extradural in location. Extradural masses arise from outside the spinal dura and may originate from the vertebral body, disc and adjacent soft tissues. On MR dura may be seen draped over the mass, and sometimes epidural fat may be seen capping the lesion.

Intradural, extramedullary lesions arise inside the thecal sac, but outside the cord and originate from the nerve roots, meninges and CSF spaces. On MRI, intradural lesions are clearly delineated by CSF and the cord is deviated away from the lesion. The subarachnoid space is enlarged up to the mass.

Intramedullary masses arise inside the spinal cord and originate from the cord parenchyma or pia. On MRI there is diffuse enlargement of the cord with gradual effacement of the subarachnoid space.

61 Answer C: Astrocytoma

The commonest intramedullary lesions are astrocytoma and ependymoma. Astrocytomas are the most common cord tumour in children and the cervical cord is the commonest location followed by the thoracic cord. Multisegmental involvement is common and they are often associated with a syrinx and cysts. Despite being low grade they tend to enhance strongly with contrast.

Ependymomas are more common in adults and occur in the conus medullaris and filum terminale. They are generally slow growing and cause vertebral body scalloping. Cysts and haemorrhage are common.

62 Answer E: Haematoma

Spinal haematomas occur due to trauma, following a procedure (typically laminectomy or epidurals), during childbirth or spontaneously, particularly in those with bleeding disorders. They are usually due to venous bleeds and are typically posterior fusiform masses. They can result in a cauda equina syndrome and require prompt neurosurgical evacuation.

Szkup P, Stoneham G. Spontaneous spinal epidural haematoma during pregnancy: case report and review of the literature. *Br J Radiol*. 2004; **77**(922): 881–4.

63 Answer C: Paget's disease

Paget's disease is characterised by abnormal and excessive remodelling of bone. The prevalence increases with age and the disease predominates in the axial skeleton. The disease occurs in three phases: osteolytic, mixed and osteosclerotic. Spinal involvement is common in the lumbar region and the vertebrae are enlarged with coarse trabeculae. Nerve entrapment and cord compression can occur. The differentials for a solitary expanded vertebra include GCT and ABC both of which are lytic and vertebral haemangiomas, which demonstrate a 'polka dot' appearance with little expansion.

64 Answer B: Von Hippel-Lindau syndrome with haemangioblastoma and renal cell carcinomas

A third of all spinal haemangioblastomas occur in patients with VHL. They are the third most common intramedullary neoplasm. They are usually intramedullary but can be extramedullary (25%) and occur most commonly in the cervical (40%) and thoracic (50%) regions. Patients present with a prolonged history of sensory and motor symptoms. They are highly vascular lesions, which are isointense on T1, high signal on T2 with multiple signal voids and bright enhancement with contrast. Low signal from haemosiderin is often seen on T2*.

65 Answer D: CMV infections can cause a brachial plexus neuropathy

CMV in the AIDS population is usually the result of reactivation. Ninety per cent of the general population have prior exposure to CMV, usually in childhood. CMV infection more typically affects the respiratory tract. Fifteen to thirty per cent of HIV patients have CNS evidence of the virus at post mortem. Brain involvement results in encephalitis, ventriculitis, infarcts or meningitis. On CT imaging there is low density diffuse white matter changes, ependymal enhancement and ring-enhancing lesions. CMV infections not uncommonly arise with other opportunistic infections such as toxoplasmosis and cryptococcosis. Diffuse periventricular calcification occurs in the congenital form and is not a feature of CMV infection in HIV.

Offiah CE, Turnbull IW. The imaging appearances of intracranial CNS infections in adult HIV and AIDS patients. *Clin Radiol.* 2006; **61**(5): 393–401.

66 Answer B: Tethered cord

Tethered cord usually presents in children with bowel and bladder dysfunction and lower limb neurology. It is slightly more common in females. Fifty per cent of patients have a hairy patch overlying the lower back. It can be associated with filum lipoma, imperforate anus, filum cysts and diastematomyelia. The main features are low-lying cord and thickened filum terminale (greater than 2 mm). Patients are treated with a decompressive laminectomy. At birth the conus medullaris should lie at L2/3 and at L1/2 at three months.

67 Answer E: Flexion extension views of lumbar spine

Pars defect is a fracture through the pars interarticularis. These are due either to a stress fracture, congenital or secondary to other condition; for example, tumours, osteomalacia or Paget's disease. Spondylolysis commonly occur at the L5 vertebra. Neurology typically occurs after a degree of spondylolisthesis. If on imaging no nerve root impingement is seen but the history is typical, this might be because the slip is unstable and so flexion extension films should be performed.

68 Answer B: Traumatic nerve root avulsion

The right T1 nerve root has been avulsed. This most commonly occurs in the cervical region following severe acute traction on the upper limb such as a fall from a motorbike. Imaging typically demonstrates an absent nerve root within the neural foramina and a pseudomeningocele. If patients are not able to have an MRI, a CT myelogram could be performed.

Sasaka KK, *et al.* Lumbosacral nerve root avulsions: MR imaging demonstration of acute abnormalities. *Am J Neuroradiol.* 2006; **27**(7): 1944–6.

69 Answer A: Tarlov cyst

A Tarlov cyst is a perineural cyst arising from the nerve root. They most commonly occur in the sacral region and can cause bone scalloping from pressure effects. It is postulated that there is a ball valve effect so CSF flows into the cyst with arterial pulsations. The spinal nerves may be visualised either in the wall of the cyst or the cyst itself. They occur in 5% of the population and are more common in women. They are usually asymptomatic but may cause symptoms such as bladder and bowel dysfunction or lower motor or sensory abnormalities.

70 Answer E: Early diastolic flow reversal

	Internal carotid artery	External carotid artery
Size	Typically larger than the ECA	Typically smaller than the ICA
Branches	No branches	Gives off multiple branches
Orientation	Orientated posterolaterally to the mastoid process	Orientated anteromedially to the face
Waveform	Low resistance	High resistance with early diastolic flow reversal
Temporal tap manoeuvre	No oscillations	Oscillations

Neuroradiology, head and neck and ENT radiology

PAPER 3: ANSWERS AND EXPLANATIONS

1 Answer C: Cementoma

Apical cysts, brown tumours, odontogenic cysts and metastasis are all lytic lesions. Cementomas arise in the apex of a vital tooth and are mixed lytic and sclerotic masses. They are often multi-centric, typically affect people aged between 30 and 40 and are more common in women.

2 Answer E: Ameloblastoma

Ameloblastoma or adamantinoma of the jaw are benign locally aggressive neoplasms. They usually affect people aged between 30 and 50 years of age and are slow-growing lesions that typically affect the lower premolars and molars. They are multilocular expansile masses and are associated with resorption of the root of the teeth.

Apical cysts are usually unilocular and dentigerous cyst are associated with the cap of the tooth. The lesion described has generally benign features and is unlikely to be a metastasis.

3 Answer A: Left optic tract

Monocular visual loss is due to a defect in the optic nerve. Bitemporal hemianopia is due to a defect at the optic chiasm level. A homonymous hemianopia is caused by a defect in the contralateral optic tract or through all the contralateral optic radiation. Right upper outer quadrantanopia is due to a defect in part of the optic radiation. Central bilateral homonymous hemianopia is due to a defect in the contralateral primary visual cortex.

4 Answer E: Swelling of the rectus muscles and levator palpebrae only

Thyroid eye disease is limited to the muscle bellies of rectus and levator palpebrae muscles and Tenon's capsule tends to be spared. This is not the case in pseudotumour. Fat haziness is seen in both thyroid eye disease and pseudotumour. In pseudotumour there is enhancement of the fat with contrast, and lacrimal gland enlargement occurs in 5% of cases.

5   Answer E: Inferior rectus

This patient has Graves' eye disease, which is an autoimmune disorder caused by long-acting thyroid simulating factor. It is commonly bilateral (75%) and results in hypertrophy of the muscle belly with sparing of the tendon insertions. The most commonly affected muscle is the inferior rectus followed by the medial, superior and then the lateral recti.

6   Answer E: Lacrimal gland

Orbital lymphoma is typically non-Hodgkin's B-cell lymphoma and occurs in middle age. It is usually associated with lymphomatous deposits elsewhere in the body. The most common site is extraconal, within the lacrimal glands. On imaging lymphoma within the lacrimal gland is usually seen as well-defined high-density mass.

7   Answer D: Melanoma

This patient has metastatic uveal melanoma. Medical students are always taught beware of the man with the glass eye and the large liver! Uveal melanoma is the most common primary intraocular neoplasm in adults. It occurs in patients aged 50–70 and is usually choroidal and unilateral. On MRI the lesion is of high signal on T1-weighted images and it is hyperdense on CT. These lesions metastasise to the lung, liver and optic nerve and prognosis is poor.

8   Answer B: DaTSCAN

Schizophrenia therapy can produce Parkinson's-like symptoms and if there are equivocal changes on the DaTSCAN, treatment should be used with caution. The only way to assess presynaptic receptors for dopaminergic uptake is with a DaTSCAN.

9   Answer B: Cystic hygroma

A cystic hygroma is the most common form of congenital malformation of the lymphatic system and usually presents within the first two years of life. On clinical examination it is a compressible mobile mass in the posterior triangle and is composed of a honeycomb of loculated cystic structures. On CT it is a well-defined mass of low attenuation, which does not appear to contain a surrounding wall and, if large, can result in mass effect. Characteristically, cystic hygromas are hypointense on T1 and hyperintense on T2-weighted MRI with no enhancement with contrast. They have been related to a range of syndromes, most commonly Turner's. It may be difficult to distinguish radiologically between a cystic hygroma and a third branchial cleft cyst. The latter possesses a thin wall, is seen just posterior to the carotid artery and a sinus opening should be visible on examination. A ranula is seen either in the sublingual or submandibular space. A thyroglossal cyst is a midline structure.

10   Answer A: Isointense to muscle on T1W MRI

Pleomorphic adenomas are benign lesions containing both mesodermal and glandular tissue. They most commonly occur in the parotid gland but can also arise within the other minor salivary glands. On CT they are generally well demarcated, homogeneous and slightly hyperdense to muscle. Typically, there is no significant enhancement post contrast. On MRI they are isointense to muscle on T1 and become hyperintense on T2-weighted images with avid enhancement post gadolinium. Adenomas of less than 0.5 cm tend to have a smooth margin while larger lesions may appear more lobulated. Eighty per cent of all pleomorphic tumours occur in the parotid gland and of these 80% occur in the superficial lobe.

11 Answer D: Fibrous dysplasia

Fibrous dysplasia is a pathology of unknown aetiology and usually occurs before 30 years of age. It involves increased proliferation of woven bone within the medullary cavity that cannot develop to lamellar bone and is most commonly monostotic but can be polyostotic. Bone expansion resulting in facial deformity can occur and malignant transformation has been described (<0.5%). If the skull base is affected the neural foraminae can become stenosed. The radiological appearances are diverse dependent on the degree of fibrous tissue produced. A CT scan characteristically reveals an expansile bony lesion that displays ground-glass density. The bony expansion can be identified as a result of widening of the medullary space with the cortex remaining intact. MRI usually shows a low signal intensity on both T1- and T2-weighted images and intense enhancement following administration of contrast. Polyostotic fibrous dysplasia is a feature of Albright's syndrome (cutaneous pigmentation, fibrous dysplasia and precocious puberty).

Paget's disease produces mixed lytic and sclerotic lesions, is more common in males, primarily involves the vertebrae and skull and occurs later in life. Ossifying fibromas are more focal, displaying discrete zones of osseous or fibrous tissue and behaving more aggressively.

12 Answer B: Inferior belly of omohyoid

The boundaries of the posterior triangle are formed anteriorly by the posterior border of sternocleidomastoid, inferiorly by the middle third of the clavicle and posteriorly by the anterior border of trapezius. The posterior triangle is bisected by the inferior belly of omohyoid approximately 2.5 cm above the clavicle, creating an occipital triangle superiorly and a supraclavicular triangle inferiorly.

13 Answer C: A mixed pattern of Alzheimer's/DLB type and vascular dementia

Alzheimer's and dementia of the Lewy body type do not have a vascular aetiology but may coexist with vascular dementia. Mesial temporal sclerosis is a form of epilepsy diagnosed clinically and is best imaged on MRI. Frontotemporal dementia presents differently and imaging shows frontal and temporal lobe changes.

14 Answer B: Luminal narrowing on left

The most common site of an extracranial internal carotid artery dissection is the segment of vessel just distal to the carotid bifurcation. The most common finding on angiography is that of a tapered luminal narrowing and associated enlargement of the diameter of the dissected vessel. If there is a severe stenosis, then a 'string' sign can be seen. An intimal flap is frequently not identified in internal carotid artery dissections and therefore the characteristic 'double lumen' sign is not usually seen. On CT the eccentric rim of intramural haematoma does not usually enhance but on MRI it can display increased signal intensity on T1-weighted images as a result of the methaemoglobin content, although fat-suppression imaging is needed in order to differentiate the intramural haematoma from surrounding periarterial fat. The rim of intramural haematoma may not exhibit hyperintensity in the first few days after dissection as it contains primarily deoxyhaemoglobin and will therefore be isointense with the surrounding muscle. Partial ptosis and constricted pupil are components of Horner's syndrome due to interruption in the sympathetic nerve supply.

15 Answer C: Drug-induced Parkinsonian syndrome

The DaTSCAN is normal hence there is no evidence of idiopathic Parkinson's disease, but this study will not exclude drug-induced symptoms, which are caused by blockade of postsynaptic receptors. The treatment of schizophrenia includes drugs, which can produce a Parkinson's-like syndrome. Early-onset Alzheimer's refers to patients under 60 years old; the symptoms and investigation are not compatible with this diagnosis. Depression is also feasible.

16 Answer A: Hyperparathyroidism secondary to parathyroid adenoma

This appearance is a 'superscan'. Causes include widespread metastatic disease, renal osteodystrophy, osteomalacia, hyperparathyroidism, hyperthyroidism, myeloproliferative disorders, Waldenström's macroglobulinaemia, mastocytosis and Paget's disease. The probable parathyroid adenoma makes this the likely cause.

17 Answer D: 24 hours

I131 has a half-life of eight days and is usually taken as an oral preparation for the treatment of hyperthyroidism. Patients are typically imaged 24 hours after ingesting the I131. Antithyroid drugs are stopped six weeks before treatment to ensure maximum uptake of I131. Patients can remain on symptomatic management, such as beta-blocker type drugs, to reduce symptoms. The peak energy of I131 is 364 keV and the absorbed dose is 50–100 cGy (rad). I123 has a half-life of 13 hours and is ingested orally; imaging is typically performed after six hours. The peak energy is 159 keV and the absorbed dose is 2–5 cGy (rad).

18 Answer C: Le Fort III

All Le Fort fractures involve the pterygoid process. Le Fort I is a transverse fracture through the maxilla, Le Fort II is more extensive and the separated fragment is pyramidal while in Le Fort III there is complete craniofacial disjunction. In practice fractures do not fit these descriptions exactly and may be asymmetrical or coexist. The classification is still in general use and aids in subsequent surgical management. In Le Fort I and II the fractured maxillary fragment is usually wired to the zygomatic arches, but if these are fractured as in Le Fort III, a more complex pin and rod fixation to the skull vault is undertaken.

19 Answer D: 3 (all three lines)

McGrigor's lines are three transverse lines visible on frontal views of the facial bones. A tripod fracture would disrupt the first line around the zygomatico-frontal suture and would disrupt the second and third lines twice. Both would be disrupted over the zygomatic arch. The second would be disrupted again at the inferior orbital rim and the third at the inferior rim of the maxillary antrum.

20 Answer A: Warthin's tumour

The description given is typical of the imaging appearance. Siladenitis is usually caused by *Streptococcus* or *Haemophilus* infections and typically produces inflammatory change within the gland and subcutaneous tissue oedema. Sialectasia does occur. Mucoepidermoid cancers are poorly defined lesions lacking enhancement which and perineural spread may be visible particularly on T2-weighted images. Sjögren's syndrome is commonly bilateral. The most common imaging feature is multiple small cysts in an enlarged parotid gland.

21 Answer A: Paget's disease

Paget's disease presents with a mixed hearing loss due to fixation of the stapes in the oval window, giving a conductive deficit and loss of cochlear bone density, producing a sensorineural deficit. Both monostotic and polyostotic fibrous dysplasia normally present as an incidental finding in a young age group with the classical ground-glass appearance on CT. The clinical picture does not fit with a potential diagnosis of osteomyelitis. Typical CT appearances of ossifying fibroma are of a cortically based lytic lesion with a thick bony rim in a young patient.

22 Answer A: A ring of low density around the cochlea

The double ring sign is due to demineralisation of the surrounding bone and is a classical finding in cochlear otosclerosis. Hypersclerosis of a poorly pneumatised mastoid is most likely to represent mastoiditis, while ossification of the oval window would support a diagnosis of fenestral sclerosis. Hypodense opacity of the mesotympanum without bony erosion is suggestive of chronic otitis media, while ossicular destruction and bony scalloping could represent cholesteatoma.

23 Answer A: Epidermoid

The most important differential for an epidermoid here is an arachnoid cyst. On FLAIR (fluid attenuated inversion recovery, i.e. a 'water-suppressed' pulse technique) sequences, an arachnoid cyst will be low signal similar to that of stationary water while epidermoids are high signal. These could also be differentiated by diffusion-weighted MR. Both an acoustic neuroma and a cystic meningioma would have areas of enhancement on T1-weighted images.

24   Answer A: Aberrant internal carotid artery

The most important feature on CT imaging is whether the lesion is of a tubular nature. This would steer you away from a diagnosis of glomus tympanicum and should prevent you a dangerous biopsy. A glomus tumour would show permeative bone changes and a dehiscent jugular bulb would also most likely show focal absence of the jugular plate.

25   Answer B: Septum pellucidum

This patient has holoprosencephaly, which is always associated with an absent septum pellucidum. Holoprosencephaly is a failure or incomplete cleavage of the cerebral hemispheres. There are three types:

- alobar – the most severe form, which typically results in death below one year of age. There is a large single ventricle with a peripheral layer of cerebral cortex. No third ventricle, falx cerebri, interhemispheric fissure, corpus callosum, septum pellucidum, olfactory or optic nerves are present. The thalami are fused

- semilobar – is a milder form and children may reach adulthood. There is a single ventricle with partially formed occipital horns and minimally developed temporal horns. There is partial fusion of the thalami, a small third ventricle and rudimentary falx cerebri

- lobar – mildest form where there is separation of the cerebral hemispheres. There are two cerebral hemispheres and two lateral ventricles. The frontal lobes are dysplastic and there is a single fused frontal horn. The thalami are separated.

26   Answer D: Ipsilateral enlargement of the choroid plexus

This child has Sturge-Weber-Dimitri syndrome, which is associated with a facial port wine stain (telangiectasia of the trigeminal nerve) and a leptomeningeal venous angioma. The leptomeningeal venous angioma is most commonly in the parietal lobe. It is associated with atrophy of the underlying cortex, thickening of the overlying skull vault and enlargement of the choroid plexus. There is gyriform cortical calcification, which can sometimes be seen on plain film. Angiomas may be seen in most visceral organs of the body.

27   Answer A: Open-lipped schizencephaly

Schizencephaly is a cleft extending from the lateral ventricle to the cortex that is lined with grey matter. There are two types of schizencephaly: open-lipped and closed-lip. Closed-lip describes the apposition of the two sides of the cleft while in open lip there is CSF separating the two sides. Schizencephaly is caused by abnormal neuronal migration due to an in utero ischaemic insult in the germinal matrix at between 30 and 60 days' gestation. Ninety per cent of schizencephaly is associated with an absent septum pellucidum. It can also be associated with abnormalities to the optic nerve in septo-optic dysplasia.

28 Answer D: Down's syndrome

Intrasutural ossicles or wormian bones are common in infancy and are considered abnormal only if >10 in number and 6 × 4mm or larger. Common conditions include rickets, osteogenesis imperfecta, pyknodysostosis, hypophosphatasia, hypothyroidism and Down's syndrome.

29 Answer A: Periventricular leukomalacia

Risk factors for germinal matrix haemorrhage are prematurity (less than 32 weeks), low birth weight, males, multiple births, prolonged labour and cyanotic heart disease. It typically occurs within the first two days of birth. The germinal matrix lies in the caudothalamic groove and is very metabolically active which makes it sensitive to low levels of oxygen. There are four grades of intraventricular haemorrhage as shown in the table below. A common finding in premature babies is flare within the periventricular white matter. Periventricular leukomalacia is the sequelae of ischaemia in the watershed areas, eventually the cystic areas are reabsorbed and ventriculomegaly occurs.

Grading	Features	Mortality
1	Flare in the periventricular region, no hydrocephalus	—
2	Subependymal haemorrhage with rupture into the ventricles	10%
3	Intraventricular haemorrhage with hydrocephalus	20%
4	Intraparenchymal haemorrhage	50%

30 Answer D: Neural tube defect

The banana and lemon sign are seen on ultrasound in patients with neural tube defects. The head appears lemon shaped at the level of the lateral ventricles due to bilateral indentation of the frontal lobe cortex, which is typically seen before 24 weeks. The banana sign is obliteration of the posterior fossa and herniation of the cerebellum.

Benacerraf BR, Stryker J, Frigoletto FDJ. Abnormal US appearance of the cerebellum (banana sign): indirect sign of spina bifida. *Radiology*. 1989; **171**(1): 151–3.

31 Answer B: Chronic subarachnoid haemorrhage

MR imaging findings of chronic subarachnoid haemorrhage are pathognomonic. T2-weighted and gradient-echo susceptibility imaging reveal characteristic hypointensity along the pial surface/subarachnoid space of the brain and spinal cord. This finding is detected classically along the surface of the brain stem and cerebellar vermis. Superficial siderosis of the CNS due to chronic, recurrent subarachnoid haemorrhage classically manifests with progressive bilateral sensorineural hearing loss, although ataxia and pyramidal signs are also observed. Underlying causes include vascular malformations, neoplasms and trauma.

Hsu WC, Loevner LA, Forman MS, *et al*. Superficial siderosis of the CNS associated with multiple cavernous malformations. *Am J Neuroradiol*. 1999; **20**(7): 1245–8.

32 Answer B: Carbon monoxide poisoning

Carbon monoxide poisoning is a leading cause of accidental poisoning. In the brain CO has a predilection for the globus pallidus. On CT there is symmetric hypodensity while on MRI the medial portions of the globus pallidus appear as areas of low signal on T1 and high signal on T2 and FLAIR images. The caudate nucleus, putamen and thalamus are occasionally involved. The differentials include Wilson's disease and cyanide poisoning.

Chung-Ping Lo, Shao-Yuan Chen, Kwo-Whei Lee, *et al*. Brain injury after acute carbon monoxide poisoning: early and late complications, *Am J Roentgenol*. 2007; **189**(4): W205–11.

33 Answer B: Low-density white matter changes within the occipital lobes

The imaging pattern of PRES is seen in eclampsia, cyclosporin toxicity following transplantation, autoimmune disorders like SLE and Wegener's and in hypertension. The exact cause is unproven but an unstable blood pressure is a frequent finding. Typical findings in PRES include reversible vasogenic oedema in the parieto-occipital, posterior frontal and cortical and subcortical white matter. The cerebellum and brainstem are less commonly involved. Haemorrhage and restricted diffusion on DWI are atypical.

McKinney AM, *et al*. Posterior reversible encephalopathy syndrome: incidence of atypical regions of involvement and imaging findings. *Am J Roentgenol*. 2007; **189**(4): 904–12.

34 Answer B: Carotid body tumour

Carotid body tumours (paragangliomas) typically present as a firm mass below and behind the angle of the jaw. They display low signal on T1 and high signal on T2 with multiple large flow voids. Avid enhancement is seen with splaying of the ICA and ECA. Up to 5% are bilateral and 6% undergo malignant change. Differentials include enhancing metastases from renal and thyroid primaries.

35 Answer A: Bilateral thalamic infarcts

Imaging features suggest deep venous sinus thrombosis. Thrombosis of the deep cerebral veins may cause relatively symmetric infarction of the basal ganglia, thalami and midbrain. Involvement of the grey-white matter may occur in a non-arterial distribution. Haemorrhagic transformation may occur and brain swelling occurs earlier than in arterial infarcts.

36 Answer C: Cerebral hypotension

Intracranial hypotension syndrome results from inadequate CSF pressure to support the brain in the skull vault, causing the brain to sag on to the skull base. The primary form probably arises from spontaneous arachnoid tears while the secondary form is associated with trauma, post lumbar puncture and dehydration. MRI is the imaging of choice and shows tonsillar/insular herniation, bilateral subdural hygromas and depression of the optic chiasm. Characteristically, diffuse dural enhancement is seen secondary to dural venous dilatation that occurs with reduced CSF volume (Monro-Kellie rule).

Sell JJ, Rupp FW, Orrison WW Jr. Iatrogenically induced intracranial hypotension syndrome. *Am J Roentgenol*. 1995; **165**(6): 1513–15.

37 Answer A: Superior cerebellar artery

The SCA is the most commonly implicated vessel in trigeminal neuralgia. Other major arteries that maybe responsible include the AICA, basilar and vertebral arteries. Vascular contact is best depicted on MR, which clearly delineates the cisternal course of the fifth nerve. In the symptomatic patient, vascular contact at the root entry zone is suggestive but not necessarily diagnostic as a high incidence of vascular contact and even deformity is seen in this region in asymptomatic patients. Treatments include microvascular decompression, radiofrequency rhizotomy and injection of the trigeminal (Gasserian) ganglion with glycerol.

Tash RR, Sze G, Leslie DR. Trigeminal neuralgia: MR imaging features. *Radiology*. 1989; **172**(3): 767–70.

38 Answer A: Cervical segment

Carotid artery dissection is known to occur after seemingly trivial trauma. Partial Horner's is present in less than 50% of patients and ipsilateral persistent headache is common. It accounts for up to 25% of strokes in the young and middle-aged patients. The extracranial portion is more commonly involved (cervical ICA at C1-C2 – 60%); dissection of the intracranial portion is relatively rare as the skull base absorbs most of the force.

39 Answer E: Endovascular stent placement

The condition described is subclavian steal syndrome, which is a term used to describe retrograde blood flow in the vertebral artery associated with proximal ipsilateral subclavian artery stenosis or occlusion. Most patients remain asymptomatic, while a few develop neurological symptoms following use of the ipsilateral arm. The left subclavian is three times more commonly involved than the right and atherosclerosis is the underlying cause. Endovascular management is common with a technical success rate of 86–100% and primary stenting of the subclavian artery is the procedure of choice.

40 Answer D: Multiple bilateral small cysts within both parotid glands

Benign lymphoepithelial cysts are painless cystic swellings of the parotid gland seen in HIV positive patients. The condition is bilateral in 20% of patients. The cysts originate from lymph nodes within the parotid gland and are typically small, multiple and in the superficial lobes. They have the typical imaging features of cysts.

41 Answer D: Friedreich's ataxia

Friedreich's ataxia is the most common inherited progressive ataxia. It usually presents before adolescence. The cerebellum is atrophied in ataxia telangiectasia and the cerebrum is atrophied in multiple sclerosis. Guillain-Barré would not produce any cervical changes.

42 Answer D: Leptomeningeal cyst

A leptomeningeal cyst or 'growing fracture' occurs in 1% of all paediatric skull fractures. It is seen in fractures associated with dural tears where arachnoid herniation and CSF pulsations produce fracture diastasis. Typical appearance is of a skull defect with indistinct scalloped bony margins usually evident two to three months after the injury. Gliosis of the adjacent brain parenchyma is common.

43 Answer B: Metaphyseal corner fracture of the tibia

The fractures considered to have a high specificity for abuse are metaphyseal fractures, posterior rib fractures, scapular fractures, fractures of the outer end of the clavicle, complex skull fractures and bilateral fractures or fractures of differing ages.

Retinal haemorrhages occur in shaking consequent to high central venous pressures. Periosteal new bone is a benign entity in infants between six weeks and six months. It occurs symmetrically in the diaphysis, never extends to the metaphysis and shows normal uptake on isotope bone scan.

Rao P, Carty H. Non-accidental injury: review of the radiology. *Clin Radiol.* 1999; **54**(1): 11–24.

44 Answer C: Thickening of the vomer

The diagnosis is choanal atresia, which is the commonest cause of neonatal nasal obstruction. This is a life-threatening condition, which is more commonly bilateral. It usually presents with respiratory distress, as babies are obligate nasal breathers. Bony septations are present in 85–90% of cases, the remainder being membranous septations. Further imaging findings include inward bowing of the posterior maxilla and narrowing of the posterior choanae to <3.4mm in a child less than two years.

45 Answer A: Progressive multifocal leukoencephalopathy

Progressive multifocal leukoencephalopathy is caused by JC virus and results in destruction of the oligodendrocytes, resulting in demyelination. It affects the white matter anywhere in the brain in HIV patients and is often bilateral but asymmetrical and is not associated with atrophy. Death typically occurs within six months. The white matter lesions do not exhibit mass effect and show minimal enhancement. Lymphoma and toxoplasmosis are more commonly discrete ring enhancing lesions. CMV typically results in patchy diffuse periventricular white matter changes. Human immunodeficiency virus produces a subacute encephalitis, which is characterised by progressive dementia.

46 Answer B: Haemorrhage on CT

Differentiating toxoplasmosis and cerebral lymphoma can be difficult as both can present as multiple ring enhancing lesions. Features that are more likely to represent lymphoma are a single lesions, subependymal spread and lesions within the corpus callosum. Features that are more likely to represent toxoplasmosis are haemorrhage on CT and high signal on T2W imaging. Toxoplasmosis has a predilection for the basal ganglia but lymphoma can also be found in this region.

47 Answer D: Craniopharyngioma

Craniopharyngiomas have a bimodal distribution with three-quarters occurring in the first two generations and one-quarter within the fifth decade. Patient's symptoms depend on the site of the tumour; for example, with diabetes insipidus when compression of the thalamus occurs or bitemporal hemianopia when compression of the optic chiasm. Tumours occur in the tuber cinereum, suprasellar and infrasellar regions. On CT tumours appear as a cystic solid midline mass with peripheral calcification and the solid portion enhances with contrast. On MRI the mass is typically high signal on T1- and T2-weighted imaging with enhancement of the solid components with contrast.

48 Answer B: Oligodendroglioma

Oligodendrocytoma is a slow-growing grade 2 cerebral tumour that is more common in men aged 30–60 years. It has a propensity for the frontal lobes and involves both the cortex and white matter. On CT there is heavy calcification within the tumour and surrounding vasogenic oedema. Erosion of the inner table of the skull occurs, thus aiding the differential from meningiomas. There is variable enhancement with contrast. On MRI the tumour is hypointense on T1W and hyperintense on T2 and FLAIR except in the areas of calcification.

49 Answer A: Overproduction of CSF

This child has a choroid plexus papilloma. They commonly occur in the lateral ventricles in children and the fourth ventricle and CPA in adults. They are commonly smooth lobulated masses which brightly enhance with contrast. Hydrocephalus is usually due to overproduction of CSF.

50 Answer A: Meningioma

All the listed tumours occur within the cerebellopontine angle (CPA). Both meningiomas and acoustic neuromas can cause expansion of the internal auditory canal and enhance brightly with contrast. Meningioma is the most likely because there is calcification within the lesion described.

	Acoustic neuromas	Meningioma
Dural tail	Rare	25%
Angle with the dura	Acute	Obtuse
Calcification	Rare	30%
Cysts degeneration	Rare	10%
IAC involvement	Common	Rare
CT features	Isodense with patchy enhancement	Isointense with bright enhancement

51 Answer C: Low signal on T1 and high signal on T2

This patient most likely has an epidermoid as it is heterogeneous, lobulated and off midline. Epidermoids are most commonly homogeneously low signal on T1 and high signal on T2-weighted imaging.

52 Answer B: Haemorrhage

Demyelisation lesions in multiple sclerosis typically occur in the periventricular region, perpendicular to the ventricle. Lesions can occur anywhere in the brain and affect both grey and white matter. Ring enhancement occurs up to six weeks after the occurrence of the plaque. Haemorrhage is not a feature.

53 Answer B: Central pontine myelinolysis

Central pontine myelinolysis or osmotic demyelination syndrome is acute demyelination secondary to rapid correction of a hyponatraemia. It commonly occurs in diabetic patients with diabetic ketoacidosis, anorexics and alcoholics. However, less common causes are SIADH, Wilson's and craniopharyngioma. Patients develop symptoms a few days following the correction of the electrolyte imbalance and presentation is varied from unconscious (locked in syndrome), spastic quadriparesis and pseudobulbar palsy or with extrapyramidal signs. High signal is seen within the pons on FLAIR and T2W usually after a couple of weeks. There may be high signal in the basal ganglia and this is typically bilateral and symmetrical. Prognosis is very poor with a mortality of approximately 90%.

54 Answer A: Optic nerve glioma

Tuberous sclerosis, neurofibromatosis one and two, von Hippel-Lindau, Sturge-Weber and hereditary haemorrhagic telangiectasia are all neurocutaneous disorders. The cutaneous lesions suggest this patient has neurofibromatosis type one (NF1). Other cutaneous manifestations of NF1 are neurofibromas and iris hamartomas. Optic nerve gliomas are seen in up to 30% of NF1. In NF2 the main cutaneous finding is café au lait spots. In patients with tuberous sclerosis there is adenoma sebaceum, shagreen patches and subungual fibrosis. In hereditary haemorrhagic telangiectasia there are cutaneous telangiectasia on the face and freckles on the lips. A port wine stain is seen in the distribution of a branch of the trigeminal nerve in Sturge-Weber.

55 Answer A: Low signal

This patient has an arachnoid cyst, which typically has similar signal characteristics to CSF (bright on T2W, low on T1W and FLAIR). On DWI the signal characteristic is similar to CSF and so is low.

56 Answer E: Congenital *Cytomegalovirus* infection

Cytomegalovirus infection affects up to 1% of pregnancies but symptoms only occur in less than 10% of those infected. There are multiple manifestations including IUGR, hepatosplenomegaly, jaundice, pneumonitis, microcephaly and chorioretinitis. Long-term neurodevelopmental sequelae are common.

Typical findings on cranial ultrasound are periventricular subependymal cysts, periventricular calcifications and hydrocephalus. *Cytomegalovirus* tends to cause periventricular calcification while toxoplasmosis causes widespread calcifications. Periventricular infarcts will not be so well defined. Tuberous sclerosis can cause subependymal hamartomas, which calcify with age, and cortical or subcortical tubers, which produce curvilinear calcifications. Rubella is much less common than congenital CMV infection.

57 Answer B: Syringomyelia

The condition described is Chiari II. This is associated with syringomyelia in 20% and hydromyelia (50%). Hydromyelia is distension of the central canal, while syringomyelia is CSF dissection through the ependymal lining to form a paracentral cavity. Imaging appearances are indistinguishable and the entity is often grouped together as syringohydromyelia. Syrinxes also occur in Chiari I and can be associated with spinal trauma, intramedullary tumours and extramedullary compressive lesions.

58 Answer D: Down's syndrome

All the options listed are associated with posterior scalloping except Down's syndrome where anterior scalloping occurs. Scalloping is most prominent with lesions that occur during growth and bony remodelling and with slow growing lesions. In NF-1 it is secondary to dural ectasia, neurofibromas or lateral thoracic meningoceles.

59 Answer B: Narrowing of the disc space with high signal in the adjacent vertebral bodies on T2-weighted images

Early diagnosis is crucial in the management of infective spondylitis. *Staphylococcus aureus* is the most common pathogen. Imaging abnormalities on X-rays are often subtle and detected late in the disease. MR findings are characteristic and consist of reduced disc space and low signal on T1 and high signal on T2 in the adjacent vertebral bodies (reflecting increased extracellular fluid in the bone marrow). Subligamentous or epidural soft-tissue masses maybe seen.

60 Answer D: Neurogenic cyst

The description above describes a chronic process resulting in bone remodelling and atrophy of the cord. Thus an epidural abscess and haematoma are unlikely. This mass is extramedullary but intradural. Although meningiomas and neuromas are intradural they are isointense on T1 hence the best answer is a neurogenic cyst. Neurogenic cyst is an intradural mass, which is commonly seen within the cervical and thoracic region. They are associated with other spinal abnormalities such as diastematomyelia and Klippel-Feil syndrome.

61 Answer B: *Tuberculosis*

Tuberculous spondylitis commonly occurs with an insidious onset in the thoracolumbar region with contiguous involvement of multiple vertebrae. Spread is usually via the haematogenous route and the vertebral bodies are involved more commonly than the posterior elements. Destruction of the vertebral body leads to vertebra plana in children and gibbus deformity in adults. Pyogenic spondylitis is the major differential which occurs more rapidly with destruction, little new bone formation and usually sparing of the posterior elements. In brucellosis, lower lumbar involvement is common and bone destruction is associated with sclerosis. Epidural extension is minimal.

62 Answer C: Residual disc material

Appearances of the post-operative spine can be challenging. In the early post-operative period, persistent symptoms are usually due to epidural haematoma, retained fragment or recurrent disc. In the subacute and chronic stage the differential is mainly between a disc and epidural fibrosis. Osseous abnormalities depend on the specific surgical procedure. Epidural fibrosis occurs commonly, enhances with contrast administration and the degree of enhancement varies with time since the operation, enhancing most strongly within a year following surgery. Neuritis, identified as intrathecal enhancement of nerve roots, is seen in approximately 20% of symptomatic patients. Early post-operative root enhancement is common in asymptomatic patients and is considered significant only if it persists beyond at least six to eight months.

63 Answer A: Haemangioma

Vertebral haemangiomas are commonly incidental findings. Pain may occur and these become symptomatic if pathologic compression fracture or haemorrhage occurs. Plain X-rays demonstrate trabecular thickening and vertical striations while a 'polka dot' appearance is seen on CT. On MRI the signal may be variable, although they are usually high on T1 and T2. The major differential on MRI is focal fatty replacement of the marrow and the distinction may be made with fat suppressed sequences. Osteoid osteoma, osteoblastoma and ABC all involve the posterior elements.

64 Answer C: MRI brain

The MRI and flexion lumbar spine films confirm that the spondylolisthesis is stable and not impinging on the nerve roots. There are now two episodes of neurology affecting different parts of the body, spaced in time, and so this patient may have multiple sclerosis. The next best test is an MRI of the brain.

65 Answer C: Paravertebral ossification

A short neck, reduced cervical movement and low posterior hair line are typical findings in Klippel-Feil syndrome, which usually affects the upper cervical region with fusion of vertebral bodies and posterior column. Other features are scoliosis, hemivertebrae, atlantoaxial fusion, rib fusion and ear abnormalities. Sprengel's deformity is often seen with this condition in 25% of cases and results in rotation and elevation of the scapula due to an omovertebral connection.

66 Answer B: Diffuse idiopathic skeletal hyperostosis

DISH is characterised by diffuse flowing ossification at the site of ligamentous and tendinous insertion points. Patients are normally over 50 and it is more common in men. Pain, tenderness and restricted movement are all common complaints. It most commonly affects the mid and lower thoracic regions and extends over at least four contiguous vertebral bodies. The pelvis can be affected with ossification of the iliolumbar and sacrotuberous ligaments.

67 Answer D: Spinal dural arteriovenous fistula

There are four types of spinal AVM: spinal dural arteriovenous fistula (Type 1), spinal cord AVM (Type 2 and 3) and spinal cord AV fistulas (Type 4). Spinal AVMs present either with progressive sensory and motor loss or acutely following a sudden bleed which has a significant mortality. Haemosiderin may be seen in the subarachnoid spaces reflecting previous bleeds. Spinal AVMs may acutely thrombose and high signal within the cord is very common. Spinal cord arteriovenous malformations are intramedullary while spinal dural and spinal cord arteriovenous malformations are extramedullary but intradural. Treatment options are embolisation, surgery or both.

68 Answer D: Tolosa-Hunt syndrome

Tolosa-Hunt syndrome is an idiopathic inflammatory disease with some similarity to orbital pseudotumour. Patients present with recurrent bouts of retro-orbital pain associated with cranial nerve palsies affecting the III, VI, V1 and VI nerves. Symptoms last for days to weeks and respond rapidly to steroid therapy. The above features are typical. Ramsay Hunt syndrome is due to herpes zoster infection involving the geniculate ganglion giving acute facial nerve paralysis, pain in the ear and a typical rash.

69 Answer C: Uniformly thick enhancing wall

Differentiating ring enhancing metastasis and ring enhancing abscesses can be difficult. Metastases typically appear as thick irregular ring enhancing lesions within the corticomedullary region. Abscesses tend to demonstrate a thinner, more uniform enhancing wall. Abscesses point towards the ventricles and can demonstrate restricted diffusion.

70 Answer B: White matter of the centrum semiovale

Human immunodeficiency virus causes encephalitis in 60% of patients with AIDS. It predominately affects the white matter, particularly the centrum semiovale and results in gliosis and demyelinating plaques. These plaques are not dissimilar to plaques in multiple sclerosis as they are in a periventricular position and high signal on T2-weighted images. Unlike plaques in MS they tend not to enhance with contrast. (Acute plaques in MS can enhance for up to six weeks after they first appear.) Generalised diffuse parenchymal atrophy is a feature.

Offiah CE, Turnbull IW. The imaging appearances of intracranial CNS infections in adult HIV and AIDS patients. *Clin Radiol*. 2006; **61**(5): 393–401.

Bibliography

GENERAL REFERENCE TEXTS

Adam A, Dixon A, editors. *Grainger & Allison's Diagnostic Radiology: a textbook of medical imaging*. 5th ed. London: Churchill Livingstone; 2007.

Brandt WE, Helms CA. *Fundamentals of Diagnostic Radiology*. 3rd ed. Philadelphia, PA: Lippincott, Williams & Wilkins; 2007.

Chapman S, Nakielny R. *Aids to Radiological Differential Diagnosis*. 4th ed. Philadelphia, PA: Saunders; 2003.

Dahnert W. *Radiology Review Manual*. 6th ed. Philadelphia, PA: Lippincott, Williams & Wilkins; 2007.

Federle M, editor. *Diagnostic Imaging: abdomen*. Salt Lake City, UT: Amirsys; 2004.

Husband JE, Reznek RH, editors. *Imaging in Oncology*. London: Taylor and Francis; 2004.

Middleton WD, Kurtz AB, Hertzberg BS. *Ultrasound: the requisites*. 2nd ed. St Louis, MO: Mosby; 2003.

Semelka RC, editor. *Abdominal-Pelvic MRI*. New York, NY: Wiley-Liss Inc; 2002.

Webb R, Brandt W, Major NM. *Fundamentals of Body CT*. 3rd ed. Philadelphia, PA: Saunders; 2006.

Weissleder R, Wittenberg M, Harisinghani M. *Primer of Diagnostic Imaging*. 3rd ed. St Louis, MO: Mosby; 2003.

ANAPHYLAXIS

Resuscitation Council (UK). *Guidelines on Emergency Treatment of Anaphylactic Reactions*. London: Resuscitation Council (UK); 2008. Available at: www.resus.org.uk (accessed 15 February 2009).

CONTRAST MEDIA

The European Society of Urogenital Radiology. *ESUR Guidelines on Contrast Media, version 6.0*. The European Society of Urogenital Radiology; 2007. Available at: www.esur.org (accessed 15February2009).

INTERVENTION

Kessel D, Robertson I. *Interventional Radiology: a survival guide*. 2nd ed. London: Churchill Livingstone; 2005.

BREAST RADIOLOGY

Kopans DB. *Breast Imaging*. Philadelphia, PA: Lippincott; 1989.

Morris E, Liberman L. *Breast MRI: diagnosis and intervention*. New York, NY: Springer-Verlag; 2005.

Roebuck E. *Clin Radiol of the Breast*. Oxford: Heinemann Medical Books; 1990.

PAEDIATRIC RADIOLOGY

Burton EM, Brody AS. *Essentials of Pediatric Radiology*. New York, NY: Thieme; 1999.

Chen H. *Atlas of Genetic Diagnosis and Counselling*. Totowa, NJ: Humana Press; 2005.

Kim D, Betz RR, editors. *Surgery of the Pediatric Spine*. New York, NY: Thieme; 2008.

Siegel MJ, Coley B, editors. *Pediatric Imaging*. Philadelphia, PA: Lippincott, Williams & Wilkins; 2005.

Staheli LT. *Fundamentals of Pediatric Orthopedics*. Philadelphia, PA: Lippincott, Williams & Wilkins; 2003.

NEURORADIOLOGY, HEAD AND NECK AND ENT RADIOLOGY

Grossman RI, Yousem DM. *Neuroradiology: the requisites*. 2nd ed. St Louis, MO: Mosby; 2003.

Hoeffner EG, Mukherji SK. *Temporal Bone Imaging*. New York, NY: Thieme; 2008.

Mancuso A, Ojiri H, Quisling RG. *Head and Neck Radiology*. Philadelphia, PA: Lippincott, Williams & Wilkins; 2001.

Mukherji SK, Chong V. *Atlas of Head and Neck Imaging*. New York, NY: Thieme; 2004.

Osborn A, Blaser S, Salzman K. *Diagnostic Imaging: brain*. Salt Lake City, UT: Amirsys; 2004.

Som PM, Curtin HD, editors. *Head and Neck Imaging*. 4th ed. St Louis, MO: Mosby; 2003.

Index

T - #0634 - 101024 - C0 - 246/174/17 - PB - 9781846193644 - Gloss Lamination